Crisis Resolution and Home Trea... ...n Mental Health

DATE DUE

Crisis Resolution and Home Treatment in Mental Health

Edited by

Sonia Johnson
Reader in Social and Community Psychiatry,
University College London

Justin Needle
Lecturer in Health Services Research and Policy,
City University London

Jonathan P. Bindman
Clinical Director, Lambeth Adult Mental Health Services, South London and
Maudsley NHS Foundation Trust, London

Graham Thornicroft
Professor of Community Psychiatry, Institute of Psychiatry,
King's College London

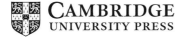
CAMBRIDGE
UNIVERSITY PRESS

CAMBRIDGE UNIVERSITY PRESS
Cambridge, New York, Melbourne, Madrid, Cape Town, Singapore, São Paulo, Delhi

Cambridge University Press
The Edinburgh Building, Cambridge CB2 8RU, UK

Published in the United States of America by Cambridge University Press, New York

www.cambridge.org
Information on this title: www.cambridge.org/9780521678759

First published 2008

Printed in the United Kingdom at the University Press, Cambridge

A catalogue record for this publication is available from the British Library

Library of Congress Cataloging-in-Publication Data

Crisis resolution and home treatment in mental health / edited by Sonia Johnson ... [et al.].
      p. ; cm.
      Includes bibliographical references and index.
      ISBN 978-0-521-67875-9
1. Crisis intervention (Mental health services)–Great Britian. 2. Home-based mental health services–Great
Britain. 3. Mentally ill–Home care–Great Britian. I. Johnson, Sonia, 1964–
      [DNLM: 1. Community Mental Health Services–trends–Great Britain. 2. Crisis Intervention–trends–
Great Britain. 3. Home Care Services–trends–Great Britain. 4. Mental Disorders–therapy–Great Britain.
WM 30 C932 2008] I. Title.

      RC480.6.C7587   2008
      362.2′0425–dc22

                                                                                            2008012846

ISBN 978-0-521-67875-9 paperback

Dedication

This book is dedicated to Anton Alexander Johnson Needle (born January 2007), whose slightly early arrival significantly prolonged its gestation but filled two of the editors' lives with joy.

Contents

Contributors

Danny Antebi is currently a consultant psychiatrist and clinical director for adult mental health working in Gwent Healthcare NHS Trust. Prior to this he was consultant psychiatrist in central Bristol with responsibility for developing services for ethnic minority populations. His clinical background is in general adult psychiatry with publications in neuropsychiatry and liaison psychiatry. He has had significant experience of medical management and service development.

Jonathan P. Bindman trained in psychiatry at the Royal Free and Maudsley Hospitals (MRCPsych 1994). He was lecturer and senior lecturer in the Health Services Research Department at the Institute of Psychiatry, King's College London, from 1997 to 2005, and was involved in the development of three crisis resolution teams within the South London and Maudsley Trust (SlaM), working as consultant psychiatrist to one of the teams from 2004 to 2007. He is now Clinical Director of Adult Mental Health Services in Lambeth, southeast London, and remains active in developing new community services.

Helen Blackwell died in October 2007 after a long struggle with distress and self-harm. She was a freelance trainer, researcher and consultant, with particular interests in self-harm, recovery and user-led services. She had worked on user-led research projects for the Sainsbury Centre for Mental Health and the Mental Health Foundation, and in the past had managed voluntary mental health services. At the time of her death, she was involved in two areas of work for the Royal College of Psychiatrists: advising the 'Better Services for People who Self-Harm' Project on user involvement, and developing user-led training in the College's Education and Training Centre. She worked for a time at Barnet Voice for Mental Health, a local service user-led organisation, where she helped to establish the user-led crisis house, Kaya House. Helen was committed to improving services for people who self-harm, to genuine user involvement and to recognising the strengths in all of us.

Christopher Bridgett is a consultant psychiatrist with the South Kensington and Chelsea crisis resolution team. After training in Oxford, he worked in London for 25 years, developing with colleagues a local comprehensive community psychiatry service as an alternative to hospital-based treatment. He is the convener of a London consultants group interested in crisis resolution and home treatment, has written on social systems interventions in crisis resolution for the Royal College of Psychiatrists and the Sainsbury Centre for Mental Health, and has run workshops for home treatment teams on the social systems approach.

Neil Brimblecombe is Director of Mental Health Nursing at the Department of Health, England and recently chaired a national review of mental health nursing. In the past, he has been a community mental health nurse in central London and worked for several years clinically in crisis/home treatment teams. He completed a Ph.D. researching crisis team assessment outcomes and has edited a book on home treatment (*Acute Mental Health Care in the Community: Intensive Home Treatment*, 2001). Neil is also visiting Professor of Mental Health Nursing at Nottingham University and Director of Nursing, Research and Development at South Staffordshire and Shropshire Healthcare Foundation Trust.

Paul Clenaghan has a Masters degree in Nursing and a Post Graduate Diploma in Health Management. He has worked in mental health for 25 years and has managed community mental health services since 1992. He currently manages mental health services in central Sydney from Redfern to Bankstown. He is a board member of an employment agency specialising in people with mental health problems. He has published articles on a range of mental health topics and areas of interest including acute care in the community and people with mental health and drug and alcohol problems.

Claudia Cooper is currently working as an MRC training fellow in health services research at University College London. She is an honorary specialist registrar for Camden and Islington NHS Foundation Trust, and she has worked in this capacity with community mental health teams for older people and adults of working age and with crisis resolution teams managing younger and older adults in crisis. Her research interests include the mental health of people with dementia and their family carers, older adult abuse, and analysis of large epidemiological surveys. She regularly teaches medical students and postgraduate courses at University College London.

Mary-Anne Cotton is a specialist registrar in psychiatry, doing, dual training in general adult and old-age psychiatry on the North London rotational training scheme. She has both clinical experience and a research interest in crisis resolution teams. Her clinical experience includes special interest sessions working with the South Camden crisis resolution team under the supervision of John Hoult. Her research interests, supervised by Sonia Johnson, include investigating factors associated with psychiatric hospital admission despite the presence of crisis resolution teams and a qualitative study exploring decision-making processes among crisis team members.

Feleena Emerton is a senior occupational therapist and deputy team leader for the Cremorne community mental health team, a community-based acute care team forming part of the Royal North Shore–Ryde mental health services in Sydney, Australia. She has worked for the past 20 years in both acute inpatient and acute community psychiatry. She was extensively involved in the establishment of an early psychosis intervention team within the community services.

Alison Faulkner is a freelance researcher, trainer and consultant, working from a service user/survivor perspective. She has over 20 years of experience as a researcher in the mental health field and has worked for a range of organisations including universities and NHS trusts, the Mental Health Foundation, Rethink and the Richmond Fellowship. She is a member of INVOLVE, which seeks to promote public involvement in research. As a user of mental health services, Alison has experience of a range of services including acute inpatient care, crisis services, psychotherapy and medication.

Martin Flowers has been a psychiatric nurse for 30 years and has worked as a clinician and manager in both inpatient and community settings. In 1998, he became involved in crisis resolution services, helping to create and manage services in Camden and Islington. He has been a fellow with the London Development Centre and South East National Institute for Mental Health in England working on the development and training of crisis resolution teams and was a community teams programme manager for the Care Service Improvement Partnership for three years. He has had an association with the practice and development department of the Sainsbury Centre for Mental Health, again being involved with the development and training of crisis resolution services. Currently he is a crisis services manager in South Yorkshire.

Harm Gijsman trained in medicine and psychiatry at Leiden University, the Netherlands. He has an M.Sc. in epidemiology from the London School of Hygiene and Tropical Medicine and a Ph.D. in clinical psychopharmacology. From 2001 to 2005 he was consultant psychiatrist with the North Lambeth home treatment team, South London and Maudsley NHS Trust. He is currently Clinical and Research Director of the Early Psychosis Program of University Medical Centre Nijmegen and Nijmegen Mental Healthcare Organisation (GGZ Nijmegen) in the Netherlands.

Helen Gilburt has a Ph.D. in biological sciences. After experiencing mental health problems herself, she has turned her research skills to working in mental health. She is currently working as a researcher at the Institute of Psychiatry, King's College London, evaluating residential and inpatient acute mental health services.

Gyles Glover trained in psychiatry and public health. He has specialised in the use of large-scale information systems documenting mental health services and their activities at a national level. He led the development of the current English NHS dataset for mental healthcare for individuals and the annual detailed inventory of mental health services. He currently works at the NHS North East Public Health Observatory.

John Hoult is a psychiatrist who has led the introduction and national dissemination of crisis resolution teams both in Australia and the UK. Following his pioneering study of the outcomes of intensive community management as an alternative to hospitalisation carried out in Sydney in the late 1970s, he worked with state governments and local services on the development and dissemination of the crisis team model, now prevalent in many parts of Australia. In the mid 1990s, he developed and led the first UK crisis resolution team, which was in Birmingham. Subsequently he went on to develop and lead crisis and assertive outreach teams in inner London and Essex. He is an advisor on service development for the National Institute of Mental Health, England and is in demand nationally and internationally as a speaker and consultant.

Sonia Johnson studied social and political sciences and medicine at the Universities of Cambridge and Oxford and social psychology at the London School of Economics before beginning her psychiatric training. She is Reader in Social and Community Psychiatry at University College London and a consultant psychiatrist in the Camden and Islington Early Intervention Service for psychosis. She has spent her career so far working in inner London, and has previously been a clinical lecturer at the Institute of Psychiatry and a consultant psychiatrist in a community mental health team in Islington. Her main research interests are in evaluating innovative services such as crisis resolution teams, assertive outreach teams and early intervention services, in women's mental health and in dual diagnosis of substance misuse and psychosis. She is lead author of two major studies of crisis team outcomes.

Brynmor Lloyd-Evans has a Diploma in Social Work and a Masters degree in Applied Social Studies from Oxford University. He has worked in London in residential care and as a community mental health team social worker and is currently a researcher at University College London, evaluating residential and inpatient acute mental health services.

Lisa Marrett qualified as a registered mental health nurse in 1990 and has a first class honours degree in sociology from the University of the West of England (1993). She has worked as a lecturer and tutor in sociology at Bath Spa University College and also Southampton University, where she studied social research methods as a postgraduate. Her clinical background is in acute inpatient care and latterly in crisis and home treatment in inner city Bristol, where she managed a crisis and home treatment team after practicing clinically in the same team for three years in a specialist post, addressing the needs of the minority ethnic service user group in the home treatment setting. Lisa now works as the Diversity Training Lead for Avon and Wiltshire Mental Health Partnership Trust.

Roberto Mezzina is one of the psychiatrists who led the psychiatric reform in Trieste, Italy's best known centre for the development of innovative community mental health services. For the past 12 years, he has led a comprehensive 24-hour community mental health centre, in which home-based crisis care is integrated with a range of other service functions. He has written extensively on community mental health both in Italian and in English, and has spoken at conferences and led workshops around the world on this theme. He is involved with colleagues in the USA, Sweden and Norway in the International Recovery Research Group, and has contributed to several initiatives of the World Health Organization.

Justin Needle is a lecturer in health services research and policy at City University, London, having previously worked at the London School of Economics. He has also taught at the University of Dundee and University College London. His research focuses on policy, practice and workforce issues relating to the allied health professions. Research projects have included a systematic review of their role in health promotion, an investigation of the scope of therapeutic practice among UK optometrists, and a cross-national comparison of the organisation and professional practice of allied health professionals across Europe. He holds degrees from the Universities of Cambridge and Dundee, and an M.Sc. in social policy and planning from the London School of Economics. He has a particular interest in the relationships between allied health professionals and broader social policy issues, such as health inequalities and social exclusion.

Stephen Niemiec has worked in psychiatric nursing for over 30 years, in New Zealand, Australia and England. In 1999, he established the Newcastle and North Tyneside crisis assessment and treatment service, which was the first city-wide service of its kind in England. The positive impacts of that service are widely known and reported in the literature. Stephen was a member of the Mental Health Taskforce for England from 2001 to 2005, an associate for the National Institute of Mental Health and Associate Director of Nursing at Northumberland,

Newcastle and North Tyneside Mental Health Trust, as well as the nurse consultant for the crisis assessment team service. Stephen then travelled widely throughout England assisting mental health trusts in their development of crisis resolution and home treatment services. In 2005, he left the UK to return to Australia, where he is now the Mental Health Nursing Advisor for Queensland Health and Associate Professor of Nursing at the University of the Sunshine Coast.

Fiona Nolan trained as a mental health nurse before obtaining a degree in politics. She has worked across inpatient and community services over the past 20 years and currently manages a crisis team in North Islington. She is the nursing research lead for Camden and Islington NHS Foundation Trust, and a nursing research fellow at University College London. She is currently completing a Ph.D. at University College London supervised by Sonia Johnson and Paul Bebbington, investigating patient satisfaction with treatment by crisis teams.

Steve Ramsey is an experienced mental health professional holding postgraduate qualifications in management. He has more than 20 years experience in the planning, implementation, training and management of community-based adult mental health services, particularly crisis resolution and home treatment services. In 2001, he established Ramsey Consulting, a company providing consultancy services in Australia and the UK. In the UK, he has been involved with the implementation, training and review of crisis resolution services in numerous trusts.

Ciaran Regan is a consultant old-age psychiatrist in Central and North West London NHS Foundation Trust. She has worked in both the UK and Australia in crisis resolution teams. Her research interests include aetiology of Alzheimer's disease, management and treatment of mood disorders, adherence to medication regimens and carer morbidity.

Simon Richards is a double-certificate registered nurse with a BA in social welfare. He has worked in healthcare for over 25 years from acute hospital settings, community crisis and rehabilitation teams and now GP Shared Care. He has been extensively trained in cognitive–behavioural therapy, particularly in family psychoeducation with Professor Ian Falloon, and in narrative and Gestalt therapies. He has presented many conference papers and has collaborated with authors in Australia on producing training texts for mental health workers. He is employed in the Lower North Shore of Sydney where he coordinates the GP Shared Care program and family programs. His current interests include metabolic syndrome, clinical supervision, family work and training of postgraduate nurses.

Alan Rosen FRANZCP, MRCPsych., DPM, MB.BS., Grad. Dip, PAS., is a senior consultant psychiatrist and Clinical Director of the Royal North Shore Hospital and Community Mental Health Services, which has won several national and regional awards. He is also an associate professor at the School of Public Health, University of Wollongong and a clinical associate professor in the Department of Psychological Medicine, University of Sydney. He is a visiting senior consultant psychiatrist for West NSW Mental Health Services and Aboriginal Medical Services. He was visiting consultant to the Psychiatric Services Project, East Timor, 2000–2002, and Visiting Fellow in Medical Anthropology, Harvard University, 2006. He is an author of the *Life Skills Profile*, a nationally mandated functional ability measure with international applications, translations and research, and of the *Australian National Mental Health Service Standards*, and has been engaged in quantitative and qualitative research on mental health service systems and psychiatric stereotypes and stigma.

Jan Scott is Professor of Psychological Medicine, University of Newcastle upon Tyne, and is a Distinguished Founding Fellow of the Academy of Cognitive Therapy. Her main research focuses on combined pharmacological and psychological treatment strategies (using pharmacotherapy and cognitive therapy) in the treatment of individuals with bipolar disorders, chronic depression and treatment-resistant schizophrenia. Her clinical practice has predominantly been based in community mental health teams and has informed her work on translating specialist extended therapies into brief interventions deliverable by mental health professionals in day-to-day practice after minimal training. Professor Scott has over 250 publications in psychiatry including papers in high-impact journals, authored academic and self-help books, training manuals and book editorships. Professor Scott was Vice-chair of the MRC Mental Health and Neurosciences Board and is an assistant editor of the British Journal of Psychiatry.

Warren Shaw is an experienced general and mental health trained nurse with postgraduate qualifications in management. He has been involved with crisis teams for the last 22 years, initially as a clinician and for the last nine years as manager in the North Coast Area Mental Health Service in NSW, Australia. He has also worked as a consultant in the UK during the last five years, undertaking staff training and service reviews of crisis resolution services in a number of trusts. He has a particular interest in the development and enhancement of skills of individual clinicians and managers, and their contribution to the functioning of the team as a whole, as well as in issues of recruitment and retention of staff.

Mary Jane Tacchi is a consultant psychiatrist in the Newcastle crisis assessment and home-based treatment service. She was instrumental in its development and in 2002 was awarded Hospital Doctor of the Year for her role in the service, which has been successful in providing a real alternative to hospitalisation and in reducing bed occupancy. Prior to taking up a consultant post, she was awarded a Mental Health Foundation Research Fellowship to explore the long-term prognosis of affective disorders and undertook a diploma in cognitive therapy. She has maintained an interest in the adaptation of this therapy model in general adult psychiatry settings. Dr Tacchi has been involved in two research studies using abbreviated models of cognitive therapy for treatment of depression in primary care and to improve medication adherence in individuals with bipolar disorders. She has published a number of papers evaluating clinical services and is frequently invited to present talks and workshops on service developments such as the crisis assessment team and the role of consultant psychiatrists in modern mental health services. She has worked with the National Institute for Mental Health in England to enable trusts around the UK to implement such services and overcome perceived barriers.

Sylvia Tang is a consultant adult psychiatrist in the Camden and Islington NHS Foundation Trust and is Medical Director for Camden and Islington Mental Health and Social Care Trust. She is a sector consultant with both inpatient beds and a community mental health team and the lead consultant for the North Islington crisis team. Her experience of working with the crisis team over the last few years has led to a close working relationship around alternatives to hospital admission and particularly early discharge from hospital.

Graham Thornicroft is Professor of Community Psychiatry and Head of the multidisciplinary Health Service and Population Research Department at the Institute of Psychiatry, King's College London. He is a consultant psychiatrist and is Director of Research and Development at the South London and Maudsley NHS Foundation Trust. He chaired the External Reference Group for the National Service Framework for Mental Health in England. His areas of research expertise include stigma and discrimination, mental health needs assessment, the development of outcome scales, cost-effectiveness evaluation of mental health treatments, and mental health services in less economically developed countries. He has authored and co-authored 20 books and over 190 papers in peer-reviewed journals.

Waquas Waheed studied medicine in Pakistan and was later trained in psychiatry in Rawalpindi, Coventry and Manchester. He is a consultant psychiatrist with the crisis resolution and home treatment team at Accrington, Lancashire. His main research interests are in the mental health of ethnic minorities, developing culturally sensitive interventions and evaluating innovative services such as crisis resolution teams.

Foreword

It is well recognised that providing good care to psychiatric patients requires a variety of services organised into a comprehensive and coordinated system. The keystone element of that system is an effective response to a psychiatric crisis.

Not that long ago, the response to a psychiatric crisis was doing an evaluation and making a disposition. Depending on the severity of the crisis, the disposition was either an appointment to an outpatient clinic or hospitalisation. The result was inadequate and patients did not get the help they needed, leading to high hospital admission rates, frequent readmissions and suffering by both patients and their families.

This volume chronicles a revolutionary change to responding to a psychiatric crisis: the introduction of the 'crisis resolution team' (CRT). The goal of the CRT is to resolve the crisis and this includes not only assessing the patient but also developing a treatment plan and delivering the services to the patient's home until the patient is stabilised. The team then takes on the responsibility for ensuring that the patient is transferred to the appropriate service for further care.

As a result of the NHS Plan in 2000, there has been a rapid and wide implementation of these teams. This much-needed book fills a gap in the available literature in this area and will be of immense help to both the clinician and the researcher. The majority of its chapters are devoted to the clinical and organisational issues and challenges that staff of CRTs confront everyday in their work. In addition, the volume also gives a history of the development of the CRT and a review of the research literature.

This scholarly volume is well organised and clearly written. Although chapters are written by various authors, a good deal of effort has gone into bringing a consistency to the chapters rarely seen in edited books.

Leonard I. Stein,
Professor Emeritus,
University of Wisconsin School of Medicine
and Public Health

Acknowledgements

We are very grateful to our editors at Cambridge University Press for their support and forbearance throughout the writing of this book, and to the contributors, most of whom were admirably prompt and helpful in submitting their chapters. Many clinical and academic colleagues and many service users with whom we have worked have contributed to the ideas in the book, but above all, we would like to acknowledge John Hoult's role. The model on which this book is based is very much a product of his innovative approach, hard work and great ability to inspire people, sustained through several decades. He has been as helpful as ever in the production of this book.

Section 1

Introduction and concepts

Introduction

Sonia Johnson and Justin Needle

Crisis resolution teams (CRTs) have risen rapidly to prominence in the UK since the mid 1990s. We will go into a good deal more detail about the characteristics of these teams in subsequent chapters, especially Chapter 6, but it is probably helpful to begin with a working definition. As currently used, the term CRT is applied to specialist multidisciplinary teams that aim to:

- assess all patients being considered for admission to acute psychiatric wards
- initiate a programme of home treatment with frequent visits (usually at least daily) for all patients for whom this appears a feasible alternative to hospital treatment
- continue home treatment until the crisis has resolved and then transfer patients to other services for any further care they may need
- facilitate early discharge from acute wards by transferring inpatients to intensive home treatment.

A note on terminology: crisis resolution team, crisis assessment and treatment team and intensive home treatment team are currently used roughly synonymously in the UK. Crisis intervention team is an older term, which originally referred to services that applied crisis intervention theory to a broad range of psychosocial crises, not only those in which admission seemed imminent (Chapter 2). In the UK, the primary care physician is the general practitioner (GP), and the UK term will be used for this role throughout the book.

Prior to 2001, only a small handful of UK centres had CRTs, generally inspired by Australian models. As mandated by the *NHS Plan* (Department of Health, 2000), almost all English catchment areas are now served by CRTs, and several thousand staff have migrated into these teams. However, in contrast to the other types of functional team introduced alongside CRTs, assertive outreach teams and early intervention services for psychosis, very little literature had been published

Crisis Resolution and Home Treatment in Mental Health, ed. Sonia Johnson, Justin Needle, Jonathan P. Bindman and Graham Thornicroft. Published by Cambridge University Press. © Cambridge University Press 2008.

about these teams at the time their nationwide introduction was required, and this gap has subsequently been filled to only a very limited degree. Thus clinicians recruited to CRTs, service managers trying to sustain them, policy makers in other countries considering whether introducing them is a good choice and mental health services researchers seeking to understand their function and evidence base have had few written sources to consult on the following types of question.

- How did the CRT model develop and what ideas about the nature of crises and how to manage them underpin it?
- How much evidence is there for the effectiveness of CRTs?
- How do clinicians in CRTs assess patients and decide who is suitable for home treatment?
- What sort of care do CRTs provide to patients whom they accept for intensive home treatment?
- How do CRTs work with other components of the mental healthcare system, such as community mental health teams and inpatient wards?
- Can CRTs be enhanced by integration with other types of acute care, such as day hospitals and crisis houses?
- How do specialist CRTs doing only short-term work compare with community mental health teams (CMHTs) whose staffing has been enhanced so that they can provide intensive home treatment in a crisis as well as continuing care?
- How should CRTs be set up and organised, and what ensures their continuing effectiveness?

This book is intended to address all of these questions, drawing on the available research evidence and, above all, on the ideas and experiences of people who have been active in the development and implementation of the CRT model. We begin with the historical context. In Chapter 2, Sonia Johnson and Graham Thornicroft describe the gradual evolution of the CRT model as part of the deinstitutionalisation movement, which has dominated mental health service development in Europe and the English-speaking world over the past five decades. They describe various precursors that have influenced the current model and identify affinities with and distinctions from other significant community mental healthcare models, such as assertive outreach teams, crisis intervention teams and mobile crisis services. In Chapter 3, Gyles Glover and Sonia Johnson describe the emergence of a more definitive CRT model based on the precursors identified in Chapter 2, and its dissemination in Australia and in the UK, especially through the work in both countries of Dr John Hoult. This chapter also describes the impact on service use in England of nationwide implementation of the CRT model: a significant reduction in admission rates appears to have ensued.

Chapters 4 and 5 discuss the research evidence base for CRTs. When CRTs first became national policy in England, studies cited in support of them were generally investigations of pioneering services carried out in the 1970s and 1980s. The use of these studies as evidence was criticised on grounds of lack of relevance to the current context. As Sonia Johnson and Graham Thornicroft describe in Chapter 4, these criticisms have some weight, as the innovative teams investigated in these classic home treatment studies tended to work over a longer term with patients rather than withdrawing following the crisis. Comparison services were also very different from modern community mental health teams. However, as Sonia Johnson and Jonathan Bindman show in Chapter 5, a more convincing evidence base is starting to accumulate, and there are now substantial grounds for believing that CRTs reduce admission rates and are probably preferred by patients to hospital admission, though other differences in clinical and social outcome have not so far been demonstrated. Many unanswered questions about CRT effectiveness remain, however, and research in this area is impeded by considerable ethical and practical difficulties in recruiting people to studies at the time of a crisis.

Chapter 6 provides the context for the clinically oriented chapters that follow by describing the core CRT model. Sonia Johnson and Justin Needle draw on the available literature on CRTs and on interviews with key experts to outline, first, the rationale for CRT development and, second, the core organisational elements of CRTs and the main interventions they deliver. They find that CRTs are more a vehicle for delivering care than a specific type of treatment. There is a general consensus that principles such as focusing on crises sufficiently severe to warrant admission, gatekeeping hospital beds and working intensively in patients' homes are important, but within this framework a variety of philosophies of care and clinical approaches to the treatment of mental illness are possible. As CRTs provide only short-term treatment to patients whose needs are often very long term, the way in which they fit into and collaborate with the wider mental healthcare system is crucial. Jonathan Bindman addresses this in Chapter 7, focusing especially on the issue of maintaining continuity of care, which is identified in several chapters as the key challenge for CRTs. Lack of continuity, for example in therapeutic relationships, is a significant potential weakness of this model, and much care needs to be taken with communication and relationships with other parts of the service system and with the patient and his/her social network if short-term crisis treatment is to be a coherent part of an effective long-term strategy.

Chapters 8 to 18 are above all addressed to CRT staff and focus on various key aspects of CRT practice. In Chapter 8, John Hoult describes the process of carrying out an assessment for CRT care, emphasising the need for comprehensive social as well as clinical assessment. Mary-Anne Cotton concludes the chapter by summarising the limited research evidence about which patient characteristics are associated with being treated at home rather than admitted to hospital. The idea of treating severely and acutely ill patients at home has from the start had opponents as well as advocates, and one of the main grounds for this opposition, as with community care in general, has been safety. Consequently, risk assessment that is as accurate as possible, both at initial assessment and repeatedly throughout the period of home treatment, is critical if CRTs are to achieve sustained acceptance and success. In Chapter 9, Neil Brimblecombe outlines a strategy for risk assessment and management in CRTs, emphasising the importance of gathering data on risk from all available sources and checking accuracy, constantly re-assessing risk and adopting a realistic approach in which hospitalisation is not seen as an outcome to be avoided at all costs. John Hoult, in Chapter 10, gives a very practical account of how to manage symptoms of mental illness, with a final section by Fiona Nolan outlining the potential contribution of psychological treatments to the work of CRTs.

As many of the contributions to the book emphasise, the CRT model is based on the assumption that social factors are of central importance in understanding and managing mental health crises, and the following two chapters are devoted to these. In Chapter 11, Jonathan Bindman and Martin Flowers argue for the great importance in CRT work of psychosocial interventions, and the need for all members of the team to be flexible and willing to take a strong interest in issues such as patients' housing, whether they have a source of money and food, and whether they have legal problems or difficulties caring for children. Chris Bridgett and Harm Gijsman focus in Chapter 12 on work with social networks, including the use of a social systems approach to crisis work, a very practical way of working where the fulcrum is the convening of a social systems meeting, attended by as many as possible of the patient's core social network.

A number of specific issues related to clinical practice are dealt with in the succeeding chapters. In Chapter 13, Mary Jane Tacchi and Jan Scott discuss the all-important issues of engagement and adherence: CRTs will not succeed in managing people at the severely mentally ill end of the spectrum if they do not have excellent skills in these areas. In Chapter 14, Alison Faulkner and Helen Blackwell emphasise the many benefits from the perspective of the service user of the availability of intensive home treatment, but also draw attention to some important pitfalls. Themes emerging from their chapter include the importance of making a range of alternatives to admission available, including residential as well as home-based services, and of continuing to try to improve the quality of care on hospital wards for those who do need to be admitted. Their accounts also make apparent the extent to which CRTs depend on good leadership and organisation and high-quality clinicians: without these there is considerable potential for disruptions in continuity of care, sometimes of a dangerous nature, and for patients to become isolated at home and experience only brief and superficial contacts with a bewildering number of staff. In Chapter 15, Fiona Nolan and Sylvia Tang focus on early discharge from hospital wards, a CRT activity that has received less attention than diversion from admission but which is especially important if length of stay as well as number of admissions is to be reduced. The chapter also includes a more general discussion of the relationship between hospital and CRT, and of ways in which this may be enhanced by integrating different components of local acute care systems. In Chapter 16, Martin Flowers and Jonathan Bindman outline strategies for managing repeat CRT users, including advance directives and joint crisis plans. They identify an important goal for CRTs, to contribute to prevention or attenuation of the severity of future crises, especially among recurrent users of acute services. Chapter 17 returns to the salience of the social for CRTs: when patients are treated in their own homes rather than in an institutional setting, their social circumstances and identities are much more visible. Danny Antebi, Waquas Waheed, Sonia Johnson and Lisa Marrett discuss needs that are specific to members of particular ethnic or religious groups, or which vary by gender or sexual orientation. While specific knowledge about minority groups can be helpful, above all CRT staff need to approach all their patients with an open-minded, curious and non-judgemental attitude and to listen to and try to understand individual accounts of experiences and identity rather than relying on stereotypes. Finally, in Chapter 18, the complex issues of coercion and compulsion in CRTs are addressed by Jonathan Bindman, who describes the ways in which CRT practice may sometimes of necessity become coercive, and the need for open discussion within CRTs of the extent to which restricting freedom is ethically justifiable.

The focus shifts in Chapters 19 to 23 to variations on and enhancements of the CRT model. Alan Rosen, Paul Clenaghan, Feleena Emerton and Simon Richards in Chapter 19, and Roberto Mezzina and Sonia Johnson in Chapter 20, describe two internationally prominent and long-established service models, the Lower North Shore mental health services in Sydney and the Trieste model, respectively, in which intensive home treatment is not the province of a specialist team but one of a range of functions of a community team that also delivers continuing care. The advantages of such systems are above all in continuity of care, but as yet relatively little evidence is available regarding how the outcomes from intensive home treatment delivered in this way compare with those of specialist CRTs. In Chapter 21, Ciaran Regan and Claudia Cooper discuss the potential application of the CRT model to older people. So far, this group seems to have been relatively little served by CRTs, even where they do not explicitly exclude those beyond retirement age, and specialist CRTs for older people are very rare. This is an issue of equity, as there is no reason why older people should not benefit from intensive home treatment. Chapter 22, by Mary Jane Tacchi, describes experiences of integrating intensive home treatment services with acute day care, thus increasing the range of available ways of caring for people in crises. Some people's home environments are such that they do not benefit from remaining in them during a crisis, and in Chapter 23, Brynmor Lloyd-Evans, Sonia Johnson and Helen Gilburt discuss the ways in which community-based crisis residential services can be combined with CRT care to offer an acceptable and appropriate alternative to admission for this group.

In the final section of the book, the perspective shifts to that of service managers and service planners considering how to set up and sustain CRTs. Chapter 24, by Martin Flowers and John Hoult, provides guidance on how to set up a team that is adequately resourced and sufficiently integrated into the local service system to meet local needs. Principles to follow in order to make sure the service survives and becomes a valued part of the local system are also set out. Key tasks in implementing the model are to recruit a staff team suited to this way of work and to provide appropriate training for them: in Chapter 25, Steve Ramsey and Warren Shaw discuss how to do this. To conclude the book, in Chapter 26, Stephen Niemiec outlines key issues in the operational management of CRTs, including ensuring the team is of adequate size, implementing shift systems and managing communication effectively.

Thus overall this book constitutes a toolkit that should go some way towards meeting the needs for information and guidance of those wishing to establish, manage, work in or investigate CRTs. Despite the paucity of previous literature describing or evaluating the CRT model, it is now relatively well established, with some consensus on its components and operational principles. However, as will become apparent in the chapters that follow, the model cannot be regarded as fixed in every detail. Different teams may follow the same organisational principles, for example rapid assessment in crisis and intensive contact at home, yet may vary considerably in the treatments they offer their patients and in the philosophy of care on which their service is based. There is still considerable scope for innovation within the framework of this model, for example in areas such as development of family interventions that work well in CRTs, and for investigation of what works best for whom in acute care systems that include CRTs. We, therefore, hope that this book will provide not only practical guidance on the current model, but also a starting point for further innovation and service development.

REFERENCE

Department of Health (2000). *The NHS Plan*. London: The Stationery Office.

2

The development of crisis resolution and home treatment teams

Sonia Johnson and Graham Thornicroft

The history of crisis resolution and home treatment teams (CRTs) has not previously been very clearly documented. This chapter fills this gap by describing the development of the CRT model, identifying its main precursors and the contributions they have made to the current model. The focus will be on services for adults of working age, and an overview will be given of the history and characteristics of the main models that have contributed to the development of current CRTs. Research evaluations of these models are discussed in Chapters 4 and 5.

Information sources used in this history

The authors carried out a literature search regarding CRTs and other forms of intensive home treatment delivered in a crisis. They looked particularly for descriptions of how the models that appeared to be CRT precursors were organised and operated, and of their origins, including any theories that had informed their development and research evidence or clinical observations that influenced them.

As relevant written sources are few, one of the authors (SJ) also carried out a series of interviews with key people involved in the development of CRTs and their precursors.[1] Box 2.1 lists these people and says a little about them. The interviews took place in the course of 2002 and 2003 in a variety of locations, including participants' offices, a conference centre, one participant's home and Terminal 3 at Heathrow airport. Two interviews were carried out by phone. All were transcribed verbatim and content analysis was used to identify the main relevant themes and historical details.

[1] These interviews also form part of the basis for Chapter 6. They are referred to in the text as 'Bracken, interview', and so on.

Crisis Resolution and Home Treatment in Mental Health, ed. Sonia Johnson, Justin Needle, Jonathan P. Bindman and Graham Thornicroft. Published by Cambridge University Press. © Cambridge University Press 2008.

Box 2.1. Interview participants

Dr Patrick Bracken. Psychiatrist. Former home treatment consultant in Birmingham, developer of the Bradford Crisis Resolution Team (in operation since 1996). Also involved in establishing the Centre for Citizenship and Community Mental Health, University of Bradford.

Mr Martin Flowers. Psychiatric nurse. First leader of the South Islington CRT, one of the early UK model services, subsequently consultant on CRTs at the National Institute for Mental Health, England.

Dr John Hoult. Psychiatrist and researcher. Has replicated the Training in Community Living model in Sydney. Subsequently responsible for the development of CRTs in locations including Sydney, Birmingham, the inner London Borough of Islington and Essex.

Dr Matt Muijen. Psychiatrist and researcher at the Daily Living Programme, London. Subsequently involved in dissemination of the CRT model as Director of the Sainsbury Centre for Mental Health, London. Now Regional Advisor for Mental Health, World Health Organization European Office.

Dr Paul Polak. Former psychiatrist. Developer of a network of innovative community services in Denver, Colorado, in the 1970s. Since 1981, founder and Chief Executive of International Development Enterprises, working on the dissemination of affordable technologies in developing countries.

Mr Steve Ramsey. Psychiatric nurse. Member of the original Sydney team and subsequently involved in development and dissemination of assertive outreach and CRT services in Sydney. Now a freelance trainer on their implementation.

Professor Alan Rosen. Psychiatrist. Involved in the Australian implementation of the Training in Community Living model. Subsequently director of Royal North Shore Hospital and Community Mental Health Services, Sydney, where crisis resolution is integrated into a case management team. Posts at the Universities of Wollongong and Sydney.

Professor S. P. Sashidharan. Psychiatrist. Medical Director, North Birmingham Mental Health Trust and Professor of Community Mental Health, University of Central England. Involved in the development of CRTs in Birmingham.

Dr Dennis Scott. Retired psychiatrist. Developer of the Barnet Crisis Service, London.

Professor Leonard Stein. Psychiatrist. Developer of the Training in Community Living model and of CRTs in Madison, Wisconsin. Emeritus professor at the University of Wisconsin and medical director of the Dane County Mental Health Center.

Defining 'emergencies' and 'crises'

Some authors draw a distinction between psychiatric emergencies and psychosocial crises (Segal, 1990; Rosen, 1997). Emergencies tend to be defined as situations in which there is a need for immediate action, generally because of a high level of risk. A definition exemplifying this is Rosen's description of an emergency as 'a life-threatening situation demanding an immediate response', often requiring the attendance of emergency services such as the police and fire brigade. Other definitions have not set the threshold for defining an emergency quite so high but have emphasised the presence of substantial risk and an urgent need for professional intervention; they have also often defined a psychiatric emergency as something that occurs only in the context of a mental illness (Katschnig and Konieczna, 1990).

In contrast, the classical use of the term 'crisis' originates in crisis intervention theory (Caplan, 1961, 1964) and describes a general human response to severe psychosocial stress, rather than a manifestation of illness. In Caplan's (1961) formulation, a crisis is

provoked when a person faces an obstacle to important life goals that is, for a time, insurmountable through the utilization of customary methods of problem-solving. A period of disorganization ensues, a period of upset, during which many different abortive attempts at solution are made. Eventually some kind of adaptation is achieved, which may or may not be in the best interest of that person and his fellows.

Crises are thus periods of transition encountered by everyone, in which the potential role for professionals is to promote an adaptive way of coping, resulting in full recovery and, ideally, psychological growth.

In clinical practice, however, it is hard to set a clear boundary between emergencies and crises. Staff in services targeting people experiencing crises, classically defined, have found that individuals of previously good psychological adjustment with no diagnosable mental illnesses rarely present to them (Katschnig *et al.*, 1993), while difficulty adjusting to psychosocial stresses often contributes to the development of situations seen as psychiatric emergencies among people with severe mental illness (Jones and Polak, 1968). The usage of these terms has, therefore, shifted, so that recent discussions of service provision and evaluation have often used the term crisis in a more pragmatic way to describe situations in which there is an urgent need for professional intervention arising at least in part from mental health problems.

Where the central goal of crisis services is to prevent admission, as with CRTs, a still narrower definition tends to be used, reflecting this goal. Crises are viewed as situations in which current clinical and social problems and associated risks are severe enough for admission to an acute psychiatric ward to be considered a potentially appropriate response (Brimblecombe, 2001a). For the most part, the service models discussed in this chapter have as their main focus crises defined in this way, as the major aim of the services is to divert people from being admitted.

The context of development of crisis resolution teams: deinstitutionalisation

The wider context for the development of various types of community-based mental health service is the process called deinstitutionalisation, which involves reducing the number of psychiatric beds (especially long-stay beds) and developing community-based alternatives. This radical shift in service provision is already the subject of an extensive literature and will not be discussed in detail in this book. In both the UK and the USA, a major shift in patterns of service provision began in the 1950s. The asylum population in the UK peaked in 1954, when there were 152 000 residents in 130 large psychiatric hospitals. Subsequently, the decline in psychiatric inpatient numbers has been steady: by 1993 there were 39 500 beds, 52% in large Victorian hospitals, and in 2005–6 there were 29 802 mental illness beds in England (Department of Health, 2007), with around a dozen of the original Victorian hospitals still open (Roberts, 2005). In the USA, the population of the state hospitals, most of which had been established in the nineteenth century, peaked in 1955. In that year, 559 000 persons out of the total population of 165 million were resident in state mental hospitals; by 1998 this had fallen to 57 151 occupied beds for a population of about 275 million (Lamb and Bachrach, 2001). Similar policies have been pursued in much of continental Europe, often beginning somewhat later: for example, France has had a national mental health service reform policy based on deinstitutionalisation since the early 1960s, the Netherlands since the early 1970s, Germany since the mid 1970s, Italy since the late 1970s, and Spain since the early 1980s.

Alternatives to acute admission: early developments

The prevailing orthodoxy favouring admission for the treatment of acute mental illness began to be questioned even in the nineteenth century. For example, John Connolly, a psychiatrist known for his campaign against the use of physical restraints, argued that some patients might be better managed at home (Connolly, 1856). A domiciliary visiting service operated from Barnhill Hospital, Glasgow, in 1880 (Brimblecombe, 2001b), and during the same decade the newly founded Mental After Care Association (renamed 'Together' in 2005) established cottage homes for the mentally ill, intended mainly to facilitate discharge from the asylums but also admitting 'some people at risk of becoming insane' (Together, 2005).

However, the first admission-diversion service to stimulate widespread interest and discussion was that established by the psychiatrist Arie Querido in Amsterdam in the 1930s (Querido, 1935, 1968). Querido was influenced by the ideas about the importance of social environment promulgated by the mental hygiene movement, which was prominent in the USA in the early twentieth century. In 1933, he became Director of the Department of Mental and Nervous Diseases of the Amsterdam Public Health Board. The Depression created financial pressure for a reduction in bed use in Amsterdam, and he was asked to make savings. He began by visiting hospitals and interviewing patients, and he concluded that admission could be avoided for some and that management at home was advantageous because the social difficulties creating the crisis were visible and amenable to intervention. He, therefore, instituted home visits by a social worker and a psychiatrist to all patients referred for acute admission. An alternative community treatment plan, sometimes involving some follow-up home visits, was formulated whenever possible. The system he established attracted considerable international attention and proved an enduring one: in the 1960s, 12 psychiatrists and 25 social workers were providing a 24-hour home visiting rota for the whole of Amsterdam (Querido, 1968).

In the UK, community mental healthcare first gathered momentum in the 1950s. Alongside the unlocking of wards and development of hostels, as well as social worker and nurse visiting schemes for discharged patients, home visits to patients referred for admission became routine practice in some areas. The 'Worthing Experiment', initiated in 1956 in Sussex, included home visits by psychiatrists and social workers to establish whether an alternative to admission could be found: Carse *et al.* (1958) reported falls of 59% and 77% in admissions to the two local hospitals serving the area. This experiment was extended to Chichester in 1957 and evaluated in a study described in Chapter 4. Other centres where home visits prior to acceptance for admission were established practice included Nottingham, Salford, Plymouth and Dingleton in Scotland (Sainsbury and Grad, 1966; Ramon, 1985; Wing, 1991).

Pioneers of specialist crisis resolution teams

The early home-visiting initiatives in the UK generally formed part of a community-oriented reform of working practices throughout the psychiatric services of a catchment area – there were not separate teams dedicated solely to managing crises and preventing admission. In the 1960s and early 1970s, specialist admission teams with a distinct identity, staff team and budget were established and evaluated in various parts of the English-speaking world.

Early developments in the USA

In 1961, Benjamin Pasamanick established a service in Louisville, Ohio, that was designed to test the feasibility of managing patients with schizophrenia at home rather than in hospital (Pasamanick *et al.*, 1964, 1967). Donald Langsley's Family Crisis Therapy service in Denver, Colorado, began operating in 1963 and aimed to prevent admission through intervention targeting the emotional difficulties of the family as a whole (Langsley and Kaplan, 1968; Langsley *et al.*, 1971). Both these programmes were selective in recruiting patients and neither involved very intensive contact, but evaluations were published (Chapter 4) and formed part of the evidence base used to argue for the feasibility of subsequent projects involving alternatives to acute admission.

The network of services developed by Paul Polak in Denver, Colorado, in the 1970s was more extensive (Polak and Jones, 1973; Polak and Kirby, 1976). Polak's work had its roots in part in British community psychiatry, as he had worked from 1964 to 1966 at Dingleton, Scotland. Maxwell Jones, pioneer of the inpatient therapeutic community movement, led the Dingleton service between 1962 and 1969, and he subsequently also worked with Polak in Denver as a consultant. During Jones's tenure, a practice developed at Dingleton of multidisciplinary home visits prior to admission to assess patients' social situations and whether they might be able to stay at home.

Polak became director of Fort Logan Mental Health Centre, Denver, in 1971. Innovations over the next five years included a team that assessed all individuals referred for admission at home and offered 24-hour home treatment whenever feasible, integration of hospital and community treatment teams, and a network of family sponsor homes in which families were paid to accommodate up to two patients in crisis, supported by the home treatment team. Distinctive characteristics of the Denver system included extensive use of volunteers, a system of staff promotion based on attainment of key skills in clinical work rather than professional qualifications, and the elimination of clinical staff offices suitable for interviewing patients so that all patient contact had to take place in homes or other community settings. This network of services endured for 10 years but withered away in the early 1980s, following Polak's departure in 1981 to work on technologies for supplying water in developing countries and the withdrawal of much state support for community mental health programmes under the Reagan administration.

The Barnet family psychiatric service

Although its resources were initially very limited, the Barnet crisis service in North London broke new ground in the UK as a specialist team with a distinct identity, dedicated to hospital diversion and the initiation of community treatment (Scott, 1980; Scott, interview). Dennis Scott, the psychiatrist who established it in 1970 at Napsbury Hospital, had trained in psychoanalysis as well as general psychiatry and was influenced more by the ideas of R. D. Laing than by any knowledge of other home assessment and treatment initiatives.

Initially, the Barnet service operated only during office hours. Patients referred for admission were interviewed at home with their families by a psychiatrist and a social worker. Their aims were to understand the family processes contributing to the crisis and to find a way of resolving it without admission. If prevention of admission seemed feasible, further meetings could sometimes be arranged during the following week, but usually visits took place no more than once a week and longer-term care after resolution of the crisis was offered in an outpatient clinic. The strength of local opposition is a striking aspect of the service's early history: in Scott's words, 'the old institution tried to terminate the existence of the team which initiated community practice' (Scott and Seccombe, 1976), with the local MP, at the instigation of Scott's colleagues, asking questions in Parliament regarding the safety of the new service. Following Scott's departure from the service (he went on to work as a group therapist using bioenergetic and transcendental models), a 24-hour service providing multidisciplinary crisis assessments continued to operate in Barnet until the introduction of CRTs.

The Training in Community Living model

The evaluation of the Training in Community Living service in Madison, Wisconsin (Stein and Test, 1980; Stein, interview), has the potentially confusing distinction of being cited as supporting evidence for two prominent service models. It is often identified as a precursor both of CRTs and of assertive community treatment (assertive outreach) teams (AOTs). There are resemblances between CRTs and AOTs: both involve intensive contact with patients in community settings and integration of treatment of mental illness with help with social and practical problems. However, the populations served and timescales are different: CRTs provide short-term treatment for mental health problems of varying type, severity and duration, while assertive outreach is a long-term approach to the care of a selected subgroup who have severe illnesses and are especially difficult to engage and treat effectively. The original Training in Community Living service had elements in common with each of these later models: as in CRTs, its patients were recruited at the time of a crisis and, whenever feasible, initial intensive home treatment was provided as a substitute for admission. However, like AOTs, the Madison team continued to treat people intensively in the community once the initial crisis had resolved, with the long-term goals of improving their stability in the community and their social functioning.

An initial pilot service in Madison had involved discharge of selected state hospital inpatients to an intensive community treatment programme. Results were promising, paving the way for introduction of the more substantial Training in Community Living programme, to which patients were recruited at the point of referral for hospital admission. Staff were available 24 hours a day and aimed to support patients in various aspects of their lives, including getting material resources such as food, shelter and medical care; coping with daily living tasks such as using public transport, preparing meals and budgeting; and job seeking and constructive use of leisure time.

A high level of staffing (14 staff for 65 patients, though the majority were nursing aides rather than professionals) allowed very intensive contact, with staff sometimes spending several hours a day with patients, especially during the initial few weeks. The evaluation of this service is described in Chapter 4.

Replication of the Training in Community Living model

A second hybrid service often cited in support of both CRTs and AOTs is that established by John Hoult in Sydney in 1979 (Hoult, 1986; Hoult, interview). Hoult had worked in Britain in the early 1970s and had visited the Dingleton service. On returning to Sydney, he became disillusioned by the very limited capacity of the community centre in which he worked for treating severely mentally ill people in their homes. Looking for alternative models, he visited Polak's service in Denver and Scott's in Barnet in 1977, and then came across an early paper on the Training in Community Living model and decided to replicate it. Alan Rosen, who had previously worked with Scott in Barnet and was recruited to work with Hoult, describes the Sydney community service as combining elements of the Barnet approach to crisis management and family work and the Madison approach to continuing care (Rosen, interview). Outcomes from both the Sydney service and the Daily Living Programme, a further replication of the Training in Community Living model carried out in London, are described in Chapter 4.

The first crisis resolution teams

The crisis resolution team in Madison, Wisconsin

The hybrid nature of the Training in Community Living programme makes it misleading to present it as a prototype of the CRT; however, one of its successors in Madison fits this bill better. In 1974, Leonard Stein moved from the state hospital where the Training in Community Living study was carried out to become director of the Dane County Mental Health Center. His brief was to set up a full network of community services for the area (Stein, 1991, 1993; Stein, interview). His most pressing task was reduction of dependence on expensive acute hospital beds. He decided that this could best be achieved by instituting a specialist crisis resolution and stabilisation service with the capacity to carry out very rapid assessments of everyone referred for hospital admission and to provide intensive community treatment for a short period. This has operated in Dane County since the 1970s. It is available 24 hours, screens all patients prior to admission, facilitates early discharges from local inpatient wards and can visit several times a day if required. Once stabilised, patients are discharged to other services for continuing care. For patients already looked after by other services, such as the local case management teams and AOTs, it fills in gaps in their availability at nights and weekends.

Crisis teams in Australia

Some features of the initial Sydney team were also subsequently incorporated in the local development of specialist CRTs (Reynolds *et al.*, 1990; Rosen, interview; Hoult, 1991; Hoult, interview). When Hoult's research study ended, resources were cut and a decision was, therefore, made to integrate the remaining staff with two existing case management teams in order to provide an intensive home treatment capacity within these teams. This service has since continued to provide an assessment and intensive treatment service to people in crisis which is integrated into a community mental health team and is described in Chapter 19.

In 1983, the Richmond Report on mental healthcare in New South Wales recommended that services modelled on Hoult's Sydney service be introduced throughout the state. Although his original team had subsequently adopted an integrated model, Hoult at this time believed that specialist CRTs, providing an initial period of intensive treatment but then withdrawing once the crisis had resolved, were more likely to produce sustained change in clinical approaches to the acutely mentally ill (Hoult, interview). This was influenced by discussions with Stein, who suggested that it was unrealistic to expect one team to provide both crisis care for a broad range of service users and intensive community continuing care for the particularly disabled subgroup requiring it. Specialist CRTs, therefore, began to be introduced across New South Wales, though full statewide implementation was not achieved as a newly elected Liberal government withdrew support from the policy in 1988.

Subsequently, crisis teams have continued operating in parts of New South Wales, bolstered since 1993 by the requirement in the Australian National Mental Health Strategy that every area should offer 24-hour access to services in the community. However, their configurations and capacities vary substantially and some have had to reduce hours or to base themselves mainly in hospital casualty departments as their resources have dwindled (Rosen, interview). In Victoria, a more prescriptive policy has been in force since 1994, prefiguring the English National Health Service (NHS) modernisation (Chapter 3) in requiring that a particular service configuration be adopted everywhere. This includes so-called crisis assessment and treatment teams, which operate 24 hours and serve adults of working age during office hours and the whole population out of hours (Carroll *et al.*, 2001). These teams resemble in most respects the CRT model subsequently introduced throughout England.

Other models of community-based crisis care

The main focus of this chapter has been on precursors to the CRT model as currently implemented in Australia and England. There have, however, been several other strands in the history of the development of alternatives to admission in the developed world over the past half-century. To conclude this chapter, we briefly describe the ones that involve specialist community teams working with people experiencing mental health crises in their own homes. As will be seen, although their origins and the names used to describe them may be different from CRTs, some of the services described as crisis intervention teams or mobile crisis services have, in fact, borne a considerable resemblance to CRTs. Other types of alternative to admission not discussed here but covered elsewhere in this book are crisis houses and other residential alternatives to admission (Chapter 23), acute day hospitals (Chapter 22) and services that integrate intensive home treatment with continuing community care (Chapters 19 and 20).

Crisis intervention services

Designated crisis intervention services have slipped out of vogue in much of the Anglophone world, but between the 1950s and the 1980s, crisis intervention theory (Caplan, 1961) underpinned the development of many services on both sides of the Atlantic. In the US heyday of the theory in the 1950s and 1960s, walk-in crisis clinics proliferated in casualty departments and, later, in community mental health centres (Wellin *et al.*, 1987). The brief psychological interventions they provided were intended, in the words of one proponent, as 'on the spot treatment for troubled feelings and the vexing ordinary problems of everyday life' (Bellak, 1960). The ascendancy of biomedical views of mental illness, failure to recruit many otherwise mentally healthy individuals to brief crisis interventions, and funding restrictions contributed to the waning of the crisis intervention model in the USA during the 1970s and 1980s. As this decline occurred, similar walk-in services based on crisis intervention theory became widespread in Europe, especially in the Netherlands and German-speaking countries (Katschnig *et al.*, 1993).

As in the USA, European services tended not to attract the generally healthy population originally envisaged (Katschnig *et al.*, 1993), and doubts were in any case increasing about whether they were an appropriate target group. Dissatisfaction also grew with the capacity of these services to prevent hospital admission. In the Netherlands, for example, walk-in mental health services providing emergency care to a wide range of people were believed to have caused a marked increase in psychiatric admissions during the 1980s (Schudel, 1995).

Such doubts about the original crisis intervention service model have meant that, even though they have retained the term 'crisis intervention' in their names, some European services have evolved towards a focus on diverting severely mentally ill individuals from acute admission and on managing them at home, thus developing an increasing resemblance to the current CRT model. For example, four mental health catchment areas in Paris are served by the Equipe Rapide d'Intervention de Crise (ERIC). This 24-hour service provides home assessments and interventions lasting up to a month. A wide range of crises, including domestic violence, are addressed by the team, which follows classical crisis intervention theory in aiming to prevent the development of chronic mental health problems among people experiencing psychosocial crises. However, ERIC resembles CRTs in aiming to assess patients referred for acute admission and to prevent this wherever possible by providing care at home instead (Robin *et al.*, 2001). Another example comes from Austria, where crisis intervention teams that work to a substantial extent in patients' homes and aim to prevent admission have been established in several regions (Haberfellner *et al.*, 1997).

Mobile crisis services

In the USA, teams described as mobile crisis services proliferated in the 1980s and 1990s. Unlike crisis intervention teams, these services have developed more as ad hoc responses to local service needs than on the basis of a defined theoretical model. At their simplest, mobile crisis services are triage services. They are often based in general hospital emergency rooms and their role is to visit patients at home when assessment in the emergency room is not feasible and to assess whether admission is required or whether some other care plan can be made. In this basic form, mobile crisis teams do not take responsibility for continuing management of the crisis but refer to other services that can undertake this (Allen, 1996).

Teams described as mobile crisis services are, however, very diverse (Geller *et al.*, 1995; Guo *et al.*, 2001), with variations in staffing, hours, where they are based and the extent to which they provide continuing treatment. Some services provide a limited number of home visits before referring on to other services if needs cannot quickly be met, while in others, such as the team serving the Lower East Side of New York (Chiu and Primeau, 1991), more prolonged home visiting has become usual. A shared characteristic of all variants of the mobile crisis service is a lack of data on their outcomes (Geller *et al.*, 1995).

Key points

- Services that offer emergency assessment and intensive home treatment as an alternative to acute hospital admission are an element in the deinstitutionalisation movement that has been in progress since the 1950s in Western Europe and the English-speaking world.
- The current CRT model has evolved rather gradually, shaped by a number of precursors in the USA, Australia and England.
- The CRTs and AOTs share some common ancestry but now serve very distinct populations (all people at risk of acute admission versus a selected subgroup with particularly high levels of need) over different timescales (short-term acute treatment over a few days or weeks versus long-term care).
- The CRTs in Europe and mobile crisis services in the USA have on the whole developed separately from CRTs in Australia and the UK, but some services bearing other names have come to bear a considerable resemblance to CRTs.

REFERENCES

Allen, M. H. (1996). Definitive treatment in the psychiatric emergency service. *Psychiatric Quarterly*, **67**, 247–62.

Bellak, L. (1960). A general hospital as a focus of community psychiatry: a trouble shooting clinic combines important functions as part of a hospital's emergency service. *Journal of the American Medical Association*, **174**, 2214–17.

Brimblecombe, N. (2001a). Introduction. In *Acute Mental Health Care in the Community: Intensive Home Treatment*, ed. N. Brimblecombe. London: Whurr, pp. 1–5.

Brimblecombe, N. (2001b). Community care and the development of intensive home treatment services. In *Acute Mental Health Care in the Community: Intensive Home Treatment*, ed. N. Brimblecombe. London: Whurr, pp. 5–28.

Caplan, G. (1961). *Approach to Community Mental Health*. New York: Grune and Stratton.

Caplan, G. (1964). *Principles of Preventive Psychiatry*. New York: Basic Books.

Carroll, A., Pickworth, J. and Protheroe, D. (2001). Service innovations: an Australian approach to community care – the Northern Crisis Assessment and Treatment Team. *Psychiatric Bulletin*, **25**, 439–41.

Carse, J., Panton, N. E. and Watt, A. (1958). A district mental health service. The Worthing Experiment. *Lancet*, **i**, 39–41.

Chiu, T. L. and Primeau, C. (1991). A psychiatric mobile crisis unit in New York City: description and assessment, with implications for mental health care in the 1990s. *International Journal of Social Psychiatry*, **37**, 251–8.

Connolly, J. (1856). *The Treatment of the Insane without Mechanical Restraints*. London: Smith, Elder and Co.

Department of Health (2007). *Hospital Activity Statistics*. London: The Stationery Office. http://www.performance.doh.gov.uk/hospitalactivity/data_requests/beds_open_overnight.htm. Accessed: 23 June 2007.

Geller, J. L., Fisher, W. H. and McDermeit, M. (1995). A national survey of mobile crisis services and their evaluation. *Psychiatric Services*, **46**, 893–7.

Guo, S., Biegel, D. E., Johnsen, J. A. and Dyches, H. (2001). Assessing the impact of community-based mobile crisis services on preventing hospitalization. *Psychiatric Services*, **52**, 223–8.

Haberfellner, E. M., Hallermann, G. and Schwarz-Traunmuller, B. (1997). Mobile crisis intervention and emergency psychiatry: experience over three years. *Psychiatrische Praxis*, **24**, 235–6.

Hoult, J. (1986). Community care of the acutely mentally ill. *British Journal of Psychiatry*, **149**, 137–44.

Hoult, J. (1991). Home treatment in New South Wales. In *The Closure of Mental Hospitals*, ed. P. Hall and I. F. Brockington. London: Gaskell, pp. 107–14.

Jones, M. and Polak, P. (1968). Crisis and confrontation. *British Journal of Psychiatry*, **114**, 169–74.

Katschnig, H. and Konieczna, T. (1990). Innovative approaches to delivery of emergency services in Europe. In *Mental Health Care Delivery*, ed. I. M. Marks and R. L. Scott. Cambridge: Cambridge University Press, pp. 85–103.

Katschnig, H., Konieczna, T. and Cooper, J. (1993). *Emergency Psychiatric and Crisis Intervention Services in Europe: A Report Based on Visits to Services in Seventeen Countries*. Geneva: World Health Organization.

Lamb, H. R. and Bachrach, L. L. (2001). Some perspectives on deinstitutionalization. *Psychiatric Services*, **52**, 1039–45.

Langsley, D. G. and Kaplan, D. M. (1968). *The Treatment of Families in Crisis*. New York: Grune & Stratton.

Langsley, D. G., Machotka, P. and Flomenhaft, K. (1971). Avoiding mental hospital admission: a follow-up study. *American Journal of Psychiatry*, **127**, 1391–4.

Pasamanick, B., Scarpitti, F. R., Lefton, M. *et al.* (1964). Home versus hospital care for schizophrenics. *Journal of the American Medical Association*, **187**, 177–81.

Pasamanick, B., Scarpitti, F. R. and Dinitz, S. (1967). *Schizophrenics in the Community: An Experimental Study in the Prevention of Hospitalization*. New York: Century-Crofts.

Polak, P. R. and Jones, M. (1973). The psychiatric nonhospital: a model for change. *Community Mental Health Journal*, **9**, 123–32.

Polak, P. R. and Kirby, M. W. (1976). A model to replace psychiatric hospitals. *Journal of Nervous and Mental Disease*, **162**, 13–22.

Querido, A. (1935). Community mental hygiene in the city of Amsterdam. *Mental Hygiene*, **19**, 177–95.

Querido, A. (1968). The shaping of community mental health care. *British Journal of Psychiatry*, **114**, 293–302.

Ramon, S. (1985). *Psychiatry in Britain: Meaning and Policy*. Beckenham: Croom Helm.

Reynolds, I., Jones, J. E., Berry, D. W. and Hoult, J. E. (1990). A crisis team for the mentally ill: the effect on patients, relatives and admissions. *Medical Journal of Australia*, **152**, 646–52.

Roberts, A. (2005). *Index of English and Welsh Lunatic Asylums and Mental Hospitals*. London: Middlesex University Web. http://www.mdx.ac.uk/www/study/4_13_Ta.htm. Accessed: 6 March 2006.

Robin, M., Pochard, F., Ampelas, J. F. *et al.* (2001). Psychiatric emergency and crisis services in France. *Therapie Familiale*, **22**, 153–68.

Rosen, A. (1997). Crisis management in the community. *Medical Journal of Australia*, **167**, 633–8.

Sainsbury, P. and Grad, J. (1966). Evaluating the community psychiatric service in Chichester. *Milbank Memorial Fund Quarterly*, **44**, 231–79.

Schudel, W. J. (1995). Acute hospital alternatives in the Netherlands: crisis intervention centres. In *Alternatives to the Hospital for Acute Psychiatric Treatment*, ed. R. Warner. Washington, DC: American Psychiatric Press, pp. 95–108.

Scott, R. D. (1980). A family-oriented crisis service to the London Borough of Barnet. *Health Trends*, **12**, 66–8.

Scott, R. D. and Seccombe, P. (1976). Community psychiatry: setting up a service on a shoestring. *Mindout*, **17**, 5–7.

Segal, S. (1990). Emergency care for the acute and severely mentally ill. In *Innovations in Mental Health Care*, ed. R. L. Scott and I. Marks. Cambridge: Cambridge University Press, pp. 104–9.

Stein, L. I. (1991). A systems approach to the treatment of people with chronic mental illness. In *The Closure of Mental Hospitals*, ed. P. Hall and I. F. Brockington. London: Gaskell, pp. 99–106.

Stein, L. I. (1993). Creating change: a case study. In *Community Mental Health Care: International Perspectives on Making it Happen*, ed. C. Dean and H. Freeman. London: Gaskell, pp. 18–34.

Stein, L. I. and Test, M. A. (1980). Alternative to mental hospital treatment. I. Conceptual model, treatment program, and clinical evaluation. *Archives of General Psychiatry*, **37**, 392–7.

Together (formerly the Mental After Care Association) (2005). *Our History*. London: Together. http://www.together-uk.org/?id=106. Accessed 22 October 2005.

Wellin, E., Slesinger, D. P. and Hollister, C. D. (1987). Psychiatric emergency services: evolution, adaptation and proliferation. *Social Science and Medicine*, **24**, 475–82.

Wing, J. K. (1991). Vision and reality. In *The Closure of Mental Hospitals*, ed. P. Hall and I. F. Brockington. London: Gaskell, pp. 10–19.

3

The crisis resolution team model: recent developments and dissemination

Gyles Glover and Sonia Johnson

As described in Chapter 2, the development of crisis services before the late 1990s was rather piecemeal. Except for the adoption of crisis teams throughout one Australian state, most of the early developments were single model services, often widely admired but little replicated. The recent NHS modernisation in England radically reversed this picture, in that the introduction of crisis resolution teams (CRTs) became government policy. The context in which this has occurred, the function that CRTs are intended to serve in modern mental healthcare systems and the implementation of this new English policy will be described in this chapter.

The first English crisis resolution teams

From the late 1980s to the late 1990s, the cornerstone of community mental healthcare in the UK was the community mental health team (CMHT). Service planners in most English catchment areas followed the pattern established by the British community care pioneers of the 1950s and 1960s: when home visits were provided in crises, this was usually the responsibility not of a distinct crisis service but of a generic catchment area service for the mentally ill. An example of a project that sought to introduce more extensive home working within this model was the introduction and evaluation by Burns and colleagues (1993) in southwest London in the late 1980s of multidisciplinary home visits for all new referrals within two weeks of referral. The CMHTs carried out these home visits, resulting in substantially lower admission rates in the group randomly allocated to this approach compared with the group who were not automatically offered assessment at home.

In the early 1990s, CMHTs were, therefore, the main providers of emergency intervention in the community. Most, however, operated only 9 am to 5 pm, five

Crisis Resolution and Home Treatment in Mental Health, ed. Sonia Johnson, Justin Needle, Jonathan P. Bindman and Graham Thornicroft. Published by Cambridge University Press. © Cambridge University Press 2008.

days a week, which limited their capacity to respond to crises and substitute for acute admission. In a few areas, doubts about the effectiveness of community management of emergencies by CMHTs led to experimentation with other models. In Birmingham, two home treatment programmes were introduced in the late 1980s and early 1990s. Dean and Gadd evaluated a programme tailored to the needs of the local Asian community – this was an integrated service offering both crisis and continuing care within a single South Birmingham sector (Dean *et al.*, 1993). Evaluation of this service is described in Chapter 4, but it was not sustained long term. Subsequently, Sashidharan and his colleagues introduced a home treatment programme to a catchment area in North Birmingham in the early 1990s that was targeted especially at young Black Caribbean men (Sashidharan, interview). Then, following a review and reorganisation of services, North Birmingham saw the introduction of a more intensive and highly staffed model of community crisis care: the Psychiatric Emergency Team established in Yardley in 1995 by John Hoult, recently arrived from Australia.

The Yardley team has been an important model for the subsequent dissemination of the CRT model in England and for the policy guidance issued by the UK Department of Health. In setting up the Yardley team, Hoult drew on his experiences in Sydney (Chapter 2) and his observations regarding organisational factors that seemed to be associated with greater effectiveness among Australian CRTs. Unlike previous Birmingham home treatment services, Yardley was a specialist team, separate from local teams providing continuing care, with functions including emergency assessments, controlling access to acute beds, providing intensive home treatment with the capacity to visit at least twice daily if needed and supporting early discharge from hospital. This model was subsequently adopted throughout North Birmingham and in other centres, including Bradford (1996) and the London Borough of Islington (1999), where Hoult worked from 1998 until 2004. John Mahoney, Chief Executive of the North Birmingham service, became joint head of mental health at the English Department of Health in 1998, enhancing the North Birmingham model's influence on national policy.

The 'crisis in acute care' and NHS modernisation

By the late 1990s, pressure for a new approach to management of psychiatric emergencies in England came from several sources. First, a small increase in the acute admission rate for adults was observed in the mid 1990s, together with a larger rise in compulsory admissions (Szmukler and Holloway, 2001). In certain areas, especially inner London, demand for acute beds considerably exceeded supply, which led to debate about whether acute bed provision had been reduced excessively. Second, dissatisfaction with the response to psychiatric emergencies, especially out of hours, was widespread among service users, carers and GPs. Third, service users' experiences of admission to acute hospital wards were frequently reported to be unpleasant: physical environments were often poor and opportunities for activity limited, and many inpatients felt unsafe, especially because they felt at risk from violence from other patients (Rose, 2001). Acute inpatient wards were also criticised for lacking clear therapeutic models for the management of crises and for limited contact between staff and patients (Quirk and Lelliott, 2001).

Each of these factors contributed to a perceived 'crisis in acute care' (Appleby, 2003). While a consensus existed among planners and providers of services that the policy of closing most large psychiatric hospitals and long-stay wards over the previous 40 years had been sensible, there was far less agreement about whether and how acute beds for management of psychiatric emergencies could be replaced by community alternatives. This was the backdrop to the NHS modernisation plans introduced between 1999 and 2002. As well as addressing this perceived deficit in acute care, the modernisation included plans to remedy the problem of difficult-to-engage, chronically ill patients through the nationwide introduction of assertive outreach teams, and to improve the prognosis of psychosis by means of early intervention services.

The first step in the development of a new policy on crisis services was the stipulation in the *National Service Framework for Mental Health* (Department of Health, 1999) that 24-hour access to emergency assessment must be available and that local services should be able to offer home treatment as an alternative to hospital admission. At this stage, no particular model of service organisation was mandated. The following year, however, saw publication of *The NHS Plan* (Department of Health, 2000), which committed the government to developing a target number of 335 crisis teams, each seeing an average of 300 people per year. The following year, more detailed guidance for their organisation appeared (Department of Health, 2001). This indicated that CRTs should comprise around 14 clinical staff (including the team leader), carry caseloads of 20 to 30 patients at a time and be available 24 hours a day, seven days a week.

Reception of the policy

A 1998 survey of chief executives of mental health trusts (Owens *et al.*, 2000) had found that 97% favoured intensive home treatment, although only 16% reported that their trusts provided it; hence this new direction was presumably well received by managers. Clinicians, by comparison, were less than unanimous. Smyth and Hoult (2000) argued that home treatment had been demonstrated to be a safe, feasible and cheaper alternative to hospitalisation, which patients overwhelmingly preferred. Pelosi and Jackson (2000) responded that the evidence was outdated (Chapter 4) and that excessive disruption to continuity of care was likely to result from CRT introduction. Four years later, Harrison and Traill (2004) reported that clinical opinion was still divided.

Monitoring

Following the publication of the National Service Framework, the Department of Health set up a system to monitor progress in moving towards complete nationwide introduction of all the new types of service. This 'service mapping' was led by one of us (G. G.) and took the form of an annual inventory of all services provided for people with a mental health problem. The 'local implementation teams' responsible for establishing the new types of service were required each autumn to appoint a mapping lead whose task was to identify all specialist services for mentally ill people within the area, irrespective of the agency running them. They had to identify, for each service, a reporter who would answer a small number of questions, indicating the size, staffing and key operational characteristics of the service. The first mapping – in many ways a pilot exercise – was undertaken in September/October 2000. The format was developed considerably during the following year and the exercise was carried out fairly consistently until spring 2006. All the data that follow are derived from this mapping.

Basic statistics are shown in Table 3.1.[1] In September 2000, only nine teams that had more than 10 staff (an effective minimum for this type of work) *and* that operated around the clock were reported. By March 2006, this had risen to 216, although we do not know exactly what 24-hour availability means in all cases: it may indicate that the CRT is fully operational and the office staffed throughout, or else that staff are on call from home for selected emergency situations only.

What is a crisis team?

Taking snapshot counts of team numbers during a period of rapid growth raises the vexed question of what counts as a team. In pure research, a detailed and specific definition would be adopted and any team failing to meet it would simply not be counted. However, working at the interface between research and service management, greater flexibility was needed. The definition of a CRT used for service mapping purposes is set out in Box 3.1. But local implementation teams were keen to show that they were implementing the new guidance, at least

---

[1] These figures are not directly comparable to the government target for reasons discussed below.

Table 3.1. Development of crisis resolution team numbers as reported in annual service mapping (England, 2000–6)[a]

	2000	2001	2002	2003	2004	2006 (Jan)
Teams	34	48	59	121	196	262
Teams available 24 hours (%)	38	44	54	61	72	97
Teams with 10 or more staff (%)	38	58	63	62	72	90
Teams with both (%)	26	35	39	48	58	82
Total staff (England)	317	573	892	1586	2985	4860

Note:
[a] Figures relate to September of the year unless indicated otherwise.
Source: Adult Mental Health Service Mapping. Durham: University of Durham and Department of Health, http://www.amhmapping.org.uk/reports.

Box 3.1. Definitions used for service mapping purposes

Crisis resolution team

A crisis resolution team (CRT, sometimes called home treatment) provides intensive support for people in mental health crisis in their own home, and stays involved until the crisis is resolved. It is designed to provide prompt and effective home treatment, including medication, in order to prevent hospital admission and provide support to informal carers. CRTs have the following characteristics:
- they are multidisciplinary
- they are available to respond 24 hours a day, seven days a week
- staff are in frequent contact with service users, often seeing them at least once on each shift
- they provide intensive contact over a short period of time
- staff stay involved until the problem is resolved
- staff in the teams are dedicated to crisis resolution and home treatment work only
- only short-term intervention is undertaken, with clients referred to other services if longer-term follow-up is needed.

Mental health crisis intervention service

A separate listing was included in the mapping for other mental health crisis intervention services that provided assessment and intervention for psychological or emotional crises but that were not intended to deliver home treatment for individuals otherwise requiring hospitalisation. Where community mental health teams provided crisis intervention and home treatment, respondents were asked to list this as one of the functions of the team rather than to identify these teams as CRTs.

in part because this was the subject of performance monitoring. They were, therefore, naturally inclined to include recently established teams that were not yet fully operational in their reporting. In practice, a senior nurse would usually be appointed first who would spend a few months recruiting staff and designing operational policies. When the first wave of staff arrived, the team would start accepting cases, though usually not at full capacity. Teams would subsequently develop in numbers, range of staff and operational hours over the next six to twelve months. In some cases, in the light of early experience, teams were either split or merged.

A second type of definitional issue arose in the early years of mapping from the existence of a number of teams providing other types of psychiatric emergency assessment or care, based, for example, on crisis intervention theory (Chapter 2). Respondents were asked to classify these as mental health crisis intervention services (Box 3.1), but some confusion is likely to have arisen in early versions of the mapping between such services and CRTs.

Crisis resolution team staff

The service mapping also requested the whole-time equivalent staff numbers, broken down by staff discipline and grade. Over the period described, team staff increased in both numbers and range. In 2000, the median number of whole-time equivalent staff per team was 6.9; by March 2006, this had risen to 16.6. Almost 5000 staff were employed in CRTs by the beginning of 2006, indicating a substantial migration within the mental health workforce, though we do not know how this may have affected other parts of the mental healthcare system in England. Table 3.2 shows the composition in terms of professional groups. Nurses remained the dominant professional group throughout, but numbers of doctors increased, while support workers, in particular the new grade of 'support time and recovery' worker, showed the most notable growth in numbers.

As described, the operational definition of a CRT for the purposes of service mapping needed to be inclusive. If a service thought it was providing a CRT, it was counted as such. In an attempt to clarify the extent to which these conformed to the *Mental Health Policy Implementation Guide* (Department of Health, 2001), the mapping asked a number of questions about fidelity to the CRT model, as it appears in this guidance (Table 3.3). One of these – the availability of staff on call 24 hours a day, 7 days a week – has been discussed above. Four other questions were asked in most years, with a fifth being added in 2006. Independent checks on the reliability of these data are not available, but they appear to indicate a shift towards teams that conform increasingly closely to the CRT model.

Table 3.2. Profile of staff working in crisis resolution teams in England[a]

	2000	2001	2002	2003	2004	2006 (Jan)
Total staff profile (%)	317	573	892	1586	2985	4860
Nurses	76.4	72.3	69.3	64.6	61.5	59.0
Social workers	6.7	8.3	10.7	9.3	11.4	8.9
Doctors	1.8	4.0	5.4	3.9	4.9	6.0
Clinical Psychologists	0.5	0.4	0.2	0.3	0.4	0.7
Occupational Therapists	3.7	3.3	1.8	2.3	2.0	2.8
Other clinical staff	3.2	2.1	3.6	9.4	9.5	12.7
Administrators and managers	7.8	9.5	9.1	10.2	10.2	9.9

Note:

[a] Figures relate to September of the year unless indicated otherwise.

Source: Adult Mental Health Service Mapping. Durham: University of Durham and Department of Health, http://www.amhmapping.org.uk/reports.

Table 3.3. Proportion of crisis resolution teams meeting each of five fidelity characteristics in each year[a]

	Percentage of teams					
	2000	2001	2002	2003	2004	2006 (Mar)
Multidisciplinary team	59	73	73	89	93	100
Staff in frequent contact with service users, often seeing them at least once on each shift	–	67	85	93	93	100
Provision of intensive contact over a short period of time	–	83	90	95	98	100
Staff stay involved until the problem is resolved	–	73	86	87	94	100
Capacity to offer intensive support at service user's home	–	–	–	–	–	97

Note:

[a] Figures relate to September of the year unless indicated otherwise. For team numbers see Table 3.1.

Source: Adult Mental Health Service Mapping. Durham: University of Durham and Department of Health, http://www.amhmapping.org.uk/reports.

Variations in style and targets

At the time the policy on crisis services was announced, it was predictable that some places would wish to modify it; it was less easy, however, to anticipate in what ways. In the event, many local implementation teams concluded that running a smaller number of larger teams offered organisational advantages. Others took the view that it was more appropriate to implement the acute home treatment function by expanding the role of generic CMHTs rather than by setting up separate teams (Chapters 19 and 20). Proponents of this approach argued that it offered greater continuity of care and that, in widely scattered rural or semi-rural communities, it minimised staff travel. The 335 team target was, however, of high political salience, so that considerable importance was accorded to target monitoring, and variations in the ways in which local areas had attempted to achieve the target resulted in some difficulties. The Department of Health derived rules for determining whether teams adopting variations on the model had met the targets. The essence of these was that alternatives were required to employ the same overall number of staff (14 per standard team) and deliver the same types of care. Under these 'flexibility' arrangements, just over half of the mental health trusts providing services successfully applied to have larger teams recognised as equivalent to more than one standard team, indicating a trend towards bigger teams that was stronger than originally envisaged. Ten local implementation teams, eight serving largely rural areas, made successful applications to get CMHTs accredited as providers of a crisis resolution function. Allowing for these variations in delivery arrangements, by January 2006 only 3 out of 173 local implementation teams were not reporting crisis service provision. The 262 actual teams noted in Table 3.1, along with elements of 34 CMHTs, constituted the equivalent of 343 standard teams.

Other targets set for acute home treatment teams in *The NHS Plan* related to their activities and the results for local services (Department of Health, 2000, Paragraph 14.31).

By 2004, all people in contact with specialist mental health services will be able to access crisis resolution services at any time. The teams will treat around 100 000 people a year who would otherwise have to be admitted to hospital, including black and South Asian service users for whom this type of service has been shown to be particularly beneficial. Pressure on acute inpatient services will be reduced by 30% and there will generally be no out-of-area admissions which are not clinically indicated.

Table 3.4 presents the available national data on service activity. For three years (2001–3), the service mapping included numbers of referrals. More recently, numbers of people referred and numbers of treatment episodes (referrals which led to the individual being taken on for care) have been monitored in the local

Table 3.4. Available data on the activity of crisis resolution teams and their impact on psychiatric admissions and occupied bed days in the mental illness specialty (710)

Year	Staff numbers	Referrals	Admissions	Occupied bed days	People referred	Treatment episodes
1998	–	–	147 577	5 310 720	–	–
1999	–	–	142 323	5 019 986	–	–
2000	317	–	139 090	5 079 720	–	–
2001	573	16 141	134 797	4 952 505	–	–
2002	892	34 568[a]	133 196	4 855 635	28 460	–
2003	1586	47 912[b]	122 403	5 341 727[c]	45 770[d]	–
2004	2985	–	117 853	5 436 282	68 760	–
2005	4860	–	–	–	–	83 800

Notes:

[a] Annualised from one quarters data.

[b] Annualised from two quarters data.

[c] Annualised from three quarters data.

[d] Not comparable with previous year because of change in method of data collection/calculation.

Sources: Adult Mental Health Service Mapping. Durham: University of Durham and Department of Health (http://www.amhmapping.org.uk/reports). *Hospital Episode Statistics.* London: Department of Health. *Local Delivery Plan Returns.* London: Department of Health. (http://www.hesonline.nhs.uk).

delivery plan quarterly returns. Hospital episode statistics are derived from the routine reporting system for admissions to hospital, which has been in place in England for many years.

The target of 100 000 people per year represents approximately the total number of individuals admitted to hospital. The number of individuals taken on for treatment by CRTs missed the target by a little over 15%. Thus the numbers treated are close to the target, although there is no basis for evaluating how many of these are people who would otherwise have been admitted to hospital: anecdotal evidence suggests that not all fall into this category and this conclusion is supported by the studies described in Chapter 5, in which a significant proportion of the control groups were not admitted. Referrals were clearly rising until 2004–5; however, for 2005, the data item collected was changed from the numbers of people referred to the number of treatment episodes.

The anticipated reduction in 'pressure on acute inpatient services' is harder to identify. The number of psychiatric admissions shows a clear declining trend, but this predates the setting up of these teams. With the exception of 2002–3, which probably has an erroneously high number of admissions resulting from the widespread reorganisation of trusts during that year, the trend from 1998–9 to 2004–5 is almost a straight line, with no apparent added impact from CRT introduction. The number of occupied bed days could be a better indication of 'pressure on beds'; unfortunately, however, in 2003–4 there was a change in the method employed for counting occupied bed days utilised by people who had stayed longer than a year. This means that the figure for 2003–4 is not comparable with that for 2002–3, although it does not explain the further rise in the following year. Consequently, it is hard to draw definite conclusions from these data. The Department of Health does not publish hospital episode statistics data broken down by service users' ethnic group, as data on this are not considered to be of sufficient quality.

Have crisis services reduced admissions?

The CRTs have an unusually clearly identifiable goal: to look after acutely ill people without recourse to hospitalisation. Detailed, geographically linked data about hospital admissions in the NHS have been available for many years. Thus the progressive introduction of CRTs and the accompanying mapping offered an unusual opportunity to evaluate the success of a major government initiative at something approaching a national level.

Glover and colleagues (2006) collated data from the mapping and the national data on admissions in order to explore whether observable local trends in admission numbers could be attributed to the implementation of CRTs. Data were analysed at the level of primary care trusts (PCTs), which cover fairly small catchment areas and tend to have a reasonably homogeneous service organisation. The main outcome measure was the number of admissions from each PCT over the six years from 1998–9 to 2003–4. The PCTs were categorised according to the year in which they first acquired a CRT (broad definitions) and according to the year in which they first had one that was available 24 hours a day (narrow definitions). They were also categorised according to the year in which they first acquired assertive outreach teams, in case this also influenced admission rates. Population size and mental health need level, as represented by the AREA index, were also taken into account.

Admissions of both men and women aged 18 to 34 showed a general sustained fall, amounting to 23% over the six-year period. As suggested by the national data above, this predated the implementation of CRTs in almost all cases. Admissions for older working age adults (35 to 64 years) showed a noticeable but much smaller (0.5%) reduction. There were CRTs in place in 34 PCTs by the time of the first satisfactory mapping in 2001; in the following two years, 14 and 51 PCTs acquired them. Corresponding figures for narrowly defined CRTs were 12, 10 and 30, respectively.

Reductions in admissions that appeared to have followed the introduction of broadly defined CRTs were seen most clearly for older working age adults, and for women. Differences were larger and more clearly statistically significant, and were also seen for young women, in the presence of narrowly defined teams offering 24-hour on call. No reductions in admissions were seen in relation to the introduction of assertive outreach teams. Overall, narrowly defined CRTs appeared to reduce admissions by slightly over 20%. Occupied bed days, however, were reduced by only a little over 10% and this result did not reach statistical significance. This last finding is important, since it raises questions about the extent to which savings from reduced inpatient provision will be available to fund teams in the long term.

The authors examined possible influences arising from alterations in bed numbers and from other alternative types of provision, such as crisis houses. It seemed unlikely that either had had a significant influence. They also considered the significance of the apparently greater effect seen for teams with 24-hour on call. They concluded that, given the nature of the study, it was impossible to say whether this increased effectiveness arose specifically from the extended service hours, or whether it might simply be that the teams with 24-hour availability tended in general also to be the ones that were better resourced and better organised.

Beyond England and Australia

This chapter has focused mainly on Australia and England, as these have been the main locations for the recent implementation and dissemination of the CRT model, and the English experience offers an illuminating national case study of the progress and early effects of its implementation. The model has, however, also attracted interest in other parts of the developed world, while in some European countries services operate that are not CRTs by name but bear a substantial resemblance to them in practice (Chapter 2). In Norway, for example, policy makers have been following the English experience with considerable interest, and all areas of the country are now required to introduce the CRT model by 2008 (Gråwe *et al.*, 2005). In Ireland, an intensive home treatment model has been implemented in a few centres that are the focus of substantial national interest, including Cavan, County Monaghan (Mental Health Commission, Ireland, 2004). Experiences of introducing the model in a variety of countries are clearly of considerable interest in understanding more about the contexts and populations in which it works best.

Key points

- Home treatment services for people with acute mental illness developed slowly in a few parts of England during the 1980s and 1990s.

- Government policy, introduced in 1998 and backed with substantial additional funding and tight monitoring of policy implementation, succeeded in changing the picture rapidly.
- By the beginning of 2006, crisis services were in place almost everywhere.
- There are some variations in the extent to which strict model fidelity criteria, for example the provision of 24-hour on call, have been followed.
- However, evidence from changes in admission patterns indicates that, overall, the introduction of CRTs has had a highly significant effect in reducing admissions, though impact on bed use has probably not been as marked.

REFERENCES

Appleby, L. (2003). So, are things getting better? *Psychiatric Bulletin*, **27**, 441–2.

Burns, T., Beadsmoore, A., Bhat, A. V. and Oliver, A. (1993). A controlled trial of home-based acute psychiatric services: I. Clinical and social outcome. *British Journal of Psychiatry*, **163**, 49–54.

Dean, C., Phillips, J., Gadd, E. M., Joseph, M. and England, S. (1993). Comparison of community based service with hospital based service for people with acute, severe psychiatric illness. *British Medical Journal*, **307**, 473–6.

Department of Health (1999). *A National Service Framework for Mental Health: Modern Standards and Service Models*. London: Department of Health.

Department of Health (2000). *The NHS Plan*. London: The Stationery Office.

Department of Health (2001). *Mental Health Policy Implementation Guide: Crisis Resolution/ Home Treatment Teams*. London: Department of Health.

Glover, G., Arts, G. and Babu, K. S. (2006). Crisis resolution/home treatment teams and psychiatric admission rates in England. *British Journal of Psychiatry*, **189**, 441.

Gråwe, R. W., Ruud, T. and Bjørngaard, H. (2005). Alternative interventions in acute mental health care. *Tidsskrift for Den norske lægeforening*, **125**, 3265–8.

Harrison, J. and Traill, B. (2004). What do consultants think about the development of specialist mental health teams? *Psychiatric Bulletin*, **28**, 83–6.

Mental Health Commission, Ireland (2004). *Strategic Plan 2004/2005*. Dublin: Mental Health Commission.

Owens, A. J., Sashidharan, A. P. and Lyse, E. (2000). Availability and acceptability of home treatment for acute psychiatric disorders. *Psychiatric Bulletin*, **24**, 169–71.

Pelosi, A. J. and Jackson, G. A. (2000). Home treatment: enigmas and fantasies. *British Medical Journal*, **320**, 308–9.

Quirk, A. and Lelliott, P. (2001). What do we know about life on acute psychiatric wards in the UK? A review of the research evidence. *Social Science and Medicine*, **53**, 1565–74.

Rose, D. (2001). *Users' Voices: The Perspectives of Mental Health Service Users on Community and Hospital Care*. London: Sainsbury Centre for Mental Health.

Smyth, M. G. and Hoult, J. (2000). The home treatment enigma. *British Medical Journal*, **320**, 305–8.

Szmukler, G. and Holloway, F. (2001). In-patient treatment. In *Textbook of Community Psychiatry*, ed. G. Thornicroft and G. Szmukler. Oxford: Oxford University Press.

Section 2

The evidence

4

The classic home treatment studies

Sonia Johnson and Graham Thornicroft

From the 1960s to the late 1980s, a series of studies, most of them randomised trials comparing groups receiving an innovative service with traditional hospital-based care, examined the feasibility of managing crises at home rather than in hospital. These studies have been highly influential, cited, for example, in the *Mental Health Policy Implementation Guide* as supporting evidence for crisis resolution teams (CRTs) (Department of Health, 2001). In this chapter, we summarise these studies and their results, and we analyse the extent to which they provide evidence for the current CRT model. Most of the studies relate to service models already mentioned in Chapter 2 and all were carried out more than a decade ago. Chapter 5 describes more recent evidence that varies in methodological quality but is more clearly related to the CRT model in its contemporary form.

Methods and aims

A literature review using the main electronic databases forms the basis for this chapter, and we also examined previous reviews of randomised controlled trials (RCTs) of crisis intervention by Joy and colleagues (2000) for the *Cochrane Library of Systematic Reviews*, and of randomised and non-randomised comparative studies on home treatment by Burns and colleagues (2001). Our aim in this chapter has been to identify all studies that compare a group cared for by an innovative service involving home-based treatment as a substitute for acute admission with a group where this was not available. We have included both studies in which patients were randomly assigned either to the experimental or control group, and those where randomisation was not used, but where a comparison took place between a group receiving home-based acute care and a group who did not.

Crisis Resolution and Home Treatment in Mental Health, ed. Sonia Johnson, Justin Needle, Jonathan P. Bindman and Graham Thornicroft. Published by Cambridge University Press. © Cambridge University Press 2008.

Our aim in reviewing these studies was to assess how far each of them contributes to the evidence that CRTs are likely to produce good outcomes in current mental health systems. In order to do this, we have considered the following questions in relation to each study.

- Is there any evidence of a difference in outcome between experimental and control services?
- Does the study yield any evidence regarding the safety of intensive home treatment?
- Is the study methodologically sound? In particular, is the introduction of the experimental intervention the likely cause of any differences in outcome found between the experimental and the control group?
- How similar is the study sample likely to be to current populations of patients presenting to crisis services in the countries where deinstitutionalisation policies have been implemented for some time?
- How closely does the experimental service resemble the current CRT model?
- How closely does the care received by control services resemble care delivered by generic community teams, for example the community mental health teams (CMHTs) available throughout the UK?

Evidence from randomised controlled trials

Table 4.1 shows the characteristics of the RCTs that we identified as comparing a group where some form of home treatment initiated in an emergency was available with a group where this was unavailable. Five of the studies were carried out in North America, two in London, one in Australia and one in India, and dates of first publication range from 1964 to 1982. Sample sizes have tended to be rather small, ranging from a total of 54 to 300, and studies have generally involved just one experimental and one control service. All the experimental services appear to have been newly established.

In terms of design limitations, two important characteristics relevant to their value as evidence for the current CRT model are shared by all or most of the studies. First, in all cases, the experimental teams continued treatment longer term following the resolution of the crisis: unlike CRTs, they did not withdraw at this stage and refer to other teams for continuing care. Second, as far as may be ascertained from descriptions, all the control services were essentially office based. Hospital care and outpatient appointments were offered, but no control team seems to have routinely visited substantial numbers of patients at home and, except in Sydney, no control service involved a community-based multidisciplinary team. In Sydney, a multidisciplinary team based in a community mental health centre was available to the control group but reportedly made little use

Table 4.1. Randomised controlled trials of home treatment as a substitute for hospital admission: study designs

Study reference (year of first main publication of results) and location	Numbers in trial	How far sample was representative of local groups with severe mental illness (study inclusions and exclusions)	Other important methodological limitations	Degree to which experimental team resembles current CRT model	Degree to which control team resemble current multidisciplinary CMHTs
Pasamanick et al. (1964) Louisville, Ohio, USA	Home treatment and antipsychotic drugs: 84 Home treatment and placebo: 59 Control: 50	Exclusions: patients with homicidal and suicidal tendencies, those without carer supervision	Reliability and validity of outcome measures uncertain; measures completed by clinicians, not independent researcher	Limited: visits from nurse only weekly, out-of-hours service answering machine only	Detail lacking, but appears limited: no evidence of home visiting or multidisciplinary team outside inpatient setting
Langsley et al. (1971) Denver, Colorado, USA	Home treatment: 150 Control: 150	Participants required to live with family within an hour's travel from hospital	Reliability and validity of outcome measures uncertain	Limited: daily visiting and 24-hour contact not provided; main element in intervention was family crisis therapy	Detail lacking, but appears limited: no evidence of home visiting or multidisciplinary team outside inpatient setting
Polak and Jones (1973) Denver, Colorado, USA		Exclusions: homicidal or suicidal patients	Some participants excluded from analysis because they did not receive home treatment: this may well bias the results in favour of home treatment	Considerable resemblance in initial care after crisis, with 24-hour service, rapid crisis response and frequent home visits; differed in continuing care longer term after crisis resolved	Detail lacking, but appears limited: no evidence of home visiting or multidisciplinary team outside inpatient setting

Table 4.1. (cont.)

Study reference (year of first main publication of results) and location	Numbers in trial	How far sample was representative of local groups with severe mental illness (study inclusions and exclusions)	Other important methodological limitations	Degree to which experimental team resembles current CRT model	Degree to which control team resemble current multidisciplinary CMHTs
Fenton et al. (1979) Montreal, Canada	Home treatment: 78 Control: 84	Exclusions: emergency presentations at weekends; homicidal or suicidal patients; not living with family; resident in Montreal for less than 6 months or not English speaker; patient or relative refused consent	High dropout: 64% interviewed at one year	Uncertain: 24-hour service available, frequency of contact not clear; differed in continuing care longer term after crisis resolved	Detail lacking, but appears limited: no evidence of home visiting or multidisciplinary team outside inpatient setting
Stein and Test (1980) Madison, Wisconsin, USA	Home treatment: 65 Control: 65	No important exclusions: sample likely to be representative of local mentally ill individuals considered for admission		Considerable resemblance in initial care after crisis, with 24-hour service, rapid response in crisis and frequent home visits; differed in continuing care longer term after crisis resolved	Limited: community mental health centre offered follow-up, but with very little use of home visiting
Hoult et al. (1981, 1983) Sydney, Australia	Home treatment: 60 Control: 60	No important exclusions: sample likely to be representative of local mentally ill individuals considered for admission	Substantial dropout at follow-up: no data available on bed use for 20 of sample	Considerable resemblance in initial care after crisis, with 24-hour service, rapid response in crisis and frequent home visits; differed in continuing care longer term after crisis resolved	Limited: very little use of home visiting

Study	Sample	Inclusion/exclusion		
Pai and Kapur (1983) Bangalore, India	Home treatment: 27 Control: 27	First episode schizophrenia only; only included if an adult family member at home most of the time	Limited: consisted of only one visiting nurse, visits on average fortnightly, no out-of-hours service	Limited: based only on hospital and outpatient clinic
Marks et al. (1994) London, UK (Daily Living Programme)	Home treatment: 92 Control: 97	Generally representative sample of local severely mentally ill individuals considered for admission, though relatively small proportion had previous history of admission	Considerable resemblance in initial care after crisis, with 24-hour service, rapid response in crisis and frequent home visits; differed in continuing care longer term after crisis resolved	Limited: multidisciplinary CMHTs not established: service largely based on outpatient appointments rather than home visiting
Merson et al. (1992) London, UK	Home treatment: 53 Control: 47	Excluded groups: those not giving informed consent before randomisation, patients already known to service or believed to require compulsory treatment	Limited: not a 24-hour service; speed of response and visit frequency appear lower than CRT model	Limited: multidisciplinary CMHTs not established; service largely based on outpatient appointments rather than home visiting

CRT, crisis resolution team; CMHT, community mental health team.

of home visits (Hoult, 1986). In the London study of Marks and colleagues (1994), a team of community psychiatric nurses was operating within the Daily Living Programme area. However, multidisciplinary teams had not yet been established, and only 9% of control group members received a home visit from a nurse during the 20-month follow-up period, while none received a home visit from a psychiatrist (Knapp *et al.*, 1994).

Other limitations are shared by some but not all of the studies. The Training in Community Living model (Chapter 2) by Stein and Test (1980) and its replications in Sydney and London (Hoult *et al.*, 1981; Marks *et al.*, 1994) have, as a major strength, freedom from narrow exclusion and inclusion criteria that might limit the extent to which their findings are representative of local clinical populations. Other studies, however, have excluded important groups such as suicidal and homicidal patients. The experimental services in all these studies, as well as in the study of Polak and Jones (1973), offered relatively intensive contact and were available 24 hours. In the other studies, details of the experimental services are often rather limited, but most appear to have offered care that was substantially more restricted in terms of hours and/or frequency of contact than the current CRT model. Other limitations relevant to some, though not all, of the studies include use of outcome measures whose reliability and validity are unknown.

Table 4.2 summarises data on outcomes from each study. Blank cells mean that the outcome in question was not measured. A wide range of different instruments was used to measure outcomes, restricting our ability to make comparisons between the studies. Several studies involved multiple follow-up points over up to 30 months. As longer-term outcomes from services providing continuing care after the resolution of the crisis are of only limited relevance as evidence for CRTs, only outcomes for follow-up points up to six months after the crisis have been included in the table. Unless otherwise noted, all the differences recorded in the table reached at least the $p < 0.05$ level that is usually used to define results as statistically significant, except in the case of cost data, where the main results are shown in the table regardless of statistical significance. Costing methods varied greatly between studies and not all conformed to current health economic practice: a simple statement about whether statistically significant cost differences were found is, therefore, often hard to extract from study reports.

Patterns in outcomes varied considerably from study to study, and many of the clinical and social outcomes measured were significant in some, but not all, of the studies. However, all the experimental services resulted in significantly lower bed use and/or admission rates than the control services, and costs were lower in all cases where they were measured. Also notable is the fact that all the significant differences on clinical and social measures that were found favoured the experimental services: in no case did a control service appear to be significantly better

Table 4.2. Randomised controlled trials of home treatment as a substitute for admission: comparison of outcomes between home treatment and control groups[a]

Study reference (year of first main publication of results) and location	Whether admitted	Bed use	Patient satisfaction with services or with life	Carer satisfaction and/or burden	Symptoms	Social functioning and/or vocational outcome	Costs	Safety	Other measures
Pasamanick et al. (1964) Louisville, Ohio, USA	Recruitment took place after admission	Proportion of follow-up period spent in community: HT with neuroleptics, 88%; HT only, 82%; C, 60%			NS	NS	Over 30 months: inpatient costs 2.6 times greater in C, group than for HT with neuroleptics	No deaths reported	
Langsley et al. (1971) Denver, Colorado, USA	HT, 13% admitted by 1 year; C, 100% admitted	HT, mean 4.0 days per patient in 6 months; C, mean 15.0 days	HT, better service satisfaction		NS	NS		HT, one death; C, 6 deaths; cause not specified	HT, better crisis management skills
Polak and Jones (1973) Denver, Colorado, USA			HT, better service satisfaction	HT, better service satisfaction					
Fenton et al. (1979) Montreal, Canada	HT, 38% admitted by 1 year; C, 100% admitted	HT, 14.5 days in 1 year; C, 41.7 days in 1 year		NS (family burden)	NS	NS	Over 2 years: HT slightly cheaper than C (means $2790 versus $3939 per patient)	Over 1 year: HT, 2 deaths (natural causes); C, 5 deaths (2 suicides)	

Table 4.2. (cont.)

Study reference (year of first main publication of results) and location	Whether admitted	Bed use	Outcomes						Other measures
			Patient satisfaction with services or with life	Carer satisfaction and/or burden	Symptoms	Social functioning and/or vocational outcome	Costs	Safety	
Stein and Test (1980) Madison, Wisconsin, USA	HT, 18% admitted by 1 year; C, 88% admitted by 1 year	HT, 5.4% of time in hospital up to 4 months; C, 20.6% time in hospital up to 4 months	NS at 4 months (life satisfaction)	NS (family burden)	HT, less severe anxiety and agitation at 4 months	HT, more time employed up to 4 months	Over 1 year: mean of $5729 and $6128 per patient for HT and C, respectively	Over 14 months: 1 suicide in each group; similar rates of violence, suicide attempts, time in prison, emergency room use	Compliance: NS at 4 months
Hoult et al. (1981, 1983) Sydney, Australia	HT, 40% admitted by 1 year; C, 96% admitted by 1 year	HT, 8.4 days per patient in 1 year; C, 53.5 days in 1 year	HT, greater service satisfaction at 1 year	HT, burden less and satisfaction greater at 4 months, although NS at 1 month	HT, less severe symptoms at 1 year	NS	Over 1 year: HT, mean $4489 per patient; C, $5669 per patient	Over 1 year: HT, C, 1 suicide, 1 natural death; similar rates of police contact; trend towards more suicide attempts in HT group (6 versus 0 in control group), but NS	

Study							
Pai and Kapur (1983) Bangalore, India	HT, none admitted; C, 100% admitted	HT, 0 days; C, mean 50 days per patient	HT, less family burden at 3, 4, 5 and 6 months	HT, symptom severity less at 3 and 6 months (but NS at 4 and 5 months)	HT, better social functioning at 3, 4, 5 and 6 months	Over 6 months: HT, total 507 rupees for 27 patients; C, 791 rupees for 27 patients	C, 1 patient excluded from study because died early in admission
Marks et al. (1994) London, UK	HT, 79% admitted by 3 months; C, 100% admitted by 3 months	HT, 13 days per patient in 3 months; C, 82 days in 3 months	NS	NS	NS	Over 4 months: HT, lower mean weekly cost per patient (£377); C, cost £716	Over 20 months: HT, 3 suicides (the first at 4 months), 1 homicide, 1 natural death; C, 2 suicides
Merson et al. (1992) London, UK	HT, 15% admitted by 12 weeks; C, 31%	HT, 1.2 days per patient in 12 weeks; C, 9.3 days in 12 weeks	HT, greater patient satisfaction at 12 weeks	Equivocal depending on method of analysis: findings either NS or favour HT	NS	Over 3 months: HT, lower total costs for group over 3 months (£56 000, for 48 patients); C, £130 000 for 52 patients	Over 3 months: HT, 1 natural death; C, 1 natural, 1 accidental death; Similar police contact rates

HT, home treatment (the experimental group receiving home treatment); C, control group; NS, not significant.

Note:

[a] Blank cells indicate the outcome in question was not measured. NS indicates that the relevant domain of outcome was measured and a difference not found at the $p = 0.05$ level. Where a better result is reported for one of the conditions, this is at at least a $p = 0.05$ level unless otherwise stated. The exception to this is the Costs column, where differences are reported regardless of statistical significance (see text).

on any of the outcomes that were measured. With regard to safety, suicide is a mercifully rare event and homicide even rarer, so it is very difficult to draw any conclusions from these relatively small studies about those events. However, scrutiny of the reported rates of adverse incidents does not suggest any obvious disparity between home treatment and control groups.

Support for the crisis resolution team model from randomised controlled trials

Returning to the questions listed at the beginning of this chapter, the extent to which there is evidence from RCTs for the current CRT model can be summarised as follows.

Is there any evidence of a difference in outcome between experimental and control services?

Findings and measures varied substantially, but overall these studies agreed in suggesting that home treatment reduced bed use. Better patient satisfaction was also found in most studies where it was measured, and no study suggested increased carer burden. Other findings varied, but it is striking that every significant finding reported favoured home treatment.

Do the studies yield evidence on the safety of intensive home treatment?

Small numbers greatly limit this, as most major adverse events are fortunately rare. As far as any judgement can be made, there was no obvious difference in adverse incidents between home treatment and control conditions.

Are the studies methodologically sound?

Some problems, such as the use of instruments without established reliability and validity, have been noted above. However, apart from rather small sample sizes and lack of power calculations, the most often quoted trials, particularly those from Madison, Sydney and London (the Daily Living Programme), were methodologically of reasonable quality.

How similar are the study samples likely to be to current populations of patients presenting in an emergency in the NHS and other modern mental health systems?

For studies that did not have too many inclusion and exclusion criteria, such as those from Madison and Sydney, the groups included in the studies were probably representative of local patients being considered for admission around the time of the study. However, most of the studies were conducted more than two decades ago and none within the past decade. Subsequent changes in service systems and the characteristics of psychiatric populations (e.g. the probable increase in comorbid substance misuse), therefore, make it very uncertain how far the findings apply to current clinical populations.

How closely do the experimental services resemble the current CRT model?

Some of the experimental services, especially in the earliest studies, resemble community mental health teams (CMHTs) rather more than CRTs when characteristics such as service intensity and hours available are compared, but others resemble CRTs more closely in these respects. However, a very important limitation in relation to their relevance to CRTs is that the services all continued care longer term after resolution of the initial crisis, generally for at least a year.

How closely does the care received by the control services resemble usual CMHT-based services in the NHS and similar service systems?

In most cases, the resemblance between study control conditions and modern mental health systems based on CMHTs appears very limited, mostly because current CMHTs are a good deal more community-based than the control services in older studies.

Non-randomised comparative studies

A second group of studies, summarised in Table 4.3, have compared a group receiving an innovative home treatment service with a group receiving more hospital-based care, but where group allocation has been determined by factors such as where they live, rather than by random assignment.

The Chichester experiment (Sainsbury and Grad, 1966) was an early study comparing a group of people who received home visits before admission (Chapter 2) with a group who did not. It prefigured some of the later studies in finding that home visits resulted in a lower admission rate (14% in Chichester versus 52% in Salisbury, where home visits were not carried out), but otherwise the experimental and control services did not bear much resemblance to contemporary CRTs and CMHTs. The two Birmingham studies are more relevant to the current context, and both found some evidence of reductions in admissions where home treatment was available. Dean *et al.* (1993) compared outcomes and costs for management by a home treatment team providing a 24-hour service in deprived inner city Sparkbrook with those for neighbouring and demographically similar Small Heath, which had a more traditional hospital-based service. The home treatment team resembled current CRTs to a substantial degree, although there is some ambiguity about the extent to which the home treatment team was separate from the CMHT that provided continuing care. A limitation of the study design is uncertainty about how similar the groups in the two areas were, especially since, in the control area, patients were included only if they were admitted to hospital. Even in this more traditional service, crises may have occurred that were considered by staff severe enough to meet the study criterion

Table 4.3. Non-randomised evaluations of home treatment: summary

Study reference (year of first main publication of results) and location	Main comparison	Outcomes	Inclusion and exclusion criteria	Methodological problems	Degree to which experimental team adhered to CRT model	Degree to which control team resembled multidisciplinary CMHT
Sainsbury and Grad (1966) Sussex, UK (the Chichester experiment)	Geographical area with practice of home visiting prior to admission versus neighbouring area where home visits not usual	Area with home visiting prior to admission: fewer admissions; similar family burden	No major exclusions: broad range of mentally ill individuals	Home treatment area had a higher overall referral rate to mental health services; not clear why	Limited: home treatment probably of low intensity	Very limited: home visiting not a usual component
Dean et al. (1993) Birmingham, UK	Geographical area with innovative home treatment service versus neighbouring area with no home treatment service	Patients in home treatment area: less likely to be admitted; more likely to be in contact with services 1 year later; relatives more satisfied; no differences in symptoms or social functioning	No major exclusions: broad range of acutely mentally ill individuals	Crises treated at home in the control group not included; strong possibility of important baseline differences between the groups compared	Considerable but more integrated with CMHT than current CRT model	Limited: control group received a mainly hospital-based service; multi-disciplinary CMHTs not available
Minghella et al. (1998) Birmingham UK	Geographical area with prototype CRT versus neighbouring area with no home treatment service	Home treatment group: less likely to be admitted; no evidence of differences in satisfaction or symptoms but small numbers followed up	No major exclusions: range of acutely mentally ill individuals, though symptom severity surprisingly low	Some evidence of difference between groups in sociodemographic characteristics at baseline	Prototype CRT: considerable resemblance to the current model	Probably considerable, though limited detail provided

CRT, crisis resolution team; CMHT, community mental health team.

of warranting admission but which were eventually managed in the community. Excluding such cases may have introduced a bias in favour of the home treatment service, which was found to result in a lower admission rate.

Still more relevant to the current context is the evaluation of Hoult's psychiatric emergency treatment service, which was introduced in Birmingham in 1994 (Minghella *et al.*, 1998; Ford *et al.*, 2001) and became a prototype for the current CRT model (Chapter 3). Comparisons were made between Yardley, the sector served by the team, and neighbouring Erdington, which was sociodemographically similar and appears to have had a multidisciplinary CMHT of some form. However, despite its relevance, the study's value was limited by substantial methodological problems, particularly by uncertainty about how comparable the groups really were. In Yardley, the CRT group consisted of people who were either admitted to acute wards or accepted for home treatment by the psychiatric emergency team, while in Erdington it again consisted just of people admitted to the acute wards. As with the Sparkbrook study, this leaves considerable room for doubt as to whether initial severity was similar, especially since comparisons of baseline characteristics were limited and analyses of outcomes did not take into account the initial characteristics of the two groups. No attempt was made to identify crises managed without admission in the control sector.

Key points

- Of the randomised and non-randomised studies investigating outcomes from precursors of CRTs, all demonstrate a reduction in admission rates when home treatment was available.
- Findings on satisfaction and on clinical and social outcomes such as symptom severity and social functioning have been more variable, although where significant findings have been reported they have all favoured the home treatment group, not the control group.
- Even though frequently cited in support of CRTs, the older randomised trials are of limited value as evidence for their introduction in modern mental health systems. This is mainly because of differences between the models they evaluated and current CRTs (especially in whether the team withdrew once the crisis had resolved), and between the control services in these studies and current mental health systems, in which even CMHTs generally work to a significant extent in patients' homes.
- Some non-randomised studies are more relevant to the current context than these older trials, but their value is restricted by uncertainties about how similar the groups being compared actually were.

REFERENCES

Burns, T., Knapp, M., Catty, J. *et al.* (2001). Home treatment for mental health problems: a systematic review. *Health Technology Assessment*, **5**, 1–153.

Dean, C., Phillips, J., Gadd, E. M., Joseph, M. and England, S. (1993). Comparison of community based service with hospital based service for people with acute, severe psychiatric illness. *British Medical Journal*, **307**, 473–6.

Department of Health (2001). *Mental Health Policy Implementation Guide: Crisis Resolution/ Home Treatment Teams.* London: Department of Health.

Fenton, F. R., Tessier, L. and Struening, E. L. (1979). A comparative trial of home and hospital psychiatric care. One year follow-up. *Archives of General Psychiatry*, **36**, 1073–9.

Ford, R., Minghella, E., Cahlmers, C. *et al.* (2001). Cost consequences of home-based and in-patient-based acute psychiatric treatment: results of an implementation study. *Journal of Mental Health*, **10**, 467–76.

Hoult, J. (1986). Community care of the acutely mentally ill. *British Journal of Psychiatry*, **149**, 137–44.

Hoult, J., Reynolds, I., Charbonneau-Powis, M., Coles, P. and Briggs, J. (1981). A controlled study of psychiatric hospital versus community treatment: the effect on relatives. *Australian and New Zealand Journal of Psychiatry*, **15**, 323–8.

Hoult, J., Reynolds, I., Charbonneau-Powis, M., Weekes, P. and Briggs, J. (1983). Psychiatric hospital versus community treatment: the results of a randomised trial. *Australian and New Zealand Journal of Psychiatry*, **17**, 160–7.

Joy, C. B., Adams, C. E. and Rice, K. (2000). Crisis intervention for people with severe mental illnesses. In *Cochrane Database of Systematic Reviews*, Issue 4, CD001087. Oxford: Update Software.

Knapp, M., Beecham, J., Koutsogeorgopoulou, V. *et al.* (1994). Service use and costs of home-based versus hospital-based care for people with serious mental illness. *British Journal of Psychiatry*, **165**, 195–203.

Langsley, D. G., Machotka, P. and Flomenhaft, K. (1971). Avoiding mental hospital admission: a follow-up study. *American Journal of Psychiatry*, **127**, 1391–4.

Marks, I., Connolly, J., Muijen, M. *et al.* (1994). Home-based versus hospital-based care for people with serious mental illness. *British Journal of Psychiatry*, **165**, 179–94.

Merson, S., Tyrer, P., Onyett, S. *et al.* (1992). Early intervention in psychiatric emergencies: A controlled clinical trial. *Lancet*, **339**, 1311–14.

Minghella, E., Ford, R., Freeman, T. *et al.* (1998). *Open All Hours: 24-hour Response for People with Mental Health Emergencies.* London: Sainsbury Centre for Mental Health.

Pai, S. and Kapur, R. L. (1983). Evaluation of home care treatment for schizophrenic patients. *Acta Psychiatrica Scandinavica*, **67**, 80–8.

Pasamanick, B., Scarpitti, F. R., Lefton, M. *et al.* (1964). Home versus hospital care for schizophrenics. *Journal of the American Medical Association*, **187**, 177–81.

Polak, P. and Jones, M. (1973). The psychiatric nonhospital: a model for change. *Community Mental Health Journal*, **9**, 123–32.

Sainsbury, P. and Grad, J. (1966). Evaluating the community psychiatric service in Chichester. *Milbank Memorial Fund Quarterly*, **44**, 231–79.

Stein, L. I. and Test, M. A. (1980). Alternative to mental hospital treatment. I. Conceptual model, treatment program, and clinical evaluation. *Archives of General Psychiatry*, **37**, 392–7.

5

Recent research on crisis resolution teams: findings and limitations

Sonia Johnson and Jonathan P. Bindman

The introduction of a government policy mandating that crisis resolution teams (CRTs) be established throughout England (Department of Health, 2000) provoked considerable dissent about whether enough research evidence supporting these teams was available to justify this requirement. This was exemplified by a heated debate in the *British Medical Journal* (Pelosi and Jackson, 2000; Smyth and Hoult, 2000; and subsequent correspondence), in which the evidence presented in favour of CRTs was described in one contribution as 'overwhelming' (Bracken *et al.*, 2000) and in another as a 'tired (and tiresome) polemic masquerading as science' (Burns, 2000). A respected commentator on community mental healthcare (Holloway, 2000) wrote:

Despite its attractions, out-of-hours home-based crisis intervention is logically a rather poor choice for mainstream purchasers and providers, given the chronic and recurrent nature of severe mental illness. The evidence base in its favour is not strong, even against the poor quality forms of 'standard care' available 20 years ago or more.

As discussed in Chapter 4, dissimilarities between current clinical populations and service contexts and those involved in the classic home treatment studies are indeed a major problem in accepting these studies as satisfactory evidence. However, while the literature on the CRT model remains limited compared with other currently favoured mental health service models such as assertive outreach and early intervention, new research evaluations with greater relevance to the current context are slowly beginning to accumulate in the new millennium. This chapter will describe these recent studies.

We will begin by describing the limited available evidence from randomised assessments of CRT outcomes, and will then discuss the evaluations of the overall impact of CRTs that have used non-randomised methods. A few further recent

Crisis Resolution and Home Treatment in Mental Health, ed. Sonia Johnson, Justin Needle, Jonathan P. Bindman and Graham Thornicroft. Published by Cambridge University Press. © Cambridge University Press 2008.

studies have examined specific aspects of CRTs, such as impact on compulsory detention rates and service user views: these will also be mentioned. Finally, we will summarise the current state of the evidence regarding CRTs and discuss some potential future research directions.

Evidence from randomised controlled trials

Randomised controlled trials (RCTs) are generally seen as the gold standard form of evidence regarding treatments in medicine, though it has been cogently argued that the complexity of interventions and the many factors that make their outcomes vary between settings limit the usefulness of this scientific method in mental health services research (Slade and Priebe, 2001). So far, the only published randomised controlled trial investigating the outcomes of CRT care in a contemporary service setting is the North Islington study, an investigation by Johnson and colleagues (2005a) of one of the teams established in inner London by John Hoult (Chapter 2).

In the North Islington study, outcomes for patients to whom the local CRT was available were compared with those using 'standard care' only. Standard care consisted of inpatient services, local community mental health teams (CMHTs) and two crisis houses. The CRT conformed closely in most respects to the CRT model described in Chapter 6, although the complexities of recruitment procedures (see below) meant that general practitioners could not refer directly to the team. All trial participants were drawn from two geographically defined sectors (small mental health service catchment areas), and the sector consultant in each was responsible for patients under the care of the CRT and of the CMHTs and inpatient services, so that people in the experimental and the control group were seeing the same psychiatrists. John Hoult was consultant in one of the sectors in the early months of the study: no significant differences were found in likelihood of admission between his and the other sector.

The investigators came to understand very clearly why so few randomised trials of crisis care for mental illness have been published in recent years, as the practical and ethical hurdles to be negotiated were considerable. In practical terms, the main challenge is that people presenting in crisis generally need to have a treatment plan made for them straight away, so there is no time to follow the usual procedures for entry into a RCT, which involve a researcher being contacted and coming to interview potentially suitable trial participants before submitting the details of those who consent for randomisation. This problem was resolved by training clinical staff to identify and recruit suitable participants, supported in the early stages of the trial by a 24-hour researcher on-call rota, staffed by the investigators. Once people had been identified as suitable, they were randomised using an automated 24-hour telephone service.

The ethical complexities of recruiting in a mental health crisis derive from the fact that many people transiently lose decision-making capacity at such a time. However, if only those who are in a position to understand the trial procedures and make a valid decision about participation were included, the sample would be very biased, as the many very unwell people who do not have capacity at the time of the crisis could not be included, even though they will often be the people at greatest risk of hospital admission. In most of the studies conducted in the 1970s and 1980s (Chapter 4), everyone referred for hospital admission was randomised at the time of the crisis without first seeking consent. This made studies feasible and meant that their samples really were typical of severely ill local people at risk of hospital admission, but it would be difficult to justify in the current climate: ethical regulation has become much tighter and, at least in principle, users' views are more important. After some debate with the local ethics committee, this was resolved in North Islington through an agreement that the following three groups could be randomised and enter the trial.

1. People with the capacity to make a decision about trial participation who gave clinicians informed consent to participate.
2. People who lacked capacity at the time of the trial, but who had been informed about it beforehand (1200 local service users were contacted before the trial began) and did not object to inclusion.
3. People who lacked capacity and who had not been contacted beforehand, but who had a carer available who was willing to give assent to participation in the trial on their behalf.

Participants were allocated at random (a process similar to a coin tossing) between the experimental group, to whom the CRT was available, and the control group, who received standard care. People in crisis who for any reason did not participate in the trial also received standard care, so that during the trial period the only people seen by the CRT were those in the study experimental group. People in groups (2) and (3) above who were allocated to the experimental group were approached again once clinicians considered they had recovered capacity and were informed of their right to withdraw from CRT care if they wished. These procedures were felt to be ethically justifiable because omission of people without capacity to consent would have led to a study sample that would have been very atypical of the usual CRT patient population, and because obtaining valid evidence about CRTs was considered especially important because of their planned nationwide introduction.

The two main outcomes on which CRT and standard care were compared were admission rates and patient satisfaction. CRT care appeared to have a very large impact on hospitalisation, with 36% (49 out of 135) of the experimental group admitted to hospital or a crisis house over the eight weeks after the crisis, compared with 69% (86 out of 125) of controls. This was statistically highly significant, as were the differences in days spent in hospital over the eight weeks and over the six months following the crisis. This large impact may have partly resulted from exclusion of some very unwell patients from the study because the procedures described above yielded no ethically acceptable way of recruiting them. The impact of the team seemed to be mostly on voluntary admissions: 18% of the experimental and 26% of the control group were compulsorily admitted under a section of the Mental Health Act, a difference which was not statistically significant. With regard to satisfaction, the CRT group were slightly more satisfied, a result that was on the borderline of statistical significance and rather more equivocal than in other investigations of home treatment (see below).

Symptoms, quality of life, social functioning and adverse incidents such as violence and self-harm were also examined using simple global indicators. No clear-cut differences were found between the two groups.

An as yet unpublished second trial was subsequently carried out by one of the authors (J. B.) and his colleagues in Inner South London, using very similar methods. A CRT closely modelled on the Islington services was established in North Southwark in 2000, with a total staff of 15 serving a relatively deprived population of 85 000. The research protocol was very similar to that applied in North Islington. During the study period, patients from the catchment area who were assessed as requiring admission were randomly allocated to either the CRT or to standard care. Standard care was assumed to consist of admission to hospital followed by community team follow-up during normal working hours, though in the event the results showed that almost a quarter of the control group were not admitted to hospital despite being assessed prior to randomisation as requiring it.

The study initially included 240 individuals (96% of those eligible), who were allocated to either the home treatment group or the hospital control group. Data about whether patients had been admitted were obtained at six months from case notes for 179 (71%). These showed that, for those allocated to CRT treatment (91), the mean number of days in hospital over six months was 25.6 and for those allocated to standard care (88) the mean was significantly greater at 43.1 days: statistically this was a significant difference ($p = 0.01$).

Though patients were interviewed at eight weeks, as in Islington, the value of the results was greatly limited by poor response rates, with only 97 subjects (39%) being interviewed. However, the results were generally consistent with those in Islington, satisfaction scores being significantly higher in the CRT group (26.6 out of 32 on the Client Satisfaction Questionnaire, compared with 22.1 for the control group; $p = 0.003$).

Non-randomised evaluations of the impact of crisis resolution teams

Non-randomised methods, generally thought to be somewhat less convincing than RCTs, have also been used to investigate the impact of CRTs. An early example of such a method being used to investigate a home treatment team that conformed in most ways to the current CRT model was the Birmingham study carried out by Minghella and colleagues (1998) and described in Chapter 4. A subsequent non-randomised comparison of outcomes with and without a CRT available was carried out by Johnson *et al.* (2005b) in South Islington prior to conducting the RCT described above in adjacent North Islington. The South Islington crisis study compared outcomes of crisis presentations identified before and after the introduction of a CRT. Following good practice guidelines for non-randomised studies, statistical adjustment was made for differences between the cohort of patients recruited before the team was introduced to the two study sectors and the cohort recruited afterwards. The CRT group were less likely to be admitted in the six weeks after the crisis, though the difference was less clear measured over six months. As in the North Islington RCT described above, the impact appeared to be more on voluntary than on compulsory admissions. Patients to whom the CRT was available were substantially more satisfied than control patients in this study: the median satisfaction score for the CRT group indicated that patients were, on average, very satisfied, whereas the median for the group recruited before the CRT began to operate indicated that they were on balance mildly dissatisfied. As with the North Islington RCT, there was little evidence of differences in symptoms, quality of life or social functioning. A trend emerged towards more violent incidents in the CRT group, but small numbers impeded interpretation, and baseline differences or greater knowledge of community incidents were both possible explanations, so that attaching much significance to this trend is likely to be unwise. Therefore, overall, the findings of this study tended to fit with those of the subsequent North Islington RCT. Whereas the methods used in the South Islington study mean that one cannot have as much confidence that the two groups were truly comparable, some data were collected about all eligible patients, so that the study group is likely to have resembled usual NHS patient populations more than the North Islington group, from which some crises had to be excluded for ethical reasons. The exclusion of some more severely ill patients from the North Islington study may go some way towards explaining why the impact on admissions seemed more marked than in South Islington.

Two naturalistic studies have observed changes in local patterns of service use with the introduction of CRTs. Jethwa *et al.* (2007) describe service use in the city of Leeds over two years before and one year after the introduction of a CRT. The service in question was a multidisciplinary team serving a population of around 750 000 people from a permanently open team base. Consultant psychiatrists, mental health nurses, social workers, occupational therapists and administrative staff were included in the team, which also had access to community-based acute day services and to a respite bed. The median number of admissions per month fell from 140.5 to 86.5 following introduction of the team. Keown *et al.* (2007) also analysed the city-wide impact on service use of CRT introduction, this time in Newcastle. They found a 45% reduction in admissions and a 22% fall in bed occupancy, although length of stay and compulsory detention under certain sections of the Mental Health Act increased. The impact of this team appeared to be principally on female admissions. Glover *et al.* (2006) have analysed national changes in the pattern of admissions following CRT introduction. Results from these analyses are discussed in Chapter 3: overall they also suggest some impact on voluntary admissions, especially on females and in areas with good model fidelity.

Investigations of specific aspects of care by crisis resolution teams

A few further studies have investigated specific aspects of CRT care, as opposed to its overall impact. The following are aspects of care that have been examined, mostly in relatively small-scale studies with limited methodological ambitions.

Effects on assessments under the Mental Health Act and compulsory admissions

Dunn (2001a,b) has published a specific investigation of the effects of CRT availability on assessments for compulsory admission. Two areas in Hertfordshire were compared, one with a seven-day-a-week community treatment team that aimed to offer an alternative to admission, the other with no such service. Adjusting figures for total local populations, fewer assessments were carried out under the Mental Health Act (1983) in the area with the CRT, and a lower proportion of the assessments that did take place resulted in detention under Section 3 of the Act, which allows compulsory admission for up to six months for treatment. A causal attribution of this difference to the availability of the team cannot very confidently be made, especially in view of the contrary findings described above, but impact on compulsory admissions is an area of interest for future investigations.

Patients' views about home treatment services

Alongside the larger studies described above, a few studies have focused mainly on patients' views about CRTs. The Bradford CRT was the setting for a survey of the preferences of patients who had experienced both home treatment and hospital admission (Bracken *et al.*, 2000). Of the sample of 96, 81% preferred home treatment. Two other UK surveys of patient views about intensive home treatment (Whittle and Mitchell, 1997; Minghella *et al.*, 1998) have resulted in response rates substantially below 50%, reflecting the difficulties posed by recruitment to research studies around the time of a crisis. Nolan (2005) carried out qualitative interviews with 20 members of the sample participating in the North Islington RCT (see above). She found that most had positive views about being treated at home rather than in hospital, but that several expressed reservations about CRT care. These included complaints about seeing too many different professionals within a short period, about lack of continuity of care and communication among CRT staff and between CRT and CMHT staff, and about very brief and superficial visits from some CRT members, in which the only objective seemed to be to ensure that patients took their medication. Hopkins and Niemiec (2007) have used qualitative methods to investigate the views of users of the Newcastle city-wide crisis resolution and home treatment service. Many aspects of the service were viewed positively, including the chance to receive treatment at home, the ease of access to the service in a crisis and the greater choice offered by the service compared with traditional services. The potential problems resulting from seeing a substantial number of different staff were felt to be overcome at least to a degree by the knowledge held within the team as a whole: seeing someone new was easier if they arrived equipped with good-quality information about current problems and plans, and if they had the skills to establish a rapport quickly. The aspect of continuity of care that did appear to be a focus for negative comments was the discharge process: the end of home treatment and handover to other services seemed often to be experienced as abrupt and unsafe.

Carers' views about crisis resolution teams

Carers' views about home treatment by the crisis assessment and treatment teams now established throughout Victoria, Australia (Chapter 2) have been surveyed by Fulford and Farhall (2001). In contrast to the enthusiasm of most carers interviewed in Hoult's initial study (Hoult *et al.*, 1983) and in a subsequent Sydney investigation of one of the first Australian specialist crisis teams (Reynolds *et al.*, 1990), views about home treatment among 77 carers who had experienced both home and hospital treatments for acute episodes were mixed, with just 55% expressing a preference for home rather than hospital treatment. Possible reasons suggested by the authors for the discrepancy between this and earlier studies were the fact that the families surveyed had all experienced several acute episodes, and the shorter period of contact with the crisis assessment and treatment teams compared with the teams in the earlier demonstration projects. However, the response rate was only 43%.

Views and experiences of staff in crisis resolution teams

The sustainability of any innovative service model in mental healthcare is dependent on recruitment and retention of motivated and skilled staff who are satisfied with their jobs. Potential threats to staff morale inherent in the CRT model include the stressful nature of clinical contacts with patients in crisis, who may pose a high risk of self-harm or violence; shift working; and lack of longer-term therapeutic relationships. However, an investigation of morale in eight London CRTs by T. Nelson, S. Johnson and P. Bebbington (unpublished data) indicated greater satisfaction and less burnout than among CMHT staff. Staff cited as particular sources of satisfaction working in a team and working short term with relatively severe problems.

Referring professionals' views about intensive home treatment services

A UK investigation of general practiners' attitudes to a new home treatment service that had been associated with reduced admission rates in rural Devon showed generally positive views, with all respondents saying that they would recommend the service to others (Whittle and Mitchell, 1997).

Implementation of the crisis resolution teams model

The goal of a national survey carried out by Onyett and colleagues (2006) was to examine how the CRT model has been implemented in England and what interventions are delivered (see also Chapter 3). A total of 243 teams were identified, operating with a relatively low median team caseload of 20. Almost all teams included nurses, the majority had support workers and just under half contained psychiatrists, but other professions were not well represented. Despite higher figures reported in national service mapping (Chapter 3), 68% reported that in practice they were gatekeepers to inpatient beds and 54% that they offered a 24-hour, seven-day-a-week home-visiting service. Around two-fifths of referred patients were taken on for continuing treatment, the main referrers being CMHTs, casualty departments and inpatient wards. Team reports of how often they provided various interventions were assessed: the most frequently provided were risk assessment, monitoring of mental state, support with self-help strategies, delivering psychosocial interventions and administering medication, with a minority of teams doing therapeutic work with families, aiming to extend social networks or offering practical help with housing or activities of daily living. Almost three-quarters of teams could initiate medication. Therefore, despite their roots in social models of treating mental illness (Chapter 2), there was some evidence that current teams tended more towards a medical than a social focus. Cited obstacles to development included problems in recruiting medical staff and social workers, and difficulties in relationships with other teams within the system and with senior medical staff.

Crisis resolution teams: the current state of the evidence

As this chapter has shown, relatively little of the research on CRTs has reached a good standard of methodological robustness, and the research design which tends to be viewed as the ideal form of evidence on health interventions, the multicentre RCT, has yet to be applied. However, some distinct trends do now seem to be emerging. One result is consistent across most of the studies, whatever method has been used, at least with relatively well-resourced CRTs that have implemented the model thoroughly. This is that CRT introduction does seem to be associated with a reduction in admissions and this has been found through application of a range of methods with varying strengths and weaknesses, suggesting it is a fairly robust result, though it is possible that it applies only to voluntary admissions. Research on service user satisfaction also tends to suggest a positive effect from CRT introduction, although this was quite a marginal finding in the RCT that is probably the most methodologically satisfactory evaluation of service user views so far (Johnson *et al.*, 2005a), and the validity of several studies has been threatened by low response rates. Beyond this, there is not as yet clear evidence of any further clinical or social benefits from CRT care, nor are there any known disadvantages. However, the body of evidence on which to evaluate impacts on outcomes other than bed use and service user views is very small. The weakness of the recent evidence regarding acute mental healthcare, despite its centrality in mental health systems, probably reflects the considerable practical and ethical difficulties encountered in conducting research in this setting, as discussed above. There is a need for innovation in developing methods for the conduct of feasible and ethically acceptable research in crises: promising directions might include greater use of deferred consent for people who initially lack capacity, and advance consent for people who may present in crisis in future.

Future directions for research on crisis resolution teams

Much remains to be done in order to achieve a comprehensive understanding of the CRT model. The following are some of the areas in which further research is desirable.

Investigation of individual patient outcomes

Further investigation of the impact on individual outcomes (such as bed use, satisfaction with services, symptoms and social functioning) of the CRT model is warranted, in particular to establish whether findings similar to those of the Islington studies are obtained in areas with different geographic, service and staff characteristics.

Investigations of the content of care and its relationship to outcomes

As discussed in Chapter 6, clinical practice may vary greatly within the overall framework of the CRT model. Further investigations of variations between patients and teams in the content of treatment provided, and of variations between CRTs in organisation and functioning, may help to develop an understanding of how this model is implemented in practice and what clinical interventions are delivered within it. This could then form the basis for comparisons of outcomes between major variants of the model, with the aim of identifying the critical ingredients that are needed for good results. Another potentially helpful research direction is to design trials of specific interventions delivered within the CRT framework: examples that could be evaluated in this way include family intervention, brief cognitive–behavioural interventions, or the use of structured relapse prevention packages or crisis plans within CRTs. For example, we do not as yet know whether outcomes from CRTs are improved if a specific therapeutic package for families is implemented by their staff.

Comparison between crisis resolution teams and intensive home treatment integrated within community mental health teams

A further question that remains unanswered is whether CRTs that work with patients only during crisis periods have advantages in terms of outcomes over CMHTs whose staffing and hours of operation have been augmented so that they can also carry out rapid crisis assessments and deliver intensive home treatment with frequent visits (Chapters 19 and 20). It may, in fact, be that the best way of delivering intensive home treatment varies from area to area, depending on the local service system and the area's demographic, geographical and epidemiological characteristics. Investigation of whether there is a difference in outcomes between these models, therefore, seems really desirable.

Further investigation of the views of service users and carers

There is considerable further scope for investigation of service user views about CRT care, especially for studies that sample from several different teams and obtain good response rates. Research on carers is still more limited: no recent studies with high response rates and well-established instruments have investigated carers' views about CRTs and whether they have any impact on carer burden. Such evidence is essential if the effects of implementation of this model are to be fully understood.

Impact within wider service systems

The introduction of home treatment is likely to have substantial effects on several elements of local community mental health systems, including inpatient services, CMHTs, casualty departments and, where they exist, residential alternatives to admission, such as crisis houses. This suggests as potential lines of enquiry investigation of the effects of CRTs on patient flows throughout the catchment area and exploration of the ways in which caseloads, working practices and demands on staff in other parts of the service system may change with the introduction of CRTs. For instance, staff dealing with inpatients may find they are now managing a smaller but more severely unwell patient group (Chapter 15). The effects of this on the functioning and outcomes of acute wards and on the experiences of staff and patients in such wards have not been investigated.

Research on well-established crisis research teams

Most of the research on CRTs relates to very recently established teams, but the organisation, functioning and outcomes of CRTs may well change over the years, and investigation of well-established CRTs is a neglected but interesting future direction. For example, examining trends in caseload size and composition, duration of contact and admission rate would be of significant interest in understanding the longer-term effects of CRT introduction. The views of service users who have experienced multiple episodes of CRT care are one interesting focus. Data on the effects of multiple episodes of intensive home treatment on various outcomes could also fruitfully be examined: while the studies described in this chapter suggest little impact on clinical and social outcomes from home treatment, some experts suggest that patients who are recurrently managed at home rather than in hospital might learn better coping skills for subsequent crises, and might also become better engaged with services and more disposed to seek help early (Chapter 6). The possibility that recurrent episodes of CRT care produce better overall engagement and better longer-term clinical and social outcomes should, therefore, be investigated.

Key points

- Recent studies in a range of UK settings and using a variety of methods suggest that CRTs have an impact on admissions.
- There is also some evidence that service users are more satisfied with them than with standard care, though better study designs and response rates are needed to be confident about this.
- Apart from these findings, there is no clear current evidence of either benefits or disadvantages to CRT care, but the evidence base remains limited.

- The practical and ethical difficulties encountered in trying to do research involving people experiencing mental health crises are likely to account for the dearth of high-quality research.
- Important questions for future research include the functioning and outcomes of well-established teams, the impact of CRT provision on carers, and whether stand-alone CRTs are preferable to augmented CMHTs that can offer rapid crisis assessment and intensive home treatment.

REFERENCES

Bracken, P., King, J., Daudjee, H. *et al.* (2000). Home treatment is an alternative to acute hospital treatment. *Electronic British Medical Journal*, rapid response. http://www.bmj.com/cgi/eletters/320/7230/305#9035. Accessed 29 June 2007.

Burns, T. (2000). Psychiatric home treatment. Vigorous, well designed trials are needed. *British Medical Journal*, **321**, 177.

Department of Health (2000). *The NHS Plan*. London: The Stationery Office.

Dunn, L. M. (2001a). Mental Health Act Assessments: does a community treatment team make a difference? *International Journal of Social Psychiatry*, **47**, 1–19.

Dunn, L. M. (2001b). Mental Health Act Assessments: does a home treatment team make a difference? In *Acute Mental Health Care in the Community: Intensive Home Treatment*, ed. N. Brimblecombe. London: Whurr, pp. 102–21.

Fulford, M. and Farhall, J. (2001). Hospital versus home care for the acutely mentally ill? Preferences of caregivers who have experienced both forms of service. *Australian & New Zealand Journal of Psychiatry*, **35**, 619–25.

Glover, G., Arts, G. and Babu, K. S. (2006). Crisis resolution/home treatment teams and psychiatric admission rates in England. *British Journal of Psychiatry*, **189**, 441.

Holloway, F. (2000). Mental health policy, fashion and evidence-based practice. *Psychiatric Bulletin*, **24**, 161–2.

Hopkins, C. and Niemiec, S. (2007). Mental health crisis at home: service user perspectives on what helps and what hinders. *Journal of Psychiatric and Mental Health Nursing*, **14**, 310–18.

Hoult, J., Reynolds, I., Charbonneau-Powis, M. *et al.* (1983). Psychiatric hospital versus community treatment: the results of a randomised trial. *Australian & New Zealand Journal of Psychiatry*, **17**, 160–7.

Jethwa, K., Galappathie, N. and Hewson, P. (2007). Effects of a crisis resolution and home treatment team on in-patient admissions. *Psychiatric Bulletin*, **31**, 170–2.

Johnson, S., Nolan, F., Pilling, S. *et al.* (2005a). Randomised controlled trial of acute mental health care by a crisis resolution team: the north Islington crisis study. *British Medical Journal*, **331**, 586–7.

Johnson, S., Nolan, F., Hoult, J. *et al.* (2005b). Outcomes of crises before and after introduction of a crisis resolution team. *British Journal of Psychiatry*, **187**, 68–75.

Keown, P., Tacchi, M. J., Niemiec, S. and Hughes, J. (2007). Changes to mental healthcare for working age adults: impact of a crisis team and an assertive outreach team. *Psychiatric Bulletin*, **31**, 288–92.

Minghella, E., Ford, R., Freeman, T. *et al.* (1998). *Open All Hours: 24-hour Response for People with Mental Health Emergencies*. London: Sainsbury Centre for Mental Health.

Nolan, F. (2005). Which patients like crisis teams and what do they like about them? In *The Sainsbury Centre for Mental Health Conference on Crisis Resolution Teams*, York, 8 September 2005.

Onyett, S., Linde, K., Glover, G. *et al.* (2006). *A National Survey of Crisis Resolution Teams in England*. London: Care Services Improvement Partnership, Department of Health and University of the West of England. Summary at http://www.nimhe.csip.org.uk/silo/files/crtexecutivesummarydoc.doc. Accessed: 4 July 2007.

Pelosi, A. J. and Jackson, G. A. (2000). Home treatment: engimas and fantasies. *British Medical Journal*, **320**, 308–9.

Reynolds, I., Jones, J. E., Berry, D. W. and Hoult, J. E. (1990). A crisis team for the mentally ill: the effect on patients, relatives and admissions. *Medical Journal of Australia*, **152**, 646–52.

Slade, M. and Priebe, S. (2001). Are randomised controlled trials the only gold that glitters? *British Journal of Psychiatry*, **179**, 286–7.

Smyth, M. G. and Hoult, J. (2000). The home treatment enigma. *British Medical Journal*, **320**, 305–8.

Whittle, P. and Mitchell, S. (1997). Community alternatives project: an evaluation of a community-based acute psychiatric team providing alternatives to admission. *Journal of Mental Health*, **6**, 417–27.

Section 3

Current practice

6

Crisis resolution teams: rationale and core model

Sonia Johnson and Justin Needle

As has been described in Chapters 2 and 3, the crisis resolution team (CRT) model has gradually evolved over the past few decades, influenced by various loosely interrelated innovations in acute community mental healthcare and promoted by a variety of interpersonal connections and international visits. Since the mid 1990s, with the nationwide implementation of CRTs in England, the model seems to have become somewhat more fixed in terms of name, organisational structure and content of interventions, but few examinations of its critical ingredients or attempts to measure degree of adherence to the model have been available. In this chapter, we aim to fill this gap by giving an account, first, of the rationale underpinning CRTs and, second, of their key organisational characteristics and components.

Information sources for this chapter

Given the previous lack of authoritative statements about the rationale and key characteristics of CRTs, this chapter seeks to strengthen the account of them by drawing on a range of expert sources. A major source is the interviews carried out by one of us (SJ) with a number of international experts on CRTs and their precursors: these interviews have already been discussed in Chapter 2 and the experts involved are listed in Box 2.1. A content analysis was carried out of these semistructured interviews. Further sources for this chapter are the writings of these experts, especially those of Hoult (Hoult, 1986, 1991; Smyth and Hoult, 2000), Stein (Stein and Test, 1980; Stein, 1991), Polak (Jones and Polak, 1968; Polak, 1971; Polak and Jones, 1973; Polak and Kirby, 1976), Scott (Scott and Ashworth, 1967; Scott, 1980), Rosen (Rosen, 1997; Rosen *et al.*, 1997) and Bracken

Crisis Resolution and Home Treatment in Mental Health, ed. Sonia Johnson, Justin Needle, Jonathan P. Bindman and Graham Thornicroft. Published by Cambridge University Press. © Cambridge University Press 2008.

(Bracken and Cohen, 2000; Bracken, 2001), as well as the NHS *Mental Health Policy Implementation Guide* (Department of Health, 2001), and other publications on CRT implementation by Brimblecombe (2001), the Sainsbury Centre for Mental Health (2001) and Crompton and Daniel (2007). Our aim is to describe the consensus that arises from these sources on rationale and key components, identifying also a few areas where the sources diverge.

The rationale for crisis resolution teams

Some innovative service models are based on an explicit theoretical framework. Early intervention services for psychosis – another of the elements in the NHS modernisation – are an example: their basis in theories about the harmful effects of long duration of untreated psychosis and the prognostic importance of the early 'critical period' is clear (Spencer *et al.*, 2001). Not so the CRT model: at least in recent descriptions of the model, little space is devoted to discussion of any underlying theory that has led to the selection of particular components as important to the model.

This lack of explicit discussion of the theoretical basis and overall rationale for the model may reflect the current status of reducing inpatient bed use as an aim: it has come to be regarded as such an obvious *desideratum* that few service planners or policy makers require much more explanation of the goals of an innovative service than that it is intended to reduce use of inpatient beds. It was not always so. In 1923, for example, the prominent psychiatrist J. R. Lord expressed his emphatic opposition to home treatment for acute illness: 'There is really very little to say in favour of home treatment, especially in the case of the poor. It is often impracticable because working class families look askance at any cessation of work on the part of the bread-winner for any reason other than physical.' His other arguments against home treatment were that the suicide risk was high and that it was 'imperative that the marital relationship should cease when signs of mental breakdown appear. It is a difficult matter to separate the sexes in a private house and home treatment may entirely fail for this reason.'

So why should a short admission to an acute hospital ward that offers medical care, intensive support and supervision from nurses and respite from life's usual stresses not be the most sensible way of managing patients who are acutely unwell and may present a risk to themselves or others? Three types of rationale for treating people intensively at home emerge from the expert sources: ethical values, clinical and research observations, and theoretical principles. These are summarised in Box 6.1 and will be explored in turn.

Box 6.1. The rationale for crisis resolution teams

Ethical values

Home treatment allows adherence to important ethical values, including respect for the dignity and autonomy of people with mental illnesses.

Clinical and research observations

- Clinical observation suggests that use of inpatient beds is inefficient when little support is available from services in the community.
- Most studies comparing home treatment with a more hospital-based comparison group have found a reduction in admissions.

Theoretical principles

- Hospital admission should be avoided if possible because it is unacceptable to many patients and may have harmful effects on them.
- Treatment in the home environment is desirable because of the very large role in many crises of difficulties in families and wider social networks.
- Managing crises in the community is an opportunity for patients to develop skills and insights that will help them to cope with their illness and with subsequent crises.
- Relationships between patients and professionals are different and less dominated by inequalities of power when crises are managed at home.

Ethical values

One strong current running through the accounts given by the experts interviewed by SJ of their reasons for establishing home treatment teams was ethical. Their commitment to introducing change had often been rooted less in theories of any kind than in their adherence to particular values and their view that previous services, especially in hospital, had not conformed to these. Principles invoked included respect for the dignity and autonomy of mentally ill individuals and the need to establish a system in which patients' rather than professionals' aspirations and values have primacy. For example, Ramsey said (interview): 'In some of the big old specialist mental hospitals, there were terrible things happening where patients were abused and maltreated and we knew we should be doing something a bit more humane and hopefully effective. I think those things drove it.' Or, more radically, Bracken (interview) commented: 'The sort of philosophy we've been trying to develop is one which recognises that psychiatry has been oppressive, that people have been damaged by their involvement with it ... What we require is an ethical base rather than a technical base. The priority in our involvement with people is respect and dignity, how people view themselves, their thoughts, how they define what's happening to them.'

Discussions of the ethical principles and social attitudes that may underlie new forms of care are rarely explicit in the scientific literature, yet such values and attitudes are likely to have an important influence on clinicians' commitment to particular models of care and on their inclination either to adhere to traditional practices or to favour innovation (Winter *et al.*, 1987).

Clinical and research observations

Another significant motivating force for innovation seems often to have been experts' observations from their own clinical experience that the services in which they worked were failing in some important way. For example, Stein has described the high readmission rate in the hospital service in which he and Test worked as the original impetus to developing a community-based model, while Hoult was frustrated by the failure of the community mental health centre in which he worked to prevent patients being admitted. As research evidence has accumulated supporting the effectiveness of acute treatment at home (Chapters 4 and 5), this has also influenced further innovations and been used in support of replications of model services and of further service development.

Theoretical principles

Thus values, clinical experience and research evidence, as well as the enthusiasm of Australians for long-haul travel, have all contributed to the development of the CRT model. Yet can it be said to be underpinned by a theory of any sort about the nature of mental health crises and the mechanisms by which the best outcomes are to be achieved in their management?

Interviewed experts varied greatly in the extent to which they described CRTs and their precursors as rooted in any particular theoretical principles. Some were reticent in ascribing any distinctive theoretical basis to CRTs and their precursors, viewing them as essentially a mechanism for transferring standard good clinical practice from a hospital into a community setting. For example Muijen (interview), discussing management of crises in the Daily Living Programme, said: 'I would not say that there was an awful lot of theory, that it was strongly based on anything like a recovery model or antipsychiatric model. It was of course very much a clinical psychiatry model, but the other thing to bear in mind is that we were faced with so many different scenarios, we very much had to think on our feet.'

At the other end of the spectrum were participants for whom managing crises at home was not an end in itself but a means to the implementation of a radically revised understanding of and approach to mental health problems. For example, Bracken (interview) commented:

> To clarify my position, home treatment has never been an end in itself. Working with people in crisis outside of the institution has always been to me simply an opportunity to try and rethink what we do with people in crisis . . . The idea of a different philosophy, different style of working, has always been top of the agenda to me – the actual specifics and logistics of home treatment have been a secondary focus.

The Bradford team's approach is shaped by the insights of 'post-psychiatry', a framework for mental healthcare that challenges the usefulness of conventional diagnosis, the assumption that the clinician's rather than the patient's point of view is privileged in assessing what ideas are rational, and the construction of 'expert' roles for mental health professionals (Bracken and Thomas, 2001). Consequently, for some of those involved in developing home treatment, it has been seen as a vehicle for radical change in the way clinical work is approached, while for others the aim is more for the approach of CRTs to be in continuity with that of the whole local service system. For example, Flowers (interview) commented: 'It should be part of the acute service, it shouldn't be so separate it's elite, it shouldn't be like that, it should be very much part of the existing services and not be seen as different or special.' Where participants interviewed did cite specific theoretical influences on their work, these were very diverse and included R. D. Laing's ideas about psychiatric diagnosis as a mechanism for scapegoating within a dysfunctional nuclear family (Scott), Franco Basaglia's 'antipsychiatric' model in Trieste (Sashidharan; Chapter 20), Caplan's crisis intervention theory (Scott, Rosen, Polak; Chapter 2), social psychological experiments demonstrating the influence of environment on behaviour (Polak), and post-war UK social psychiatric research demonstrating the adverse effects of institutionalisation and the social influences on mental illness (Hoult, Stein, Sashidharan). Despite this diversity, some common themes can be identified in accounts of the reasons for setting up home treatment services. In particular, the following four principles appeared to be shared by most of the people interviewed.

1. Hospital admission can be harmful and unacceptable to patients

One justification for CRT care shared to some degree by all was that home treatment is desirable because hospital admission can be harmful to some aspects of patients' functioning, and also because many are dissatisfied with it. More specifically the following views were held.

- Hospital admission disrupts all aspects of patients' daily lives and may thus damage their social networks and social functioning: '[Treatment at home] is also a learning experience, and it's in their social context and allows them to maintain their normal life. They have got things like going to college or work and perhaps they can manage that, and it's not quite so catastrophic as a long inpatient stay' (Flowers, interview).

- Institutionalisation has been shown to have harmful effects, including a passive approach to life and more severe negative symptoms (Wing and Brown, 1970).
- Hospital admission is an unpleasant and alienating experience for many. Two of the experts interviewed (Bracken, Sashidharan) felt this was especially salient for certain ethnic minorities. For example, home treatment in Birmingham was established especially to meet the needs of the local Black Caribbean population (Bracken, interview):

> In Birmingham at that time, All Saints Hospital, the institution that was delivering care, was literally back to back with Winson Green Prison. The two institutions were one in the cultural geography of West Birmingham for the Black population. They saw All Saints Hospital, where there had been a number of high profile deaths of young black men, and the idea was that you can't develop a trusting engaged mental health service for this community and continue to do it from the institution.

- Being admitted to hospital results in even greater stigma than being diagnosed as mentally ill. Rosen (interview) described the hierarchy of stigma in which psychiatric admission is almost at the pinnacle:

> There is a stepwise stigmatisation which occurs – first of all when they go from their GP to a psychiatric service, in a psychiatric service they are somehow devalued a bit. Then if you see a psychiatrist you're devalued a bit more, then if you take medication, that's another step. And to go to hospital that's worse and [even worse] if you have to go to hospital on an involuntary basis . . .

2. Difficulties in families and wider social networks play a very large role in many crises

Most expert sources agreed that this is one of the main justifications for acute home treatment. Some had developed specific theories about the relationship between family and social factors and crises. For example, Polak's research studies, carried out with Maxwell Jones at Dingleton and in Denver (Chapter 2), involved examining, first, the extent of agreement between patients and professionals about the antecedents of crises and, second, the degree to which major social stressors could be identified in the lives of individuals presenting for acute hospital admission. He concluded that clinicians tended systematically to overestimate increases in symptom severity as causes of crises and to overlook their social precipitants (Jones and Polak, 1968; Polak, 1970). A disadvantage of hospital settings is that they tend to result in a focus on the individual rather than on the role in crises of families and wider social networks. For example,

Hoult (interview) described why he was dissatisfied when working in a service where admission was the usual response to crises among people with psychosis.

I was working in a community mental health centre, there were people I would work with and we'd try and be exploring their family problems and we could see there were problems … They'd get into hospital on a weekend or in an evening, and they'd stay for weeks, and the hospital would be taking a quite different approach to what we wanted to do. And then we'd go round again and try to deal with what we thought was a family problem, and the family would say, look it's all right now, we'll call you when we need you, he just needs to take the medication and it'll be all right. So it was fairly unsatisfactory.

3. Managing crises in the community is an opportunity for patients to develop skills and insights that subsequently remain valuable

This idea was again expressed by several experts. An important observation underlying it was that patients do not seem to find it easy to transfer new daily living and problem-solving skills that they have learnt in hospital or another institutional setting to community living (Stein and Test, 1980). Rather, new skills seem to be sustained better if they are learnt in the environment in which they will need to be applied in future; consequently, crises managed at home are more likely to result in patients acquiring new skills that can be applied to future crises.

4. Relationships between patients and professionals are different when crises are managed at home

Another view recurrently expressed by the interviewed experts was that part of the value of home treatment is that relationships established between patients and professionals are more equal and based on negotiation and partnership than when patients are admitted (Ramsey, Flowers, Bracken, Sashidharan, Muijen, Rosen). For example, Ramsey (interview) commented:

Unlike the hospital you're on their terms. The amount of power that you and the client have got is much more even than in the hospital. You're on their turf; you're there because they agree that you're there and that impacts on the relationship in an enormous way. It means that they're much more confident because it's their living room. They have considerably more control over what happens because they can ask you to leave … And so it's much more of a collaborative relationship.

This change in relationship was seen as justifying intensive home treatment not only on ethical grounds but also because of its beneficial effects on patients' long-term willingness to engage with services when experiencing future crises. Thus a patient who has experienced effective home management of a crisis may be more willing to seek help at an early stage and remain engaged with services when warning signs of another crisis emerge.

The core crisis resolution team model

This section again draws on the expert sources described at the beginning in Chapter 2 to identify the key features of the CRT model. In general, we have accepted components of the model as supported by expert consensus if at least seven of the nine interviewed experts saw them as essential or highly desirable for the effective implementation of the model.[1]

Target group for crisis resolution teams

The main target group for CRTs is people who, in the absence of the team or another highly intensive community alternative, would be admitted to an acute hospital bed. Identifying this group is sometimes straightforward, but a question that will sometimes arise is how imminent admission has to be for CRT involvement to be appropriate. There is some potential conflict between the goal of detecting an evolving crisis early enough to make community intervention more likely to succeed, and the requirement that crises be of sufficient severity to warrant admission. Therefore, it is probably appropriate for CRTs also to become involved with people for whom admission may not occur immediately without the team's intervention, but who are currently deteriorating significantly and appear very likely to require admission in the coming days and weeks unless intensive home treatment is initiated. A good relationship between the CRT and CMHTs and other local secondary services will facilitate identification of this group. If another less intensive intervention, such as weekly contact with the CMHT worker, a change in medication or attendance at a day service, has potential to halt the deterioration, then this rather than CRT intervention should initially be introduced. Sometimes the CRT may also be asked to provide intensive home treatment to someone who has had a severe untreated illness for some time, but who has previously resisted any intervention and has not quite seemed to reach the threshold for compulsory detention. In such cases, CRTs may feel that their involvement is justified if a severe mental illness such as schizophrenia would remain untreated without their intensive intervention and supervision of treatment.

As people admitted to inpatient units for the most part suffer from mental illnesses of substantial severity, it follows that CRTs will also focus on people with such disorders. In terms of the range of diagnoses included, the *Mental Health Policy Implementation Guide* (Department of Health, 2001) has suggested the exclusion of people with a sole diagnosis of personality disorder, but, as discussed

---

[1] Dr. Scott's interview was not included in this assessment of consensus on key characteristics because of the considerable differences between the team he established and modern CRTs, and because he had only limited experience of CRTs and current mental health service systems.

in Chapter 10, this seems questionable as some such individuals do appear to engage with brief episodes of CRT care and to avoid hospitalisation in this way. People with drug and alcohol disorders and no other major psychiatric disorder are a more obviously appropriate exclusion but, given the high rates of comorbid disorders on inpatient units, CRTs will necessarily be managing many people with 'dual diagnosis' of severe mental illness and comorbid substance misuse.

Most innovative service developments and research in this area have related to adults of working age (18 to 65 years), and the *Policy Implementation Guide* suggests that the service should be available for people aged 16 to 65 years, also indicating that people with learning disabilities and organic disorders should be excluded. However, as discussed in Chapter 21, the exclusion of older people raises substantial issues of equity in that there is no reason to believe that home treatment is less effective for them and, indeed, some grounds for suspecting that it may be more effective and appropriate. Likewise, the exclusion of people with learning disabilities, especially those at the less severe end of the spectrum, may be difficult to justify in the absence of evidence about whether or not they are likely to benefit (Hassiotis *et al.*, 2000). Policy in both of these areas should ideally be informed by research about the best ways to manage crises and should offer alternatives to admission for older people and people with learning disabilities. Until such evidence becomes available, pragmatic decisions will need to be made locally about whether CRTs should work with these groups, probably influenced by the other services available to them, the expertise available in the CRTs, the scope for joint working with specialist older people's services and those for learning disability, and the capacity of the CRTs.

Key organisational features

Box 6.2 summarises a set of organisational features of CRTs that are supported by expert consensus.

Multidisciplinary working is important not so much because the roles of different professions are different – much crisis work may be appropriate for someone from any professional background – as because a mixture of perspectives gives the team as a whole a broad approach, conferring 'hybrid vigour' (Rosen, interview) and ensuring a focus on both clinical and social aspects of patients' difficulties. The *Policy Implementation Guide* suggests that psychiatric nurses, psychiatrists, occupational therapists, social workers, psychologists and support workers should all be included in the team, though in practice nurses appear to be the dominant group and occupational therapists and psychologists relatively rare birds in this context (Chapter 4), even though the contribution of each profession is potentially significant (Chapter 10). The experts interviewed (mostly themselves psychiatrists) agreed on the need for psychiatrists to work

> **Box 6.2. Key organisational characteristics of crisis resolution teams**
>
> - A multidisciplinary team capable of delivering a full range of acute psychiatric interventions in the community.
> - Intensive home treatment offered rather than hospital admission whenever feasible.
> - Low patient–staff ratios allow visits two or three times daily when required.
> - Availability over 24 hours (though staff may be on call from home during the night).
> - For patients already on the caseload of other community services (e. g. CMHTs), the team works in partnership with these services.
> - Team approach, with caseload shared between clinicians and at least daily handover meetings for review of patients.
> - Psychiatrists are part of the team.
> - Rapid emergency assessments, with response within an hour when this is needed.
> - Gatekeeping role: team controls access to all local acute inpatient beds.
> - Intensive home treatment programme is short term, with most patients discharged to continuing care services (if needed) within six weeks.

within the team if a realistic alternative to acute admission were to be provided, though in practice a variety of models are in use for psychiatrist involvement and evidence on which is best is not available (Chapter 7). Chapter 25 discusses further the recruitment of CRT staff teams.

Capacity to visit at least twice a day is also identified as important by most expert sources, though Stein and Rosen commented that daily visits were probably more usual in the services they knew. Advantages of initial twice-daily visiting are:

- the opportunities for comprehensive initial assessment
- intensive monitoring of adherence and initial responses to medication
- ability to tolerate higher levels of risk because it is constantly monitored and reevaluated
- intensive building of relationships between staff and patients and carers.

Twenty-four hour availability, at least in the form of a telephone number that patients and carers can call to speak directly to a staff member, is highly desirable if patients who would have been admitted in the absence of the team are to be managed at home (Flowers, interview):

If you're going to take people on who would be in hospital, the carers need to be able to contact you at any time, or the hostel – that availability is key or you can't do it. You can't just say sleep well, we'll be back tomorrow – people are going to say, no, we can't cope with that. You have to be able to say we are available – often then people don't ring because it calms them down.

Whether outcomes differ between services where staff working the night-time shift are based in the CRT and offer a full home-visiting service and those where they are on call from home has not been established: the former arrangement seems more likely to result in prompt assessment of all new referrals.

Control over who can be admitted to inpatient beds – or 'gatekeeping' – is also supported by a strong expert consensus, with CRTs seen as much less able to reduce admissions if they do not automatically assess every potential admission for suitability for home treatment.

A team approach was seen as essential, as 24-hour cover obviously cannot be sustained by an individual staff member, and service users need to develop a relationship with the team as a whole rather than solely with particular individuals. Among the experts consulted, views varied as to whether a particular individual within the team should take on a coordinating role for care during the crisis, as is recommended by the Department of Health (2001). For example, this is not routine practice in the State of Victoria's crisis assessment and treatment teams, as such a role is seen as out of keeping with the very short timescale of the team's involvement and the limited contribution a single individual within the team can make to a particular patient's care (Carroll *et al.*, 2001). With large teams, even if there is no crisis coordinator, it is desirable to organise visits so that patients have a relatively large amount of contact with certain staff members, allowing therapeutic relationships to develop. Handover meetings should occur at the beginning of each shift. Generally, the handover between morning and afternoon shifts will be the most extensive, involving substantial discussion of each patient currently on the caseload. Handover meetings and good-quality record keeping are crucial to ensuring continuity of care, especially if there is no system of having a lead crisis coordinator.

Given the short-term involvement of the CRT, it is also crucial that relationships are maintained through the crisis period with those responsible for providing long-term care, for example CMHT care coordinators (the professionals within the CMHT who have responsibility for continuing support and monitoring of a particular patient and for ensuring that care plans are in place). A weekly joint review with the care coordinator during the period of CRT care is ideal, and care coordinators should certainly not be seeing patients any less frequently than usual while they are under the care of the CRT. Care coordinators will often be the clinicians who know the patient best, and they should be actively involved in planning their care during the crisis. Often it will also be beneficial if they are actively involved in delivering some of the interventions, such as psychoeducation and family work, as they can then build on these after the crisis period. Towards the end of the crisis period, the CRT will gradually reduce the frequency of visits and hand over to the team responsible for continuing care: except with some especially complex difficulties, the period of crisis care will not usually exceed about six weeks.

Core interventions

A core range of interventions to be delivered by CRT staff is again identifiable as supported by expert consensus, although the content of some of these interventions has not been specified in great detail. Box 6.3 summarises these core interventions.

Box 6.3. Core crisis resolution team interventions

- Comprehensive initial assessment, including risk, symptoms, social circumstances and relationships, substance use and physical health status.
- Engagement: intensive attempts to establish a therapeutic relationship and negotiate a treatment plan that is acceptable to patients.
- Symptom management, including starting or adjusting medication.
- Medication administered to patients in the community and their adherence encouraged and supervised, twice daily if needed.
- Practical help: support with resolving pressing financial, housing or childcare problems, getting home into a habitable state, obtaining food.
- Opportunities to talk through current problems with staff, brief interventions aimed at increasing problem-solving abilities and daily living skills.
- Education about mental health problems for patients and social network.
- Identification and discussion of potential triggers to the crisis, including difficulties in family and other important relationships.
- Relapse prevention work and planning for management of future crises.
- Discharge planning beginning at an early stage, so that continuing care services are available as soon as the crisis has resolved.

One principle recurrently expressed by experts concerning the range of interventions that should be available was that they should as a minimum match those which can be delivered in hospital (Sashidharan, interview):

When we started off with this business more than 10 years ago now, the emphasis was on saying that we can do everything that's being done in psychiatric hospitals, but we don't need a hospital for that. The only thing that we can't do is actually to lock people up. Apart from that custodial angle to psychiatric care, I would say that everything that's possible within the acute treatment or management of severe mental illness we can and must do within home treatment.

Therefore, one requirement is an initial assessment at least as comprehensive as that available in hospital, including physical examination and investigations where indicated. The physical health of the mentally ill has recently been identified in UK policy as an unjustifiably neglected area (Department of Health, 2006), and ensuring that adequate systems are in place for assessing this satisfactorily is a particular challenge for CRTs: good links with general practitioners are helpful, but they are likely also to need to have some facilities for carrying out physical health assessments and investigations themselves. Risk assessment is obviously a further key area of assessment and may need to be repeated every few hours where people at relatively high risk are managed in the community. Assessment in general is discussed further in Chapter 8 and risk assessment and management in Chapter 9.

Management of acute symptoms also follows good clinical practice as adhered to in hospital wards (Chapter 10). Some of the experts interviewed expressed reservations about making medication too central to crisis team work, but all sources agreed that teams should be able when needed to deliver each dose of medication and encourage the patient to take it. An area in which details of the CRT model are somewhat vague and a clear consensus yet to be established is the role of specific psychological interventions, for example targeting particular symptoms. The *Policy Implementation Guide* (Department of Health, 2001) suggests that 'a range of therapies' should be available from the team, but agreement does not seem to have been established on specific brief interventions that should be a routine part of CRT care. Several interviewees mentioned, however, that staff who happened to have training in interventions such as cognitive therapy for psychosis or massage for stress relief were encouraged to use these; as discussed in Chapter 10, further research is highly desirable on the use of brief interventions in areas such as promoting adherence, managing anxiety symptoms and reducing substance misuse. An important question regarding more complex psychological and social interventions is whether these are best provided within the CRT, where intensive contact may offer a good opportunity for engagement, or by CMHTs and other longer-term services, where the timescale for intervention is less restricted. General emotional support and opportunities for patients to talk through their difficulties are, however, key components of the work of a CRT with all patients.

An intensive approach to engagement and to negotiating a shared set of aims and a treatment plan with services users and their social networks is a further standard intervention. With patients who are ambivalent about engaging with them, CRTs will draw on the approaches characteristic of assertive outreach teams (Burns and Firn, 2002), emphasising flexibility and persistence in the ways in which they try to establish and maintain contact, and making their interventions more acceptable by basing them as much as possible on patients' own views about what their main difficulties are. Chapter 13 discusses further the ways in which CRTs promote engagement and adherence.

A strong expert consensus also supports help with immediate practical and social problems as a key component of CRT care, reflecting the view that social triggers are very significant to crises. Successful home management requires patients to have food, a habitable home and a way of addressing very immediate social problems, such as severe debt or threat of eviction, which are often a higher priority than symptoms from patients' perspectives (see Chapter 11). For example Flowers (interview) commented:

> You need to be able to address practical stuff – you need a float, a hundred pounds or so in petty cash, it's really important for sorting gas and electric, taking them home, making sure they've got money for the meters – you can't leave people if it's cold and dark . . . Going to the shop is part of the treatment too. You need staff who recognise that going to Sainsbury's is part of the job.

Again reflecting the roots of CRTs in the idea that crises should be understood in their social context, working with families and social networks is also a key component, although a clear consensus is not yet apparent on which interventions should be routinely provided (interventions with the social network are discussed further in Chapter 12). Educating families about their relatives' mental health problems, involving them in care planning and giving them practical and emotional support in their roles are the main carer-focused interventions specified in the *Policy Implementation Guide* (Department of Health, 2001) and are supported by expert opinion. However, those interviewed varied in the degree to which they advocated more extensive work using more structured approaches with families and social networks. Work with social networks was identified as an element in crisis work that could easily fall by the wayside, despite its importance: five of the interview participants felt that CRTs risk becoming little more than medication-delivery services if they are hard pressed and if training and leadership in working with social systems and social problems are not given high priority.

Education for patients about their mental health problems, structured work on relapse prevention and the identification of early warning signs of relapse, and formulation of plans for management of future crises are emphasised strongly by the *Policy Implementation Guide* (Department of Health, 2001) and by some, though not all, of the sources on which this chapter draws. Structured relapse-prevention work, advance directives and crisis cards (Chapter 16) are elements of care for severe mental illness that have recently attracted increasing interest and an accumulating evidence base. There are variations in views about whether these should primarily be seen as the task of CRTs or of the teams that provide longer-term care: a joint approach to tasks such as developing relapse-prevention plans may often be helpful.

The current status of the crisis resolution team model

Although there is relatively little published literature devoted to the rationale for, and essential components of, CRTs, a degree of consensus has emerged.

With regard to its rationale, the model cannot be seen as clearly derived from a set of theoretical principles, having developed through processes that have included clinicians and managers trying to find pragmatic ways of resolving difficulties encountered in their local services, to provide care more economically or to meet the needs of particular minority groups. Nonetheless, there are some precepts, such as the importance of social factors in triggering and perpetuating crises, that attract widespread agreement from relevant experts and are thus potentially useful in constructing a supporting rationale for the model. It should be noted, however, that these ideas provide general support for managing crises as much as possible at home rather than through hospital admissions, but they do not specifically imply that such home treatment should be delivered by short-term specialist teams rather than as one of the functions of general community teams that also provide longer-term care.

There also seems to be a consensus among experts on certain organisational and operational principles for CRTs, including providing treatment as far as possible in community settings, extended-hours availability and frequent visits, and on a set of core interventions that include help with pressing practical and social problems, inclusion of informal carers in treatment plans and ensuring that medication is taken consistently and correctly. There is much that is not specified, however, and a variety of theories about mental health crises and the best ways to manage them can be accommodated within this framework, from radical approaches such as post-psychiatry to approaches that differ relatively little from those of modern inpatient units. For example, there is agreement on the desirability of supporting and involving carers, but the content of interventions to be carried out with them has not been specified in any detail and the overall CRT model can accommodate both teams in which family intervention is confined to simple education and practical support and those which use much more formal and structured family interventions.

The current CRT model is probably more appropriately seen as a model specifying how services should be organised rather than as a treatment model. There is considerable scope for investigation of whether outcomes are influenced by variations in treatment practices within the model and of whether there are essential characteristics required for CRTs to achieve good outcomes, including the key question of whether a separate team is needed or whether this approach to care is feasible within a multifunction CMHT (Chapters 19 and 20). A firm consensus did not emerge from the interviews with experts on this issue. Three of the eight interviewees who expressed a view about this believed strongly that a separation between crisis care and continuing treatment was needed to maintain the intensive nature of home treatment and the required focus on comprehensive community assessment. The rest saw this as an as yet unresolved issue, with several identifying a need for further research; For example, Stein (interview) commented:

It's a very important question and one where I don't think we have the data to support one decision over the other. I can give you some important factors to think about, which is that there is a human tendency to work with people who are most like yourself . . . and I just think that's why I believe in specialised teams, that if you get a group of people together who are interested in working with severely mentally ill patients that are not easy to work with, then you don't get creaming, you can't take the easy ones and sort of slough off the other ones. But it's an open question, I mean it's a research question.

In response to the question, 'Do you think it needs to be a separate service from the CMHTs?', Muijen replied, 'No, I don't think so at all. I think there are a number of functions that need to be delivered, and at the moment there is too much splitting up of them between teams.'

Key points

- Although the CRT model has become more fixed in terms of name, organisational structure and content of interventions, few examinations of its rationale and core characteristics have been carried out. This chapter draws on international expert opinion to help to fill this gap.
- Three types of rationale for intensive home treatment emerge from expert sources: ethical values, clinical and research observations, and theoretical principles.
- Four theoretical principles were identified: hospital admission can be harmful and unacceptable to patients; difficulties in families and social networks play a large role in many crises; managing crises in the community is an opportunity for patients to develop valuable skills; and relationships between patients and professionals are different when crises are managed at home.
- The main target group for CRTs is people with severe mental illness who, in the absence of the team or other intensive community alternative, would be admitted to hospital. Official guidance in the UK excludes people over 65 years and those with learning disabilities, which raises substantial issues of equity.
- Organisational features of CRTs supported by expert consensus include provision of treatment in community settings; multidisciplinary working to ensure a focus on both clinical and social problems; the capacity to visit at least twice a day; 24-hour availability; control of access to inpatient beds; a team approach; and maintaining relationships with those providing long-term care.
- Core interventions supported by experts include comprehensive initial assessment; intensive attempts to establish (and involve patients and carers in)

treatment plans; symptom management, including starting or adjusting medication; administering medication and ensuring it is taken consistently and correctly; education for patients and social networks; and help with practical and social problems.

- Though the CRT model is not clearly derived from theoretical principles, the relevance of social factors is widely accepted and provides a rationale for the model.

- Further research is needed into whether outcomes are influenced by variations in treatment practices and whether there are essential characteristics required for CRTs to achieve good outcomes, in particular whether this approach to care is feasible within a general team providing longer-term care.

REFERENCES

Bracken, P. (2001). The radical possibilities of home treatment; post-psychiatry in action. In *Acute Mental Health Care in the Community: Intensive Home Treatment*, ed. N. Brimblecombe. London: Whurr, pp. 139–62.

Bracken, P. and Cohen, B. (2000). Home treatment in Bradford. *Psychiatric Bulletin*, **23**, 349–52.

Bracken, P. and Thomas, P. (2001). Post-psychiatry: a new direction for mental health. *British Medical Journal*, **322**, 724–7.

Brimblecombe, N. (ed.) (2001). *Acute Mental Health Care in the Community: Intensive Home Treatment*. London: Whurr.

Burns, T. and Firn, M. (2002). *Assertive Outreach in Mental Health: A Manual for Practitioners*. Oxford: Oxford University Press.

Carroll, A., Pickworth, J. and Protheroe, D. (2001). Service innovations: an Australian approach to community care – the Northern Crisis Assessment and Treatment Team. *Psychiatric Bulletin*, **25**, 439–41.

Crompton, N. and Daniel, D. (2007). *Guidance Statement on Fidelity and Best Practice for Crisis Services*. London: Department of Health/Care Services Improvement Partnership.

Department of Health (2001). *Mental Health Policy Implementation Guide: Crisis Resolution/Home Treatment Teams*. London: Department of Health.

Department of Health (2006). *Choosing Health: Supporting the Physical Needs of People with Severe Mental Illness – Commissioning Framework*. London: Department of Health.

Hassiotis, A., Barron, P. and O'Hara, J. (2000). Mental health services for people with learning disabilities. *British Medical Journal*, **321**, 583–4.

Hoult, J. (1986). Community care of the acutely mentally ill. *British Journal of Psychiatry*, **149**, 137–44.

Hoult, J. (1991). Home treatment in New South Wales. In *The Closure of Mental Hospitals*, ed. P. Hall and I. F. Brockington. London: Gaskell, pp. 104–14.

Jones, M. and Polak, P. (1968). Crisis and confrontation. *British Journal of Psychiatry*, **114**, 169–74.

Lord, J. R. (1923). Lunacy law and institutional and home treatment of the insane. *Journal of Mental Science*, **69**, 155–62.

Polak, P. (1970). Patterns of discord. Goals of patients, therapists, and community members. *Archives of General Psychiatry*, **23**, 277–83.

Polak, P. (1971). Social systems intervention. *Archives of General Psychiatry*, **25**, 110–17.

Polak, P. and Jones, M. (1973). The psychiatric nonhospital: a model for change. *Community Mental Health Journal*, **9**, 123–32.

Polak, P. R. and Kirby, M. W. (1976). A model to replace psychiatric hospitals. *Journal of Nervous and Mental Disease*, **162**, 13–22.

Rosen, A. (1997). Crisis management in the community. *Medical Journal of Australia*, **167**, 633–8.

Rosen, A., Diamond, R. J., Miller, V. and Stein, L. I. (1997). Becoming real: from model programs to implemented services. *New Directions for Mental Health Services*, **74**, 27–41.

Sainsbury Centre for Mental Health (2001). *Mental Health Topics: Crisis Resolution*. London: Sainsbury Centre for Mental Health.

Scott, R. D. (1980). A family orientated psychiatric service to the London Borough of Barnet. *Health Trends*, **12**, 65–8.

Scott, R. D. and Ashworth, P. L. (1967). 'Closure' at the first schizophrenic breakdown: a family study. *British Journal of Medical Psychology*, **42**, 13–32.

Smyth, M. G. and Hoult, J. (2000). The home treatment enigma. *British Medical Journal*, **320**, 305–8.

Spencer, E., Birchwood, M. and McGovern, D. (2001). Management of first-episode psychosis. *Advances in Psychiatric Treatment*, **7**, 133–40.

Stein, L. I. (1991). A systems approach to the treatment of people with chronic mental illness. In *The Closure of Mental Hospitals*, ed. P. Hall and I. F. Brockington. London: Gaskell, pp. 99–106.

Stein, L. I. and Test, M. A. (1980). Alternative to mental hospital treatment. I. Conceptual model, treatment program, and clinical evaluation. *Archives of General Psychiatry*, **37**, 392–7.

Wing, J. K. and Brown, G. W. (1970). *Institutionalism and Schizophrenia*. Cambridge: Cambridge University Press.

Winter, D. A., Shivakumar, H., Brown, R. J. *et al.* (1987). Explorations of a crisis intervention service. *British Journal of Psychiatry*, **151**, 232–9.

7

The crisis resolution team within the community service system

Jonathan P. Bindman

Though the model of home treatment presented in this book is fairly clearly defined (Chapter 6), in practice the functioning of a team will be dependent on the context in which it operates. This includes the demographic and geographical nature of the area, and also the service context – the other services available to people in a mental health crisis, to which the crisis resolution team (CRT) must relate. The relationship between the CRT and inpatient wards and casualty departments will be considered in Chapter 15, and the clinical and operational details of referral and assessment processes in Chapters 8 and 26. In this chapter, a broader perspective is taken on the way in which CRTs fit into catchment area community mental health service systems and on the problems that may arise. The need for the CRT to have multiple interfaces with other teams and parts of the service has consequences for continuity of patient care, and these consequences are discussed and some practical proposals made for dealing with them. In the initial part of the chapter, the main focus is on working with the community mental health teams (CMHTs), which take responsibility for assessments not deemed to be crises and for continuing care of most severely mentally ill service users. Some specific issues regarding other types of recently introduced functional team, particularly early intervention services and assertive outreach teams (AOT), will then be considered.

Referrals to crisis resolution teams from primary care

An important decision for CRTs is whether to be directly accessible to referrals from primary care. General practitioners (GPs) are likely to appreciate having direct access to CRTs, and accessibility and availability of rapid crisis assessment will be promoted by such access. However, although this has not been

Crisis Resolution and Home Treatment in Mental Health, ed. Sonia Johnson, Justin Needle, Jonathan P. Bindman and Graham Thornicroft. Published by Cambridge University Press. © Cambridge University Press 2008.

systematically evaluated by research studies, acceptance of referrals directly from GPs may increase the proportion of assessments that do not result in acceptance for home treatment: this may appear inefficient if resources are scarce. If direct referrals are accepted, strategies need to be found for helping GPs to understand the role of the service as well as possible, particularly that its primary goal is diversion from admission rather than resolution of psychosocial crises. If they are not accepted, alternative care pathways need to be developed that allow seriously ill service users first seen in primary care to access services swiftly.

Referrals from other parts of the community mental health service system

As described in Chapter 8, CRTs will usually operate a two-stage process for accepting referrals from other parts of the service, consisting of a screening process applied to referrals received by phone, fax or email, followed by a face-to-face assessment interview.

Screening

The team must decide what level of information to require when a referral is made. It is tempting to insist that referrers should always provide detailed information including demographic details, a full description of the presenting crisis, the social context and the previous psychiatric history, with information on current involvement with services and prescribed medication, forensic history and a detailed risk assessment, and also that they have assessed the client's willingness to accept treatment at home. While such a detailed initial assessment will certainly make life easier for the CRT, it may appear hopelessly impractical for the referrer. If the client is being referred by a CMHT care coordinator who knows the client well, or if the service is one of those fortunate few that have information systems which allow up-to-date information to be easily obtained wherever the client may present, asking for such information is undoubtedly useful. However, in many situations setting stringent criteria for an initial referral will simply create a barrier to rapid and appropriate referral of people in crisis. The CRT needs to adapt its procedures to the needs of its referrers, and if they include casualty departments faced with clients who give partial information, duty workers in CMHTs who have limited personal knowledge of the clients, staff working out of hours with no access to records, or staff working with incomplete or unreliable information systems, the CRT must compromise and take a flexible approach to accepting partial information. A minimum level of acceptable information will need to be agreed with referrers if excessive time is not to be wasted carrying out face-to-face assessments on people who turn out to be unsuitable for home treatment for trivial or avoidable reasons (such as being from the wrong catchment area, or being too intoxicated to assess). Such a minimum might include home address (or responsible catchment area according to local protocols if of no fixed abode), basic demographic details and a narrative account of what is known about the presenting crisis, the mental state and whatever risk criteria are felt to justify hospital admission.

Assessment

The process of carrying out an assessment interview is described in Chapter 8. The present chapter focuses on those aspects of the assessment that concern the relationship between the CRT and other services. If the client is referred by a CMHT, then there may be the option of a joint assessment, which should be preferred whenever possible. Clients presenting via other routes such as casualty may also be known to a CMHT, and again a joint assessment may be feasible. Even when a client is assessed and accepted out of hours, it may be best to accept them on a provisional basis pending a joint assessment with their care coordinator at the earliest possible opportunity.

There are obvious advantages of a joint assessment, such as allowing exchange of information and developing a mutually agreed plan of treatment with an agreed end-point. Additionally, however, a joint assessment is an opportunity for the acceptance criteria for the CRT to be explained and agreed in dialogue. While it might appear that a CRT can set out clear criteria for acceptance that will make it fairly straightforward to decide who should be accepted, the reality is somewhat different. The central criterion most commonly adopted for the CRT to accept referrals from other parts of the service is that the client 'would, without the involvement of the CRT, require admission to hospital' (Chapter 8). This has the advantage of being a relatively simple definition that is easy to communicate to other professionals. However, the criterion that the patient *'would ... require admission to hospital'* is not without difficulties. The decision that someone is in need of hospital admission is, in fact, a rather subjective one, and professionals often differ in their perception of the risks (of self-harm or harm to others) associated with a crisis, and also in their beliefs about the benefits of admission.

Differing perceptions of risk are a common source of dispute between CRTs and referrers. Two types of dispute can be distinguished. In one, the referring clinician has a genuine belief that the risk associated with the crisis is high enough to justify admission, while the CRT takes a different view on the interpretation of the clinical situation. In the other type of dispute, there is probably little disagreement about the actual risk, but there is a difference in the willingness of the professionals concerned to accept the risk associated with deciding not to admit. This situation is particularly likely to arise when the referrer does not come from the service that is providing the beds and, therefore, has no incentive to take responsibility for a level of risk which the same clinician might accept to protect his or her 'own' beds. A situation then arises in which a referrer suggests that the alternatives are to admit the patient or for the CRT to provide treatment, while the CRT takes the view that neither is necessary and the patient could be discharged home for some less intensive form of follow-up.

Problems in agreeing on the need for hospital admission can also arise because of different views about the benefits of admission, though this is perhaps a less common source of difficulty than the issue of risk. However, a problem can arise because, if strictly applied, the criterion has an inherent paradox, which is that those clinicians who believe that hospital admission is seldom helpful will judge most clients in crisis as not requiring it and, therefore, exclude them from the treatment at home which they believe is more appropriate. Such clinicians are put in an awkward position if asked by the CRT, 'Will you admit this client to hospital if we do not accept him?' The honest answer might be, 'No, but I still think the client will benefit from your service'.

A further problem can arise in interpreting the central criterion because of its hypothetical nature. It involves a speculation about what would be necessary if the CRT were not to provide care, which inevitably gives rise to a possible source of disagreement. Randomised controlled trials of CRTs have clearly demonstrated that a significant minority of clients referred to CRTs as 'requiring hospital admission' are not, in fact, admitted if, as a result of randomisation, home treatment is not offered (Chapters 5 and 8). Their need for admission is hypothetical and disappears once the option of CRT is withheld. Consequently, CRTs may suspect that some referrals are described as being in need of admission only to access home treatment, and there is no real intention to admit. This is not actually surprising: the threshold for a hypothetical admission will always be lower than for a real admission, which will require the referrer to negotiate other barriers (such as finding a scarce bed or detaining a reluctant patient).

While CRTs may at times become frustrated by what appears to be manipulation of their acceptance criteria to make life easier for referrers, there is an alternative view of the situation. This is that the referrer is attempting to apply another criterion altogether, which is whether the client can benefit from intensive home treatment, regardless of whether hospital admission is at issue. Though such a criterion appears less clear-cut than the requirement for hospital admission, it may be a better basis for dialogue between referrer and CRT in individual cases, and if this is explicitly acknowledged it may be easier to reach agreement than by arguing about whether the client 'really needs to be admitted'.

A similar point can be made about yet another problem with the criterion, which is whether it applies only if *immediate* admission is necessary or whether it is acceptable to refer a client from a CMHT to a CRT on the grounds that admission will be needed in the near future if intensive home treatment is not provided. Though such a referral can easily be dismissed on the grounds that it is speculative and the referrer should try again when the patient is actually in need of admission, again there may be a legitimate argument that some admissions are predictable in advance and the CRT may have a useful role in averting them. However, this argument cannot be taken too far since, at any point, a significant minority of any CMHT's caseload will be regarded as at elevated risk of relapse, and daily visits are not a realistic option for most of them, even if some might benefit.

Gatekeeping

As described in Chapter 6, the power to 'gatekeep' is regarded as essential to CRT function within the care system, and should be supported by hospital policies requiring that all admissions be cleared with the CRT. This puts the CRT in a position of considerable power, which must be used with care. Other teams may have a strong view that a particular client needs inpatient care, perhaps on the basis of a history of successful inpatient treatment, or having failed to work with the client in the community despite making reasonable efforts. While it is important that the CRT attempts an assessment wherever possible, including in some situations where the referring team does not appear to believe home treatment is likely to succeed, if the CRT appears to be operating a veto on admission without adequately explaining their position, this may cause resentment. Though the CRT is better resourced to manage patients in the community, in some cases their insistence on doing so may be seen as an implied criticism of the efforts made by the CMHT. If staff in a CMHT believe that the CRT is inappropriately thwarting their reasonable attempts to admit, the CMHT may, in turn, attempt to undermine the CRT. Staff in the CMHT may attempt to bypass the CRT and access beds directly by negotiating with inpatient teams or bed managers, may draw attention to CRT failures to avoid admission (of which there should always be plenty) and may cause difficulties when the CRT attempts to discharge the patient ('he's not ready, if you discharge him he'll have to go into hospital').

Criminal justice system referrals and assessments for compulsory admission

If a CRT is to function effectively as a gatekeeper, it must be in a position to assess potential admissions to acute beds from all sources. This includes those referrals which come via the police and those which are identified by other services as needing assessment for compulsory admission. However, this presents CRTs with a problem because the level of concern about risk is likely to be higher in such cases, and referrers may be less likely to regard community treatment as an option.

Though some clients referred by the police are very disturbed, others have problems that are amenable to crisis resolution and it is well worth ensuring that CRTs are routinely involved in their assessment. Clients referred for compulsory admission by community teams present more difficulties. Community assessments may be difficult to organise and involve a number of different personnel including police, ambulance crew, and the mandatory social worker and doctors, in addition to CRT and community team staff. In these circumstances, particularly if access to the client's home involves forced entry or the client is aroused and distressed, it can feel very difficult for CRT staff to insist on being involved in the assessment. If the CRT staff decide they wish to offer home treatment to the client, they may be faced with considerable scepticism from everyone else involved. In the face of these pressures, it is tempting for the CRT to allow a situation to develop in which they do not attend compulsory assessments, or they rely on community teams to tell them which assessments they need not bother to attend. However, this is unsatisfactory. As explained above, there may be a number of reasons why CMHTs would like to bypass CRT involvement with their clients, and if compulsory assessment allows this, it may be over-used. A compromise might be to insist that all compulsory assessments must be discussed with the CRT, but to allow the CRT to make a decision in a proportion of cases, in discussion with the referrer, that community treatment is an unlikely outcome and the assessment need not be attended; however, the potential cost of such a compromise in terms of loss of a comprehensive gatekeeping role needs to be considered.

Resolving disputes

A number of areas of possible dispute between referrers and CRTs have been described, but the extent to which such arguments happen in practice will depend on several factors. The most important is probably the degree of pressure experienced by the CRT, the CMHTs and the inpatient services. When beds are scarce, the CRT has a 'full board' of clients and the CMHT is too busy to provide greater input to deteriorating clients, tensions between the services may rise and arguments about referral criteria may break out. Sometimes the opposite applies, however, and busy teams 'just get on with it', saving time-consuming wrangles about 'who does what' for periods when they are less busy!

The structure of the services may also tend to promote good agreement between teams. If a CRT relates to only one CMHT, a single casualty department and a single inpatient unit, and is located in the same place as these other services, good working relationships can develop, both informally and by attending meetings together. Arguments about referral criteria can then be easily resolved. A CRT serving multiple sites and teams will have less opportunity to achieve stable relationships, and disputes may break out periodically, or distrust of the CRT and conflict over referrals may become entrenched. As with all teams, personal rivalries and ancient disputes may affect team relationships if inadequately managed.

Possible solutions are not hard to suggest, though they require constant effort to implement in practice (see also Chapters 24 and 26); examples include good communication by telephone and email; timely use of information systems; regular meetings between teams to discuss referrals and resolve disputes; good personal relationships between 'opposite numbers' in different teams, so that a quick phone call can be made to head off a developing dispute; colocation; and developing efficient service structures that minimise the number of team interfaces.

Discharging patients from the crisis resolution team

Clients will be discharged from a CRT to a range of follow-up options, and there will be some who need no further contact with a psychiatric service and can be discharged to primary care. However, given that clients will usually be discharged from the CRT within a few weeks of a significant mental health crisis, the majority will be discharged to a CMHT or specialist service, and again issues arise at the interface that may be resolved by a mixture of policies and protocols and good relationships and communication strategies. Most CRT clients will fall into two groups: those already in contact with a mental health team, from which they are referred to the CRT and to which they can return, and new clients to the services, who need to be accepted by the CMHT at the point of discharge from the CRT.

As a matter of policy, if a client has a care coordinator before coming to the CRT, the care coordinator should be encouraged to remain involved with the client during the period of care from the CRT, and to agree a discharge plan with the CRT at an early stage in the crisis so that discharge is straightforward as soon as the crisis is resolved. This often works well, and most care coordinators are keen to remain involved with their clients and to accept them back promptly. However, tensions can arise between professionals over treatment. Clients can express strong preferences for one team or the other (perhaps resenting CRT intrusiveness, or welcoming the higher level of support), and care coordinators can – sometimes quite understandably – see the period of CRT care as an opportunity for a break. Additionally, it is not uncommon for crises to arise at times when clients are in the process of being transferred between care coordinators, care coordinators are on holiday or off sick, or there are difficulties in the relationship between the client and care coordinator (or consultant or service generally). Under these circumstances, the CRT may find that it has difficulty engaging with a CMHT partner to discuss treatment plans or discharge. There may also be different views of appropriate timescales: a care coordinator might respond to a request to carry out a joint visit and agree discharge by suggesting a meeting in two weeks, while the CRT wishes to discharge at a day's notice.

With clients who come into contact with the service for the first time via the CRT, the CRT should refer to the appropriate CMHT at an early stage so that a joint visit can be arranged, a care coordinator allocated and a discharge plan made at the earliest appropriate stage. Difficulties may arise if the CMHT and CRT take a different view about the need for follow-up, or the CMHT is under pressure and does not allocate a care coordinator promptly.

To some extent problems can be addressed by policies that state clearly that the CRT should communicate promptly with the CMHT, that known clients should be accepted promptly by the CMHT as soon as discharge is requested and that CRT clients who are new to the service should be allocated with the same priority as inpatients. However, as with all team interfaces, policies will not ensure effective joint working without good personal communication.

Functional services and crisis resolution teams

The CRT is one of three types of functional service (i.e. services that serve a specific demographic or clinical group, or that are defined by offering a particular form of treatment) that are now mandatory throughout England and that are also increasingly prevalent in other countries. The other two are assertive outreach services (Burns and Firn, 2002) and early intervention services for psychosis (Birchwood *et al.*, 2000). The interface between CRTs and these two types of service and the ways in which overlap may occur will now be discussed.

Assertive outreach

A full description of assertive outreach services is beyond the scope of this chapter, but broadly these are services that are aimed at patients with:

- a severe mental illness, perhaps defined by a diagnosis of psychosis
- an enduring illness, typically involving a criterion of a long period in contact with services or a number of previous hospital admissions
- previous difficulties in engaging with services.

The AOT itself will usually have:

- a defined, relatively small caseload
- a team-based approach, with more than one member of the team being involved with each client
- the ability to maintain contact with patients flexibly and to go to patients who will not come to them.

Furthermore, extended hours working is common. It can be seen that these features may overlap with those of the CRT to some extent. While the CRT will be unsuitable for some clients who are very resistant to engaging, others may still accept CRT involvement in crisis. As far as the characteristics of the team go, CRT and AOTs may have rather similar team-based approaches and flexible working styles. Even the crucial distinction that an AOT will have long-term clients and CRTs will not may become quite blurred when the CRT has repeated involvement with a client in successive or prolonged crises.

The AOTs value continuity of care and usually try hard to maintain their relationship with clients through periods of relapse. For this reason, they are unlikely to refer to the CRT unless absolutely necessary and referrals are likely to be carefully considered. Additionally, care coordinators in AOTs are likely to be able to maintain a higher level of contact with their clients during the period of CRT care than CMHT staff. Sometimes the only reason why an AOT needs to refer to the CRT is that they cannot be available at night or weekends. A potential solution to this is a period of joint working, with the CRT being involved on weekends while the AOT resumes daily visits during the week.

Early intervention services for psychosis

Early intervention services for people with first-episode psychosis vary considerably in their configuration and staffing, and in the intensity of care they can deliver. The better-resourced services tend to adopt an assertive outreach style of working with patients who are more difficult to engage. As with AOTs, they may see clients very frequently, sometimes as often as five times weekly, during periods of relapse. Therefore, they are likely to have a high threshold for CRT referral and to be referring clients whose needs they see as pressing and severe when they do refer. Their policy will usually be to remain in frequent contact through the crisis, so that the working relationship between CRT and staff in the early intervention service will need to be especially close and well organised for the two teams to collaborate effectively. A further distinctive aspect of early intervention services is that one of their central aims is to engage with potentially eligible patients at the earliest possible stage in their pathway into mental health services. Consequently, CRT staff should refer new presentations of psychosis to the early intervention service immediately they become aware of them. Medication management is an area in which there is some potential for disputes if the CRT and early intervention service do not have a strong working relationship and a clear shared understanding of good practice in first-episode psychosis. Early intervention services generally initiate medication at lower doses than are typical in established psychosis, as people experiencing a first episode are particularly likely to recover on lower doses and are especially sensitive to side effects (Remington, 2005). Staff in early intervention services may feel that CRTs overmedicate their client, while CRTs may consider that the early intervention service is impeding effective and quick treatment of positive psychotic symptoms. As with all such disputes, clear mutual understanding and excellent communication will be needed for good joint working.

Continuity of care and crisis resolution teams

Though research has not, on the whole, demonstrated that continuity of care reduces service use, every clinician knows how much easier and more efficient decision making is with a client one knows personally and has seen before both in crisis and in recovery. Clients also value continuity and often express frustration at having to relate to new staff who do not know them. Referral from a CMHT or specialist service to a CRT involves a break in longitudinal continuity (continuity over time), with all the disadvantages for patient care that implies: clients must relate to new staff (often in large numbers) when at their most vulnerable; the CRT will be making decisions about clients with whom they are not really familiar; and there is a risk of poor decision making, causing distress to the client, and precipitating disengagement or worsening the client's mental state. Cross-sectional continuity (continuity at a point in time) will also be affected as the CRT may, at least initially, not have adequate relationships or communication with the client, the carers or the GP.

While solutions to these problems are inevitably rather partial and not guaranteed to succeed, they are based on a simple principle – that continuity of care is extremely important for services and for clients.

Improving longitudinal continuity

Longitudinal continuity can only be achieved by working with the client until the job is done and having a properly arranged handover, which may take time. This can cause tension with the aim of CRTs to work for limited time periods and keep up turnover.

Improving cross-sectional continuity

Close relationships must be developed between CRT staff and staff of other teams. This will be assisted if the services are aligned as much as possible (e.g. one CRT serving one or two sectors or inpatient wards will function better than one which serves the clients of multiple sectors and wards). It will also be helped by colocating CRT team bases with CMHT bases or on the same site as wards. Within sites or buildings, there may be ways of maximising the opportunities for corridor or canteen interaction, or ensuring that where formal meetings must take place they can do so with the minimum of travelling.

Communications are important. Telephone contact is seldom as good as face-to-face contact but is still essential, both at the point of initial referral and throughout the period of CRT care. It is common for patients to be referred to the CRT without the direct involvement of CMHT care coordinators, perhaps because they attend casualty or are referred out of hours, but contact with the person who knows the patient best is essential. There are numerous barriers to effective communication, such as unrecorded or out-of-date phone numbers, incompatible shift patterns, or care coordinators being on leave with no cover arrangements.

Information technology must be used effectively and can enhance communication of the information needed for good decision making.

Clear structures are vital: regular meetings, named individuals responsible for liaising with other teams, and clear transfer protocols (though these will never be a substitute for good working relationships, and will tend to be subverted or ignored if the underlying relationship is not working).

For repeat service users, there are further challenges in ensuring continuity of approach through recurrent crises (these are discussed in Chapter 16).

Key points

- The development of CRTs has led to the creation of new interfaces within mental health services.
- This gives rise to many sources of tension between professionals and also has potential to cause a loss of continuity of care for clients.
- These problems can be partly alleviated by adopting clear referral criteria, policies and protocols, and explicit communication structures.
- However, personal communication between professionals and good interpersonal relationships are also essential if the disadvantages to client care of the loss of continuity are to be outweighed by the benefits of receiving specialist treatments when needed.

REFERENCES

Birchwood, M., Fowler, D. and Jackson, C. (2000). *Early Intervention in Psychosis: A Guide to Concepts, Evidence and Interventions*. Chichester: John Wiley.

Burns, T. and Firn, M. (2002). *Assertive Outreach in Mental Health: A Manual for Practitioners*. Oxford: Oxford University Press.

Remington, G. (2005). Rational pharmacotherapy in early psychosis. *British Journal of Psychiatry*, **187**, S77–84.

8

Assessment of crises

John Hoult and Mary-Anne Cotton

A comprehensive assessment of the nature of a crisis needs to include not only the individual's mental state but also their domestic circumstances and social network. A key outcome of this assessment is determining who is suitable for home treatment. This chapter is in two parts. In the first, John Hoult provides clinical guidance on the process of taking and accepting referrals, information gathering and the issues most important for initial decision making. In the second, Mary-Anne Cotton then reviews the literature on the factors relevant to determining suitability for home treatment.

Taking and accepting referrals

Who is suitable for referral to a crisis resolution team?

In England, the *Mental Health Policy Implementation Guide* for the 335 CRTs set up by the Department of Health (2001) states (p. 11) that the services should be for those 'with severe mental illness (e.g. schizophrenia, bipolar affective disorder and severe depressive disorders) with an acute psychiatric crisis of such severity that without the involvement of a CRT hospitalization would be necessary'. While we agree that this group of patients is the main focus of crisis resolution teams (CRTs), the list of individuals for whom the guidelines say the service is not appropriate is too extensive. People with an exclusive diagnosis of personality disorder do get into acute crisis and often do get admitted to hospital; however, CRTs can usually prevent this with brief intervention. Another example where CRTs can be helpful is with people who have self-harmed and been taken to the accident and emergency (A&E) department, and whose problems are such that the liaison staff become justifiably worried about sending the person home

Crisis Resolution and Home Treatment in Mental Health, ed. Sonia Johnson, Justin Needle, Jonathan P. Bindman and Graham Thornicroft. Published by Cambridge University Press. © Cambridge University Press 2008.

alone. A brief intervention by the CRT prevents admission and can ensure adequate follow-up. The prime focus of these teams remains, however, the group identified by the guidelines.

The CRTs are also very useful for allowing early discharge of their target group from inpatient units (Chapter 15). They can provide more intensive monitoring and support at the patient's home than the community mental health teams (CMHTs) and they can ensure that medication is being taken and the patient is adjusting to discharge.

Who can refer to a crisis resolution team?

The individuals and organisations who refer people to CRTs are listed in Box 8.1. It is not advisable to accept direct referrals from the public, or self-referrals from CRT-naive patients, as it is likely that the service would become over-burdened with inappropriate referrals. If, however, the person has been recently discharged from the CRT then they or their carers can recontact the team. After a period of six months, these patients should first seek the advice of their general practitioner (GP), the CMHT or, occasionally, the A&E department for initial assessment, prior to referral back to the CRT.

Box 8.1. Who refers to crisis resolution teams?

The commonest referrers are:
- GPs
- CMHTs
- A&E departments
- psychiatric outpatient departments
- psychiatric inpatient wards (referring patients for early discharge).

Less-frequent referrers are:
- social services departments
- alcohol and drug services
- police.

The referral process

The referral should be done by phone or face to face, otherwise vital details will be overlooked. A CRT should be wary of referrals made by referrers who have not seen the person recently, and the CRT should always try to get the referrer to see the person first if at all feasible, since this often reveals that there is, in fact, no crisis. Teams need a printed referral form, which should be used to record basic personal information and a number of other details (Box 8.2). As much information as possible should be obtained at this stage. Offering to carry out a joint assessment with the referrer is good practice.

> ## Box 8.2. Information that should be recorded on the referral form
>
> The basic information that should be recorded is:
> - the time of referral
> - the referrer's name, address and relationship to the patient
> - the GP's details
> - care coordinator's details, if patient is known to a CMHT
> - the urgency of the referral and how quick the response needs to be
> - the referrer's expectations of the team
> - A *brief* history.
>
> The history, while brief, should include:
> - the reason for the referral
> - the nature of the main problem, if different from above
> - events leading up to the referral
> - the main symptoms
> - any past history
> - drug and alcohol history
> - risk factors
> - social supports and networks, with contact details for the main individuals
> - current medication.

Accepting the referral

Each shift should have a nominated senior clinically qualified member of staff responsible for accepting referrals. If this person is out on a visit and the referral is urgent, then they should be contacted either by pager or mobile phone and informed that a referral needs to be taken. Once the referral has been accepted, it should be decided who needs to attend, and when and where the assessment should take place.

Some referrals require a very rapid response, though most do not. It is best to spend some time gathering information about the person rather than rushing straight to see him or her. In the event that the referral is inappropriate it may be possible to offer the referrer an alternative course of action over the phone; however, if this meets resistance it may be better to accept the referral, conduct the assessment and then provide feedback and advice to the referrer. A CRT should be wary of accepting too readily everything related by the referrer, especially if it is second-hand information.

The assessment process

Prior to going out on the assessment

As much information as possible should be collected before a team member goes out on the assessment. One of the early pioneers of CRTs always taught new teams to 'make three phone calls before going out on an assessment'. The more prepared a team is before the assessment, the better informed it is and the more options are open to it (Case study 8.1). Potential sources of information are:

- care coordinators in the CMHT, if the person has one
- inpatient wards, if previously known to them
- discharge summaries and case notes
- psychiatrists, if the person has one
- GPs
- relatives/significant others in their social network.

Of course one should respect confidentiality, but this should not be used as a reason for not attempting to obtain information. Members of the person's social network will often be well aware of the problems occurring and their input will be very helpful.

CASE STUDY 8.1. INFORMATION GATHERING PRIOR TO ACCEPTING A REFERRAL

A 35-year-old man, recently arrived in town, was referred by a CMHT member who had seen him only once. The referral stated that he had become suicidal and angry and was hearing voices. According to previous discharge summaries, he had a past history of stabbing someone.

The members of the CRT were apprehensive about going to visit this man because of his anger and history of violence. However, they traced several previous hospitals to which he had been admitted and learned that the stabbing incident had happened many years previously and been repeated from discharge summary to discharge summary, without being described. There was no history of recent violence. A phone call to his mother in another city revealed that the stabbing had happened 15 years before in a fight, in self-defence, and that there had been no subsequent violence. From a phone call to his present partner, the CRT learned that he was angry with the Benefits Agency because of their inability to solve his benefit problems. She also confirmed that no physical violence had occurred in the time they had been together. The CRT then visited. He was happy to see the team, cooperated well with them and displayed no anger towards them.

This story illustrates three important points: first, CRTs should gather as much information as possible before visiting; second, incomplete or even false information can be recorded in case notes and risk assessments and be carried forward without being checked; third, it is important to ascertain the context in which the events occurred.

Who should be present at the assessment?

At the stage of information gathering, decisions need to be made about who should be present at the assessment. There is no hard and fast rule about this and each assessment has to be evaluated according to the nature of the referral and the person to be assessed. It is important to establish if there is any risk involved in seeing the person. If the person is well known to the service and there is little risk, then only one CRT member need attend, but in most cases a joint assessment is advisable. It is often not necessary to have a psychiatrist present at the initial assessment as long as the person is seen by one relatively soon after being accepted. It is always useful to have the referrer present and also the care coordinator, if available. In England, if it is a Mental Health Act assessment, then an approved social worker and two doctors must be present, in which case it is a good thing for one of the doctors to be a member of the CRT. Having members of the person's social network present during the assessment is most helpful, for reasons which will be outlined below. There is the potential for too many people to be present at the interview, so judgements need to be made. Sometimes the person is assessed alone while members of the social network wait in another room to be interviewed before everyone is brought together.

Where should the assessment be held?

If it can be arranged, the assessment should take place in the person's own home, though there are times when there is no choice about the setting, for example the A&E department or the police cells. People are at their most relaxed and least defensive in their own home, and the team can also assess the environment in which they will be treated. Usually it will also be easier to meet the relatives and other important members of the social network at the person's home. Teams must resist getting into the habit of asking that the person go to the A&E department and then assessing them there. Not only is the assessment likely to be more valid in the person's own home, but an expectation will also have been created that admission is likely if they attend A&E.

Carrying out the assessment

Assessment of a crisis is in many ways very similar to any other psychiatric assessment. On arrival, the team members should introduce themselves and explain the purpose of their visit. Sometimes the person may refuse to be interviewed and the team has to negotiate their way in. This is one reason why sufficient details need to be gained prior to the visit; if, for example, the person denies the behavioural disturbances alleged against him or her, and no details are available, then the team will struggle to make progress. The presence of the referrer is a good way to overcome this.

As with any history, it is important to clarify what the main problem is, and who has it. Not infrequently, it is not the person being assessed who has the problem (especially if the person is manic), but the referrer. Understanding this helps to direct the assessment. Obtaining the individual's history follows the usual format of psychiatric histories, including carrying out a mental state examination. As well as obtaining a history, talking to the family, carer and social network provides information that can range from helpful to vital; a different perspective is brought to the history and sometimes hidden issues and secrets emerge.

The team observes the quality of the relationship with the social network and what the expectations are of the team. The home environment can also give an indication of what the team needs to offer. Are there essentials such as food, electricity and bedding? Is the place a disorganized mess? Is the neighbourhood dangerous?

Because it is anticipated that the person will be treated at home, a detailed risk assessment is needed. The issues which this should address are described in Box 8.3.

Box 8.3. Issues that should be addressed in a risk assessment

Main risk factors, including:
- challenging behaviours
- chaotic, intrusive or disorganised behaviours
- ideas of suicide or self-harm
- self-neglect
- the presence of drug or alcohol misuse
- interpersonal conflicts
- child care issues
- environmental hazards or problems
- unwillingness to cooperate.

Factors that modify the above risk factors, for example:
- the degree to which social support can be mobilised
- the person's desire to remain at home and avoid hospitalisation
- the extent to which the CRT can engage the person and secure their willingness to cooperate
- the CRT's ability to respond quickly to emergencies
- the CRT's ability to monitor the person's behaviour
- the anticipated effect of medication on the person's behaviour and illness, and the ability of the CRT to ensure that their medication is taken.

It should be noted that the availability of the CRT is in itself a significant risk-modifying factor.

How do assessments by a crisis resolution team differ from other types of psychiatric assessment?

There are a number of differences between CRT and other types of assessment.

1. They usually happen when one or more people are in a state of crisis. There are tensions and heightened emotions, a fear that matters are getting out of control, and coping mechanisms are strained. Sometimes there has been disturbed,

even challenging, behaviour. There is an expectation that the team should do something to fix the situation, and do it quickly.

2. They do not usually take place in a hospital or clinic, but on the person's own territory, where staff have to observe the person's rules rather than vice versa. But while staff have less control, the advantage is that the person and their social network are less guarded and will reveal more of themselves.

3. Because of differences 1 and 2, CRTs have to be more flexible. The person may not be at home when staff arrive, so they will have to come back later or be prepared to go to where the person is, such as at a friend's house or in a cafe. Staff might need to negotiate with the person for some time to gain access to the home. They may need to put up with some abuse. The usual comforts and security of a hospital are sometimes missing; there may, for example, be no furniture, electricity or heating in the home.

4. The CRTs are much more likely to involve the social network in the assessment. The reasons for this have already been discussed, but the advantages cannot be stressed too strongly.

5. Assessments by a CRT will usually take a lot longer than those carried out in hospital or by community mental health teams. If the team is to treat someone at home safely and adequately, they will need to assess the risk factors properly, as well as the factors that modify the risks and the person's willingness to cooperate. In addition, CRTs need to undertake planning for immediate management and then initiate it. All of this can take two to three hours. But it is by no means time wasted, especially if there is resistance from patient and family to being admitted, for while the whole process is going on the team builds up a therapeutic alliance with them.

6. The CRT should attend each assessment with the expectation that they will be able to manage and treat the patient at home, no matter how disturbed they sound from the history given by the referrer. It is this attitude that distinguishes a good CRT from one that is just a funnel into hospital. Even with disturbed and seemingly uncooperative patients with psychosis, the team should spend a lengthy period trying to engage with them and finding areas where common ground can be established so that a therapeutic alliance can develop. A good CRT will strive to achieve this, not simply assume straightaway that admission is the only solution.

Some difficult groups

As mentioned above, everyone in crisis is potentially suitable for home treatment by a CRT and a decision cannot be made until the person has been assessed. From experience, there are two main groups who are more difficult to manage at home.

These are people who are disorganised, intrusive and/or have disturbed or aggressive behaviour, but who:

- will not or cannot engage, despite the team having spent a lot of time talking, so the team is not able to work with them; the majority of this group suffers from schizophrenia
- will engage but for a number of reasons their behaviour does not settle quickly enough; the majority of this group suffers from a manic illness.

Sometimes the treatment given simply does not work fast enough and the burden on the carers becomes too great, or the patient's behaviour becomes too risky. In other cases, the patient is rarely home at the agreed time to receive supervised medication and meet with the team. In all cases, it is important to note that it is the patient's *behaviour*, not their diagnosis, which results in home treatment not being possible.

There are a few other groups for which home treatment by the CRT is too difficult. These are people who:

- misuse drugs or alcohol to such an extent that safe management becomes too problematic
- have severe depression that fails to improve quickly enough with treatment, and whose behaviour is too much of a burden for their carers (it is, however, uncommon to have to admit people with depression)
- make demands for admission accompanied by threats to behave in such a disturbed manner that the CRT is forced to go against their judgement and acquiesce; such situations are rare and patients who do this usually have a diagnosis of personality disorder.

Good CRTs rarely need to admit people who are suicidal. A lengthy, detailed and sympathetic assessment helps to engage the person, and the offer of help to deal with their problems engenders hope.

Factors relevant to determining suitability for home treatment: a review of the literature

A comprehensive literature search was carried out in order to identify all papers that compared people accepted for home treatment or crisis intervention with those admitted to hospital. All retrieved papers were assessed and their results, the robustness of the methods used and the statistical analyses were examined. More details of this review have been published by Cotton *et al.* (2007).

Limitations of the literature

The literature examining features associated with hospital admission despite the availability of a CRT is limited. When searching, therefore, it was necessary to use a broader definition of crisis treatment. This, however, makes it difficult to draw generalisable conclusions and gives rise to the following limitations.

Mixture of services models

The main problem in summarising the literature is that it concerns a wide variety of service models offered as less-restrictive alternatives to hospital. Fewer than half of the papers identified appeared to investigate crisis/home treatment teams with configurations and intervention profiles that adhered to current CRT practice (Dean and Gadd, 1990; Bracken and Cohen, 1999; Brimblecombe and O'Sullivan, 1999; Guo *et al.*, 2001; Brimblecombe *et al.*, 2003), and some provided too little information on the alternative under investigation to judge how similar it was to the current CRT model (Schnyder *et al.*, 1999; Abas *et al.*, 2003). The remaining four papers investigated a variety of alternatives to hospital: two investigated residential housing projects (Segal *et al.*, 1996; Walsh, 1986); one looked at an outpatient service (Slagg, 1993); and one explored a service that consisted of a hybrid between day hospital and home treatment (Harrison *et al.*, 2001; see also Chapter 22). It was also unclear in those papers investigating crisis teams whether the teams were gatekeepers for hospital beds (Chapter 6). This would influence how proactive the home treatment team might be in attempting to prevent hospital admission.

Statistical analysis

Only half of the papers conducted a regression analysis, a type of analysis that allows identification of factors which still seem to influence likelihood of admission when all the other factors are taken into account. Some papers investigated very small numbers of patients, which casts some doubt on the validity of the findings.

Outcomes

Four papers investigated outcomes other than admission to hospital. In three papers, there was no analysis of patients at initial assessment, only of failures of the intervention (Walsh, 1986; Brimblecombe and O'Sullivan, 1999; Brimblecombe *et al.*, 2003). One study looked at acceptance to home treatment rather than admission to hospital; however, those not accepted to home treatment will include people whose difficulties were not severe enough to warrant admission or intensive home treatment (Harrison *et al.*, 2001).

Comparability of variables

The variables that were investigated varied considerably from study to study, and most did not investigate a full set of those likely to influence admission, nor did they all measure all the factors in the same way, creating difficulties in comparing and combining results from different papers.

Summary of results

No very definite consensus emerged from the literature about which factors influenced the likelihood of being admitted despite the availability of a less-restrictive alternative. This is probably a consequence of the methodological reasons outlined above. The factors that were most often associated with a greater likelihood of hospital admission are shown in Box 8.4.

Box 8.4. Factors associated with hospital admission despite the presence of a 'less-restrictive alternative'

The following factors make hospital admission more likely:
- *mode of referral*: referral via the legal system (e.g. police stations, courts), referral outside normal working hours, referrals other than self-referrals
- *symptom severity*: having greater symptom severity, having psychotic symptoms
- *comorbid features*: current history of substance misuse, primary or secondary diagnosis of personality disorder
- *past history*: previous history of hospital admission
- *sociodemographic features*: male, living alone
- *uncooperativeness*: with attempts to assess and treat in the community.

Risks

Features such as suicidal intentions and risk to others were not commonly found to be risk factors. Although these features were cursorily mentioned in a few papers, severe suicidal ideation was found to be significantly and independently associated with hospital admission in only one paper (Brimblecombe *et al.*, 2003). This was a well-conducted study and should perhaps be given greater weight than the others. No papers offered a statistical analysis of whether risk to others was a significant factor in determining the decision. Two papers do, however, cite this as a reason given for admission to hospital (Dean and Gadd, 1990; Abas *et al.*, 2003). There was little mention of other risk factors such as self-neglect or risk from others. These omissions do seem odd but may be because such factors were subsumed under differently classified variables, such as symptom severity or cooperativeness/engagement.

A recent study (Cotton *et al.*, 2007) has investigated factors associated with admission in the areas served by three inner London CRTs. The sample was drawn from the Islington and Southwark CRT studies described in Chapter 5 (Johnson *et al.*, 2005a,b). It included 358 patients and looked at a comprehensive set of the variables previously identified as potentially important influences on decisions to admit. A regression analysis allowed identification of factors that were independent influences on hospital admission when adjustment was made for all the other factors. Patients who were uncooperative with the initial assessment, those at risk of unintentional harm to themselves (such as through self-neglect or reckless behaviour), those with a history of previous compulsory admission and those assessed in casualty were all significantly more likely to be admitted. Furthermore, one CRT was substantially more successful at treating patients at home than the other two. This last finding could be a consequence of differences in setting as well as different styles of management, team dynamics and thresholds for admission.

Inconsistencies

There are several inconsistencies in the findings of different papers, including variations in whether symptom severity and substance misuse were found to be important predictors of admission. These probably result from different patient profiles in different studies, although overall the studies seem to suggest that people with drug and alcohol problems complicating other problems were probably more likely to be admitted as inpatients.

Conclusions from the review

The literature available allows a few tentative conclusions to be drawn about the factors that may be important in determining whether people are admitted despite the availability of a CRT. More and stronger studies are, however, needed before this work can really be used effectively as an aid to decision making and as a clear indication of what works for whom in managing mental health crises. This is not surprising since, as was discussed in the first part of this chapter, each situation has subtly different complexities and in most cases decisions can only be arrived at after in-depth assessment. Factors such as team resources and management play a major role. Building up rapport and gaining the person's trust is paramount and may be the distinguishing feature that enables successful home treatment for someone who poses a high risk. It is sometimes very clear that a person needs admission to hospital; in most cases, however, there is an argument that intensive home treatment should be carefully considered before making arrangements for admission.

Key points

- Findings from the limited literature on patients who are likely to fail home treatment are inconclusive, though candidate factors include referral via the legal system, uncooperativeness, substance misuse and past history of admission.

- Risk factors alone do not determine whether someone will be suitable for CRT intervention: if sufficient risk-modifying factors – such as good social support and willingness to engage – are present, even relatively high-risk patients may be treated at home by a CRT.
- Assessments should include gathering information from a wide range of sources.
- Building rapport and engaging with patients and their social networks is one over-arching factor that seems from a clinical perspective to lead to successful home treatment.
- If there are doubts about a person's suitability, a trial period of CRT intervention can allow for continued assessment of the situation and may lead to a successful outcome.

REFERENCES

Abas, M., Vanderpyl, J., Le Prou, T. *et al.* (2003). Psychiatric hospitalization: reasons for admission and alternatives to admission in South Auckland, New Zealand. *Australian and New Zealand Journal of Psychiatry*, **37**, 620–5.

Bracken, P. and Cohen, B. (1999). Home treatment in Bradford. *Psychiatric Bulletin*, **23**, 349–52.

Brimblecombe, N. and O'Sullivan, G. (1999). Diagnosis, assessment and admission from a community treatment team. *Psychiatric Bulletin*, **23**, 72–4.

Brimblecombe, N., O'Sullivan, G. and Parkinson, B. (2003). Home treatment as an alternative to inpatient admission: characteristics of those treated and factors predicting hospitalization. *Journal of Psychiatric and Mental Health Nursing*, **10**, 683–7.

Cotton, M. A., Johnson, S., Bindman, J. *et al.* (2007). An investigation of factors associated with psychiatric hospital admission despite the presence of crisis resolution teams. *BMC Psychiatry*, **7**, 52.

Dean, C. and Gadd, E. (1990). Home treatment for acute psychiatric illness. *British Medical Journal*, **301**, 1021–3.

Department of Health (2001). *Mental Health Policy Implementation Guide*. London: Department of Health.

Guo, S., Biegel, D., Johnsen, J. and Dyches, H. (2001). Assessing the impact of community-based mobile crisis services on preventing hospitalization. *Psychiatric Services*, **52**, 223–8.

Harrison, J., Alam, N. and Marshall, J. (2001). Home or away: which patients are suitable for a psychiatric home treatment service? *Psychiatric Bulletin*, **25**, 310–13.

Johnson, S., Nolan, F., Hoult, J. *et al.* (2005a). The outcomes of psychiatric crises before and after introduction of a crisis resolution team. *British Journal of Psychiatry*, **187**, 68–75.

Johnson, S., Nolan, F., Pilling, S. *et al.* (2005b). Randomised controlled trial of care by a crisis resolution team: the North Islington Crisis Study. *British Medical Journal*, **331**, 599–602.

Schnyder, U., Klaghofer, R., Luethold, A. and Buddeberg, C. (1999). Characteristics of psychiatric emergencies and the choice of intervention strategies. *Acta Psychiatrica Scandinavica*, **99**, 179–87.

Segal, S., Watson, M. and Akutsu P. (1996). Quality of care and use of less restrictive alternatives in the psychiatric emergency service. *Psychiatric Services*, **47**, 623–7.

Slagg, N. (1993). Characteristics of emergency room patients that predict hospitalization or disposal to alternative treatment. *Hospital and Community Psychiatry*, **44**, 252–6.

Walsh, S. (1986). Characteristics of failures in an emergency residential alternative to psychiatric hospitalization. *Social Work in Health Care*, **11**, 53–64.

9

Assessment and management of risk

Neil Brimblecombe

The assessment and management of risk is central to mental health practice. This is true in all areas, but especially so in acute settings where risk to self or others is a common concern. The role of crisis resolution teams (CRTs) in England is to assess individuals in a crisis situation and offer home treatment as an alternative to hospital admission where possible. When home treatment is contemplated, risks of suicide, aggression, severe self-neglect and reckless behaviour need to be carefully assessed and decisions made about whether home treatment is likely to be safe. Strategies for monitoring and minimising risk in community settings need to be put in place to enable safe, but responsive, care to be provided. This chapter summarises research on risk in home treatment services and provides guidelines for assessing, monitoring and managing risk to service users, carers, professionals and the community.

Evidence

The CRTs act as gatekeepers to inpatient services (Department of Health, 2002) and hence work with individuals who, by definition, are potentially in need of high levels of support and care and are likely to present high levels of risk to themselves or, more rarely, to others. There is no evidence to date of increased risk of suicide or violence associated with the use of crisis services as opposed to more traditional approaches such as hospital admission. A *Cochrane Review* of the limited number of studies of crisis services for those with severe mental health problems showed no difference in death rates compared with those receiving traditional inpatient care (Joy *et al.*, 2004). The majority of (largely descriptive) studies of services similar to those crisis/home treatment services currently in place in England also typically show no increased risk (Brimblecombe, 2001),

Crisis Resolution and Home Treatment in Mental Health, ed. Sonia Johnson, Justin Needle, Jonathan P. Bindman and Graham Thornicroft. Published by Cambridge University Press. © Cambridge University Press 2008.

although drawing conclusions about such relatively rare events as suicides is inherently difficult without very large samples.

Working with service users and carers

At the centre of any assessment of risk must be the relationship with, and information gathered from, the service user and any carer who is involved. Although crisis services may see many people who, by reason of their mental state, may not be able to give a full account of their current situation, the principles should always be that:

- assessment is a shared process between the professional and the service user
- the service user is an expert in their own feelings and experiences.

Working in such a way requires a range of skills, attitudes and knowledge from the crisis team assessor, including:

- good interpersonal and negotiation skills
- positive user-centred attitudes
- specific understanding of the effects of mental health problems
- an understanding of factors related to increased risk
- an understanding of the potential benefits and limitations of both home and inpatient treatment
- an understanding of legal and professional accountabilities.

Who assesses?

As CRTs are multidisciplinary and usually take a generic approach to assessments, so the professional background and experience of the assessor will vary. Team-based training, good supervision structures and systems for learning from adverse events are essential to ensure that all members of the team have the skills and confidence to assess risk in acute situations. However, variability in assessments will be reduced and the confidence of the assessor increased if assessments are carried out by pairs of professionals whenever possible, and particularly if there is concern about risk. This gives the advantage of having more than one clinical opinion, as well as reducing any risk to staff in an unknown setting. It can be particularly valuable to have another professional who is already engaged with the service user present, for example a general practitioner or community mental health nurse. This is of potential value in:

- reducing the anxiety of the service user, making an accurate assessment more likely
- assessing any changes in the way that the service user presents compared with their usual, or best, level of functioning

- sharing specific information about previous incidents of self-harm or aggression that may not be available to the assessor from other sources
- sharing current concerns about risk
- sharing any other relevant information that their more in-depth knowledge of the service user's circumstances may give them.

Similarly, friends, relatives and carers have much to offer in providing valuable information about any issues of risk. While confidentiality may prohibit the assessors from divulging personal information about the service user, it will rarely prevent them from asking questions of others or listening to their views and concerns.

Assessment tools and note keeping

Assessment tools provide a standardised approach to assessment and recording and establish a minimum standard of data gathering. They can offer many advantages over an unstructured approach to risk assessment, such as:

- evidence of change over time
- prompts to encourage a full assessment
- evidence that a full and appropriate assessment has taken place.

A range of standard tools is available to support clinicians in carrying out risk assessments, particularly in assessing the risk of suicide and self-harm (Lewis and Roberts, 2001) (Box 9.1). Though such tools may be reliable (i.e. different clinicians produce similar measurements when using them) and have concurrent validity (i.e. they produce similar results to other tools when measuring similar things), they do not have established ability to predict outcomes in short-term care. Their principal value is, therefore, to ensure that a full clinical assessment is carried out and recorded.

> ### Box 9.1. Practice example: risk assessment tools
>
> The crisis services in South Essex Mental Health Trust utilise the FACE assessment tool (http://www.facecode.com). The Risk Profile details key aspects of risk to self or others, including risk history, current warning signs and risk management plan. This nationally developed tool is used throughout local services, facilitating clear communication of risk.

Research has shown previously that community mental health services in England do not tend to use standardised assessment tools derived from research, but most do use locally derived forms (either computerised or paper based) that prompt staff to ask about and record risk information in a systematic way

(Higgins *et al.*, 2005). Informal contacts with a significant number of crisis services in England suggest that CRTs also tend not to use standardised assessment or risk assessment tools, but that most do utilise the tool or form in common use across their own trust. This has the advantage that other parts of the mental health service are likely to be familiar with it and this will facilitate information sharing. Local training is also commonly available. The disadvantages of taking a purely local approach rather than using standardised assessment tools are that local systems are generally not supported by evidence, depth of assessment of particular risks or areas of functioning may be lacking and they are less useful for communicating risk to services outside the local area.

It is important that assessments, as well as plans and subsequent actions taken, are clearly defined and recorded. Although practice should not be defensive, it should be *defensible*, and clear evidence should be available that the team:

- tried to identify risks
- weighed them up
- put in place a reasonable plan
- carried out the plan
- reassessed at frequent intervals, including responding rapidly and appropriately to changing circumstances or information.

Principles for risk assessment and risk management: self-harm and violence

All risk assessment needs to identify any factors present that are statistically proven to be significantly associated with increased risk. Table 9.1 lists selected factors associated with increased risk of suicide or harm to others.[1] The mere presence of one or more such factors is not, however, sufficient grounds on which to base a clinical decision. As predictors, all of these factors are, on their own, weak. Previous suicide attempts, for example, are by far the best single predictor of future suicide but only 1% of those who are admitted to an accident and emergency department following an act of self-harm are likely to take their own life in the following year (Hawton, 1987). It is clear that an actuarial approach to risk assessment needs to be supplemented by exploration of the meaning of current and previous events (Case Study 9.1). For example, if there has been a previous suicide attempt, how similar is the current situation? What is different? Was the previous attempt 'serious' in terms of intent? How did the service user cope following the last attempt? Do they have any new social supports that were

---

[1] For summaries of risk factors see, for example, Nestor (2002), Hawton *et al.* (2005), Saunders and Hawton (2005) and Gillies and O'Brien (2006).

Table 9.1. Selected factors associated with increased risk of suicide or harm to others

Suicide	Risk to others
Previous self-harm or suicide attempts	History of violence
Being male	Substance misuse
Substance misuse	Morbid jealousy
Physical illness	Clouding of consciousness and confusion
Loss in childhood	Escalating conflict with specific individuals
Lack of employment	Persecutory delusions with fear of imminent attack
Being young, Asian and female	Sustained anger or fear
Previous aggressive behaviour	Plans for, and/or fantasies of, attack
Access to means	Impulsivity
Recent clinical improvement	History of threats
Recent contact with GP	Involvement of close relative or companion in conflict arising from delusional convictions

CASE STUDY 9.1. ACTUARIAL AND CIRCUMSTANTIAL FACTORS

John is a 30-year-old farmer with a history of a serious suicide attempt by hanging two years previously. This was linked to a period of depression arising after the death of a family member. He has become depressed again. The crisis team assessed John and noted factors related to an increased risk, including age, gender, occupation, previous history and low mood, but noted that his circumstances were markedly different from those at the time of his previous suicide attempt. He now has a child and, despite his current very low mood and thoughts of death, he is clear that he could never kill himself as this would cause lasting harm to his son.

not previously available? Asking the service user specific questions regarding risk is almost always the best way to gather information. There is no evidence that asking about thoughts of self-harm increases risk (Hyman, 1994).

One factor that should always be taken into account when assessing any form of risk is the use of illegal substances and/or alcohol. This is common in people with severe mental health problems (Department of Health, 2002). Such use is potentially a significant additional risk factor, increasing risk in all categories. Specific questions should be asked about this issue, while making it clear that such questions are perfectly standard and that any information received will be treated confidentially. As with so much else in the process of assessment, the interpersonal abilities of the assessor are key to the service user feeling comfortable enough to disclose. Even when substance use is disclosed, its extent is often understated. Encouraging service users to talk about their substance use by methodically working through an average day or week is more likely to produce accurate information.

Previous history of self-harm should be addressed as a related, but sometimes distinct, issue from suicidal thoughts and acts. Many individuals who self-harm do so as a means of coping with feelings and may be anxious that their self-harm will be misinterpreted as either suicidal features or 'attention-seeking' behaviour. Previous contact with services may have led them to expect that they will be criticised for such actions or forced to desist from them in the absence of other coping mechanisms. Whilst self-harm may escalate into suicide attempts or create risk of severe physical damage, trying to understand the meaning of self-harming to the individual may be more important than simply trying to prevent it in the short term.

Other risks

While risk of suicide and violence to others tend to receive greatest attention in assessments, many people with severe mental health problems are also at heightened risk of:
- violence or abuse from others, including financial exploitation
- non-deliberate self-harm, such as self-neglect or a decreased awareness of environmental risk and concern for safety
- physical illness.

A particular challenge for community services that aim to offer a direct alternative to hospital admission is to ensure that an adequate physical health assessment is carried out. It is clearly established that people with severe mental health problems are at increased risk of serious physical health problems (Disability Rights Commission, 2006), which may be caused or exacerbated by psychotropic medication (and associated weight gain), self-neglect, poor nutrition, stress or substance misuse.

Hospital admission or home treatment?

Where risk to self or others has been identified through assessment, a decision is required as to whether this can be managed with reasonable safety at home through intensive home treatment or requires hospital admission. To make this decision, it is necessary to be clear about what can and cannot be offered in a community setting. In community settings there is:
- no 24-hour instant availability (although this may be mediated by the presence of a carer)
- no 'specialing': direct one-to-one observation is not possible over an extended period of time

- less control over the environment than in hospital
- a need for at least partially successful negotiation with service user and others to make care plans work.

It is also important to recognise that admission to hospital may not, in any case, have the effect of eliminating, or even reducing, risk. The experience of hospital admission can be distressing and stigmatising in itself, and suicides are still relatively common in inpatient settings. Risk may simply be delayed, as suicides are also relatively common in the period immediately following discharge from a ward (Appleby *et al.*, 2001). The risk of aggressive or violent behaviour may be increased by a compulsory admission, or by the stresses of a crowded ward environment.

A key component of good practice is realistic attitudes from staff members. A clear part of the rationale for CRTs is to prevent hospital admission, and reducing admissions is likely to be a key audit indicator for any assessment of a service. Additionally, crisis team members are likely to have clear views as to the preferability of home-based over hospital-based care. It is important that team members do not allow either external pressures or personal enthusiasm unduly to influence practice. Hospital admission is an appropriate course of action where it is the best way to meet an individual's needs, especially where significant risk is present. Even the most successful CRT must expect to admit a substantial proportion of the clients it assesses, and appropriate admissions are not 'failures'.

Risk as part of the wider assessment

Risk is just one factor that needs to be taken into account when deciding whether home treatment can take place (Brimblecombe, 2001). Other factors include:
- likely compliance with any home treatment plan
- support from family and/or others
- need for specific hospital-based treatments
- availability of other community services
- acceptability of home treatment to the client.

Risk management plans

To as large a degree as possible, risk management plans need to be negotiated and agreed. Although crisis team workers will have their own professional anxieties and concepts of healthy behaviour, these need to be mediated by what is meaningful and tolerable for the service user.

Clear care plans are also vital to ensure that a team, with a number of workers providing care over 24 hours, works in a consistent and coherent manner. Providing a copy of the care plan for the service user and/or carer can be helpful and should be portrayed as part of a collaborative process, whereby the team should rightly be held to account if it does not provide what it has planned.

Some risk management strategies

Emergency management

Service users and carers should be clear as to what action to take in an emergency situation. This can include the provision of emergency phone numbers and the identification of short-term coping strategies, such as staying with a trusted neighbour until the CRT arrives. The circumstances that should lead to the police being called can be discussed.

Identifying stressors and early signs

The CRT can work with the service user and carer to identify behavioural and psychological signs that a dangerous event may be more likely, for example becoming increasingly angry about the noise from a neighbour or having more frequent fantasies about death. Such indicators can be linked with specific actions, such as phoning the CRT or engaging in a proven distracting activity.

Structuring time

Having a structured day with activities negotiated and agreed provides a supportive structure for individuals with intrusive or distressing thoughts. Some crisis services have access to acute day-care provision that offers structured activities, which may be helpful for distraction, or occupational therapy, which may also provide rewarding experiences or opportunities to develop life skills.

Acting as 'care coordinator' to provide comprehensive services

In a complicated health and social care system, it is vitally important that someone takes on the role of coordinating care packages. This may be carried out by a professional who is already involved, such as a key worker in a community mental health team, or by a crisis team member. If the former, it is essential that good communication is maintained and that a clear plan is shared between the teams involved.

Risk minimisation

While it is not possible to manage environmental risks to the same degree at home as in a ward setting, CRTs can help to reduce overall risk by identifying such risks. For someone at risk of impulsive or accidental overdose, it is often possible to negotiate for the team to hold their medication for them and reintroduce it in a structured way as control is regained. Box 11.1 (p. 140) suggests some other risks associated with the home environment that can be addressed by the CRT.

Continued risk assessment

Risk assessment is a continuous process, not a single event. Close monitoring of risk is essential and needs to be incorporated within care plans. Levels of risk are likely to fluctuate and may necessitate changes in approach or levels of input from the crisis team, or even brief periods of hospital admission at times of particular risk (Brimblecombe, 2003). Care plans need to be flexible, and a willingness to adapt to changing circumstances is essential.

Managing risk to staff

Any plan to provide care in a home environment needs to consider potential risks to staff. Such risks may arise from service users themselves, from carers or friends, or from visiting a risky neighbourhood after dark. Lone-worker policies need to be in place in organisations to help to fulfil the employer's duty of care to its staff. Training is also increasingly becoming available to help staff to develop 'de-escalation skills'. However, each situation is different and requires flexible thinking by the team. Risk may be reduced by meeting in a location other than the service user's home. Visiting in pairs and considering the gender of workers may be appropriate. Where a risk to staff emerges during an episode of care, the care plan must be reconsidered by the team, taking all factors into account.

Advance statements

Where service users are temporarily unable to engage fully in discussion about their management plans, the existence of a previous statement about what they would like to happen in such circumstances can be extremely valuable. This allows the use of their expertise and ensures that actions carried out on their behalf are acceptable.

Key points

Risk assessment and management in crisis settings is a challenging endeavour. It can be made safer for both service users and professionals by ensuring that:

- A collaborative approach is taken with service users.
- Carers can provide vital information and support in both assessing and helping to manage risk.
- Methodical assessments address specific issues of risk, judged within the individual context of the service user's life.
- The assessment involves the gathering of adequate information, whenever possible from a range of sources, concerning previous incidents of risk and current concerns.

- Clear recording is made of any assessment and plan, including frequent reassessments.
- The safety needs of staff are specifically addressed where potential risk is identified.
- The benefits and limitations of hospital admission are understood.
- A wide range of flexible risk management approaches is potentially available in response to individual need.

REFERENCES

Appleby, L., Shaw, J., Sherratt, J. *et al.* (2001). *Safety First: Report of the National Confidential Inquiry into Suicide and Homicide by People with Mental Illness.* London: The Stationery Office.

Brimblecombe, N. (2001). Intensive home treatment for individuals with suicidal ideation. In *Acute Mental Health Care in the Community: Intensive Home Treatment*, ed. N. Brimblecombe. London: Whurr, pp. 122–38.

Brimblecombe, N., O'Sullivan, G. and Parkinson, B. (2003). Home treatment as an alternative to inpatient admission: characteristics of those treated and factors predicting hospitalization. *Journal of Psychiatric and Mental Health Nursing*, **10**, 683–7.

Department of Health (2002). *Mental Health Policy Implementation Guide: Dual Diagnosis Good Practice Guide.* London, Department of Health.

Disability Rights Commission (2006). *Equal Treatment: Closing the Gap.* London, Disability Rights Commission.

Gillies, D. and O'Brien, L. (2006). Interpersonal violence and mental illness: a literature review. *Contemporary Nurse*, **21**, 277–86.

Hawton, K. (1987). Assessment of suicide risk. *British Journal of Psychiatry*, **150**, 143–53.

Hawton K., Sutton L., Haw C., Sinclair J. and Deeks J. (2005). Schizophrenia and suicide: systematic review of risk factors. *British Journal of Psychiatry* **187**, 9–20.

Higgins, N., Watts, D., Bindman, J., Slade, M. and Thornicroft, G. (2005). Assessing violence risk in general adult psychiatry. *Psychiatric Bulletin*, **29**, 131–3.

Hyman, S. E. (1994). The suicidal patient. In *Manual of Psychiatric Emergencies*, 3rd edn, ed. S. E. Hyman and G. E. Tesar. Boston: Little Brown.

Joy, C. B., Adams, C. E. and Rice, K. (2004). Crisis intervention for people with severe mental illnesses. *The Cochrane Database of Systematic Reviews*, Issue 4, CD001087. Oxford: Update Software.

Lewis, S. and Roberts, A. R. (2001). Crisis assessment tools: the good, the bad, and the available. *Brief Treatment and Crisis Intervention*, **1**, 19–28.

Nestor, P. G. (2002). Mental disorder and violence: personality dimensions and clinical features. *American Journal of Psychiatry*, **159**, 1973–8.

Saunders, K. and Hawton, K. (2005). Suicide prevention and audit. *British Journal of Hospital Medicine*, **66**, 627–30.

10

Symptom management

John Hoult and Fiona Nolan

Crisis resolution teams (CRTs) are required to address and alleviate the symptoms of the full spectrum of psychiatric disorders. In this chapter, John Hoult discusses the assessment, management and monitoring of symptoms by the multidisciplinary team, including the management of agitated and suicidal patients, and particular considerations relating to prescribing and monitoring medication in crises. The role of psychologists in CRTs and the potential of brief psychological interventions are then described by Fiona Nolan.

The phases of symptom management

Managing symptoms at home with a CRT is in most ways similar to managing symptoms elsewhere, so the similarities will not be mentioned here. Going into the full details of management of specific mental illnesses is beyond the scope of this book, and we assume that teams will be aware of current good practice guidance, such as the NICE guidelines for management of a variety of disorders (http://www.nice.org.uk). Chapter 8 provides a description of how assessment of people in crises differs from assessments elsewhere. In what follows, there will be a brief mention of the assessment phase, but more emphasis will be given to how to plan care and manage people with the more common types of symptom within the CRT.

The planning phase

While the assessment is going on, staff silently wonder what they can do to treat the person at home. Options start to formulate in their minds, changing as information emerges. By the end of the history taking and assessment, a couple of options will have crystallised, and the possible resources required to implement

Crisis Resolution and Home Treatment in Mental Health, ed. Sonia Johnson, Justin Needle, Jonathan P. Bindman and Graham Thornicroft. Published by Cambridge University Press. © Cambridge University Press 2008.

them will have been considered. Occasionally, the CRT will encounter a lot of drama while doing an assessment. Patients with manic disorders, borderline personality disorders and challenging behaviour can be intrusive, demanding, disorganised or abusive, and this can result in heightened emotions among members of the social network who are present. The CRT staff must not allow themselves to be rushed into decision making by all this; they need to stay calm and keep everyone talking in the expectation that the drama will blow itself out (as it usually does). Even the stormiest scenes can subside, allowing rational planning for home treatment to proceed. Staff should have some idea of the expectations of the person in crisis, and of the social network. What follows – and the order in which steps are taken – depends on the CRT's assessment of the situation. This is a fluid process and can require skilled judgement, which comes with experience.

The CRT members generally explain to the patient and the social network how the team operates, its availability and what it can do. They ask them for their opinion as to what they would like to happen, and what they think the options are. Staff then put forward the options they have formulated. They explain the consequences of those options. They emphasise the team's ready availability and ability to support, treat and monitor intensively. Sometimes the person, or members of their social network, may be wary about home treatment as they may not have experienced it before and have previously been used to admission as a matter of course. In such cases, a detailed explanation of the team's experiences with similar patients can help. Sometimes clients will express fears or raise objections to home treatment: it is helpful to deal with these one by one in a systematic way. If the person has not been sleeping, explain how medication will ensure sleep. If their behaviour has been disturbed, explain how the team can effectively deal with that, and how frequent monitoring allows new plans to be quickly implemented. For patients and carers who are particularly apprehensive, a useful technique is to keep asking them what other problems they foresee, and then explain how the team can address these problems.

When treating someone in crisis at home, much more than symptoms must be addressed: practical problems such as food, electricity, money, accommodation and other environmental factors may need to be included in plans, either immediately or within a day or so (Chapter 11). Plans need also to include dealing with interpersonal problems (Chapter 12), since symptoms do not exist in a vacuum but are affected by stressors involving others. Support for the social network has to be considered. Medication has to be planned for in most cases.

Finally, the degree of supervision and monitoring by the CRT (and perhaps the social network) has to be agreed on. All too often, in spite of the CRT's best efforts, case notes are not available and no-one who might know the person can be contacted. Naturally, this is most likely to happen on Friday nights! A diagnosis may be difficult to establish. The team has to do the best it can at the time and gather the required information as soon as possible.

The immediate implementation phase

The main aims of the immediate implementation phase are:

- calming disturbed behaviour and emotions
- establishing a therapeutic relationship
- ensuring short-term community survival, e.g. food, accommodation, etc.
- giving explanation, reassurance, advice and guidance to the patient and his/her social network.

Once the plan is agreed on, everyone must be clear about it, and about how they can contact the CRT in an emergency. This in itself is often an important part of symptom management, allaying everyone's understandable anxiety. The CRT need to make sure that the person and those in their social network are aware of the team's capacity to respond quickly if necessary and to visit frequently. Once again, the order in which interventions are done is a matter of judgement and will depend on the nature of the situation.

Medication

In almost all cases, medication will be needed as the crisis will involve disturbed emotions and sometimes disturbed behaviour. Families and social networks can be quite fraught. If home treatment is to be effectively implemented, then the CRT must calm the situation as quickly as possible. Lorazepam 1–2 mg will be sufficient to calm most patients; sometimes an antipsychotic such as risperidone or olanzapine needs to be added. The CRT must wait 30 to 45 minutes after first administration to see that the medication is working and that there are no untoward effects. It is important that the patient sleeps, especially on the first night, otherwise the team will start to lose credibility. Sleeping tablets in an effective dose are, therefore, also essential in many cases.

Staff from the CRT need to monitor the taking of medication for most patients in the initial phase. Often they need to watch the medication being swallowed, just as happens on the ward. If patients have their own medication and there is likely to be confusion about what will be taken, the team needs to take it away and administer it as directed. Sometimes medication administration can be entrusted to the family under the guidance of the team.

If the patient is in any way disturbed, then the team needs to visit at least twice a day initially to monitor the symptom severity, particularly the behavioural disturbance, as it is this that determines the person's capacity to survive in the community. Medication levels should be adjusted up or down according to response and the presence of side effects. It is important to avoid over-sedating if possible.

Housing problems

As well as being important in their own right for a person's community survival, housing problems can also affect symptoms. Immediate attention to them will sometimes improve rapport with patients and has even been the key to engagement with them (Chapter 11). For people who have lost their accommodation, some CRTs are fortunate to have access to a crisis house (Chapter 23). Other innovative teams have placed the person in a motel, private hotel or bed and breakfast facility for a few days until alternative accommodation can be arranged. The suitability of these options obviously depends on the level of disturbance that has happened and may possibly happen.

Address, remove or reduce stressors

Usually stressors are interpersonal in nature. The team has to reduce conflict (and occasionally over-protectiveness) by whatever means are available: advice, explanation, separating combatants by moving someone (usually the patient) to other accommodation. Crisis theory proposes that when people and their social networks are in a state of crisis they are also at their most susceptible to help and most willing to change (Chapter 2). The CRT members are in a unique position to take advantage of this: they will often witness the conflicts taking place or hear people say things in the heat of the moment and, while the team may not be able to do much during the initial interview, the fact of having witnessed these events gives an easy opportunity to address them constructively within the next few days. This opportunity is usually lost when a person is admitted to hospital: the staff who witnessed the conflict will not be the staff who subsequently deal with the patient; the latter will not have a proper understanding of the nature and intensity of what happened, making denial by the patient or social network easier. In addition, members of the social network will often only see junior staff on the ward. The CRT members, therefore, have the opportunity to change interpersonal relationships for the better (Chapter 12).

Give explanations, advice and guidance

Explanations, advice and guidance are often neglected in other situations, but become much more important in the context of home treatment. Patient, family and carers need to know what has gone wrong, what is likely to happen, what they should do if something else goes wrong and how they should handle the situation. The CRTs have to explain things and give advice for the immediate future.

They must make sure that everyone understands the care plan and knows how to contact them and what their response will be.

Supervision and monitoring

In many cases the person being cared for by the CRT would otherwise have been in hospital. Initially, the team must visit frequently if there has been any disturbance or threat of disturbance. On the first day, a visit at about 9 pm to make sure that the situation remains calm and to administer night sedation does wonders to reassure everyone – patient, social network and team. A visit early the next day (at 8 or 9 am) has a similar effect. After a day or two of frequent and unrushed visits, even sceptical relatives lose their apprehension and are won over to the benefits of home treatment.

Support for the social network

Supporting the social network ought to be obvious but too often is neglected. Acutely disturbed behaviour has its effect, and not just on the patient; the social network can be in crisis too and needs help in understanding and carrying on, especially if it is continuing to care for the patient in conjunction with the team.

The medium-term implementation phase

Within a few days, the condition of most patients begins to stabilise: the disturbed behaviour will have settled, a regular sleep pattern will be established, a therapeutic relationship formed. The diagnosis will often become clearer once information (e.g. from case notes, discharge summaries, stories from previously unavailable care coordinators or people in the social network) becomes available. The team will get a better idea of not only the problems that need to be dealt with but also the supports and resources available.

Ongoing support

Just being there, visiting often and being readily available gives patients and families a great sense of security. Having someone to talk to, someone they can ask the many trivial questions that need answers or someone to get advice from are matters that can seem trivial to health professionals but are very important to patients and carers.

Supervision and monitoring

In the early part of this phase, this probably needs to be continued. As time progresses, people who are on twice-daily visits can drop down to once per day. The important thing is to make sure that symptoms do not suddenly worsen without the CRT being aware of it and being able to respond immediately.

The practice of taking medication to the patient daily or twice daily is as important in making sure that monitoring occurs as it is in ensuring that medication is taken.

Medication

The first few days often require frequent adjustment of medication in order to ascertain the right dosage: not so much that the person is disabled by side effects; not so little that symptoms (especially disturbed behaviour) are not brought under control. Factors that may result in medication changes include clarification of diagnosis, initial side effects and information about the patient's previous response to medication.

During the acute phase, the patient may have been given an explanation about their medication. If so, they are very likely not to have understood or retained it. In the medium-term implementation phase, the explanation should be repeated to both patient and family so that they are more likely to retain it. As the behavioural disturbance settles, medications such as lorazepam, which are useful in calming the disturbance, should be reduced and then discontinued, sleeping tablets likewise. With continued improvement, there comes a time when medication management gets handed back to the patient. Dosette boxes, with compartments for the tablets to be taken on each day, are often very useful in preventing confusion and helping to monitor the taking of medication.

Practical problems

If there were practical problems that needed attention in the immediate implementation phase, then they will still need attention in this phase. By now, the more immediate problems will have been fixed to some degree, but accommodation and benefits issues will have come to the fore. Sometimes a flat will have become a chaotic mess and will need to be cleaned. Repairs may have to be organised. Other tasks include sending the patient for blood tests and X-rays, organising appointments with and taking them to see general practitioners (GPs), medical clinics or dentists, and helping them to get clothing. Doing these activities with the patient helps to cement the therapeutic relationship.

Exploring the social network and addressing problems

At this time the CRT needs to be seeking out and meeting with significant others in the patient's social network who have not yet been spoken to. Neighbours, clergy, more distant relatives and ex-partners may each have something useful (and occasionally quite important) to tell the team, or may be able to help with management. Where there are relationship problems, the team needs to explore these, finding out how they affect the patient and trying to deal with them. This usually involves meetings with the patient and members of the social network.

While not all team members may have the skills to do this, it is vital that at least some staff are able to handle such situations: if the problems do not get dealt with, they can prevent full recovery and are likely to trigger further relapses. Staff in a CRT, like all staff, find it difficult to do social systems intervention; it often gets ignored and only when the patient does not improve as expected do they finally get around to trying to deal with it.

Involving the community mental health team

If the patient is on the caseload of a community mental health team (CMHT), the care coordinator should be notified at the earliest stage, and should be asked to do a joint visit with CRT staff and to remain involved with the patient throughout the duration of CRT management. The CRT should not make significant changes without consultation with the care coordinator. For patients not known to their local CMHT who are likely to need continuing care, the CRT should contact the team early in this phase and request that a care coordinator be nominated to meet with the patient and CRT staff. This provides an opportunity for the care coordinator to get to know the prospective patient and start forming a relationship prior to the CRT ceasing its involvement.

The late implementation phase

It is important to reiterate that the CRT should stay involved with the patient until the crisis has resolved. This means that:

- the person's behavioural disturbance has gone
- psychotic and other symptoms have gone, are steadily diminishing or have stabilised
- medication is now at maintenance levels and is being taken reliably
- the CRT has reduced its visits to perhaps only twice weekly
- practical problems have been sorted out or solutions are in hand
- education about the illness has been undertaken
- the social system has been assessed and informed, and either problems have been dealt with or plans for further interventions are clear
- a good link has been established with the CMHT, a care coordinator has met several times with the patient and social network, and there are clear plans for ongoing management.

Managing particular presentations

Different symptoms and presentations require different approaches, which are described in this section. The general principles of management described above apply to all of these symptoms.

Challenging behaviour/threats of violence

The CRT will almost always be made aware by the referrer of behavioural problems and threats. Preparatory work is very important to get the exact details of the threats and behaviours: when they happened, what they were, whom they were directed against, how serious the event was, was anyone harmed, and how certain of the facts is the referrer? Often reports of violence or threats of it get exaggerated, people over-react and the over-reaction itself worsens the situation. The exact details should be elicited, if at all possible, others who might have more details should be contacted. Old notes should be checked and care coordinators consulted. Are there people, such as a partner, relative or friend, who might accompany the team to help to assess safely? Are there people who should not go because they might inflame the situation? Might the police be needed? (They rarely are, and their presence may escalate the tension or increase the likelihood of compulsory treatment, but sometimes they are necessary.) It is better to keep down the numbers at the assessment. In advance, potential appropriate medication can be identified and taken to the assessment so that it can be administered straight away. At least two staff should go.

At the house or flat, reasonable safety precautions should be taken without making these obvious. The following approach is advised. Stay calm and avoid confrontation. *Be prepared to spend a lot of time on the interview – do not rush things*. Explain who you are, who asked you to come and why you have been asked to come – do not try to hide these details. Take a long history, going into a lot of detail: as well as making sure that you have got the story right, it calms things down and gives you time to build rapport. *Keep talking*. If necessary, get an account from whomever else is present. The two stories may differ, and you will have to try to square them, or work out which is the more credible.

As the assessment goes on, possible management strategies begin to form. It is ideal when a management plan flows naturally from the ongoing discussions and is accepted by the patient, but usually this does not happen. There comes a time when plans have to be put to the person and to the relevant others who are present. Sometimes staff may need to withdraw so that they can agree on a plan. Sometimes several options can be given to the person to get across the idea that their point of view is not being ignored, and that they still have some power in the decision-making process. There are times when the options come down to either taking medication from the staff and accepting frequent monitoring or going to hospital compulsorily. Critics complain that this is tantamount to blackmail, but, in truth, if the team considers that without home treatment the person will have to be admitted, it is a statement of fact. The presentation of such options may result in increased emotional tension but this has to be weathered; compromises may have to be negotiated and, it is hoped, a plan will finally be accepted by all concerned.

Medication will usually be required and here the value of having had the foresight to bring some to the assessment becomes apparent. It can happen that, at the end of a long interview, there is a brief window of time when the person will accept medication, and the CRT will need to be alert to this window and take the opportunity it presents. A delay in giving medication may result in refusal later, leading to further lengthy negotiations, or else admission. Ensuring that the person has a good night's sleep is vital, as is getting control of any disturbed behaviour; failure to do either will seriously jeopardise home treatment efforts. Antipsychotic medication and anti-anxiety drugs such as lorazepam, used in combination, calm most people. Once medication has been administered, the team needs to stay with the person until it is clear that the situation has calmed and looks like it will remain that way in the immediate future.

Management is never just about medication. Social matters certainly need considering, though most will not need to be attended to immediately. Family members, if present, do need advice, guidance and explanation. In addition, they may have a lot to contribute to management, in particular in monitoring the situation.

Early reassessment is also vital. Sometimes a staff member will need to stay with the person for many hours after the initial dose of medication; sometimes the team can leave but will need to re-attend within a few hours. If the medication has been given at night and the person goes off to sleep, the situation can be left until the next day, but the team may well need to attend first thing in the morning in case the disturbed behaviour starts building up again. Carers must have the team's contact details and be reassured that they can phone at any time of the day or night to speak to a team member.

Suicidal patients

It should be rare for a CRT to admit suicidal patients just because they are suicidal. Almost every suicidal patient is engageable, so the team's task is to engage the patient, offer him/her hope and then do their best to resolve whatever problems triggered the suicidal ideas. Almost all suicidal patients are depressed in one way or another. The commonest groups referred to CRTs are people in accident and emergency (A&E) departments who have overdosed in reaction to a temporary stressful situation, people with various depressive disorders and people with borderline personality disorder (see below). People who have taken overdoses in response to acute social stress usually only encounter the CRT once, when being assessed for discharge from A&E.

As always, the starting point for management is getting a good, detailed history, exploring the triggers of the suicidal ideas, the various problems the patient has and the nature of their social supports. During this process, rapport builds up. The team needs to know why suicide seems the only solution, how strong is the suicidal urge, how solvable are the person's problems, and what resources can be mobilised to help them. Often the question 'Do you really want to die or do you want your problems solved?', asked towards the end of history taking, is the one that opens the door to home treatment. Most patients want their problems solved. When they say so, the way is open for the team to give hope and offer to work with the patient to deal with their problems. The team members need to give the patient confidence that they will be able to fix these problems.

Mobilising social support is a big help in managing the suicidal patient, but people providing such support will themselves need support from the team. Monitoring appropriate to the perceived risk may be needed: the house or flat should be checked to ensure that there is no potentially lethal medication lying around and the team needs to dispense medication and monitor whether it is being taken. If possible, the less-toxic antidepressants should be prescribed so that any further overdose will not prove fatal when medication control is handed back to the patient. Sleep needs to be ensured, and benzodiazepines may be needed for a short time to deal with any associated anxiety.

Severe depression

A person with severe depression may be so agitated or so slowed down that getting a history takes forever, or just may not be possible. The presence of the social network is very important in these cases. Planning management may be similarly difficult, especially if the person is almost mute and/or indecisive. The CRT and social network may have to decide on management plans for the person and tell him/her what is going to happen.

Very often it is members of the social network who have contacted the mental health services; in most cases they will be willing to monitor the person and (later on) medication, provided that they have had adequate explanation and instruction and know that the CRT can be readily contacted, and will come if needed.

The obvious medications are antidepressants and sleeping tablets (almost certainly the person will not have been sleeping). If the person has psychotic symptoms, an antipsychotic drug is needed. Sometimes an anti-anxiety drug is also needed to deal with anxiety and agitation. Getting the person to take and swallow the tablet can take infinite patience and much coaxing and cajoling; for example, their depressive delusions may be that they are guilty of unpardonable sins and that the CRT and the family are the agents who will justifiably kill them with their tablets. Whatever medication is given, the person must get off to sleep that first night, both for their own sake and to reassure the family. For those people who have lost a lot of weight, a dietary supplement should considered until their appetite is restored.

If suicide is still a risk, necessary precautions must be taken, such as ensuring that the means of acting on suicidal ideas are removed and a close watch is kept on the person. *The CRT must not forget that it is when depressed patients begin to improve that they can succeed in killing themselves.* Patient and family need explanation, education, guidance and reassurance, and the feeling that they are well supported, particularly in the first week or so. The team must make sure that the burden to which the family have agreed is tolerable. Occasionally it may be necessary to admit the patient if there is little sign of improvement and the burden becomes too great.

Luckily, most severely depressed patients improve fairly quickly and are very grateful for the help given. Some take longer, and arranging for the person to go to a day hospital can give the family welcome relief. Support for everyone still needs to be kept up. Some people make minimal improvement and the 'pros and cons' of hospitalisation have to be debated. Depressed people are the ones most likely to benefit from swift access to psychological services provided the area is lucky enough to have this.

Manic symptoms

Most manic patients will cooperate with the CRT and be happy to be treated at home. The trouble is that they are full of energy and want to be out doing things, so it can be a big job to locate them and medicate them. With manic patients, the team needs to get control of the over-activity as soon as possible. Initially, it is better to over-sedate rather than under-sedate them.

Once agreement is reached on a management plan, the person needs to be medicated as soon as possible. Anti-manic drugs such as lithium and valproate can be started at the initial meeting, but they take too long to exert their effect so other drugs are needed. An antipsychotic such as risperidone or olanzapine acts quickly and should be given. So should lorazepam, since a response to it is usually seen within 45 minutes. Not infrequently, the patient will go to sleep with this medication – a welcome outcome.

The assessment and planning phases can be full of hilarity, abuse and drama, the last when patients realise that they are going to have to accept treatment. The plans need to include the place of treatment and the degree of monitoring that is required. Sometimes patients get shared amongst relatives and friends on a shift system. These carers will need a lot of support from CRT. If there is no support network volunteering to do the job, then the CRT must be prepared to do a lot of monitoring and people who are more disturbed may need to be admitted.

The team should wait to see how the initial dose has worked and, if it has not calmed the over-activity much, then the team doctor (or whichever doctor is present) will have to consider an increased dose. The aim is sedation, and if it cannot be achieved quickly then home treatment probably will not last long. The patient will need to be visited again within a few hours of being sedated, to make sure the situation remains calm and to give further treatment if needed. The CRT should administer all medications at this stage and make sure they are being swallowed. Just before the evening shift finishes work, staff should visit and administer sufficient medication to try to ensure the patient gets a good night's sleep. Frequent visiting, sometimes several times daily and at length, is needed until it is clear that the over-activity is diminished. Sending the patient to a day hospital can alleviate the burden on the family and allow them to get on with their usual activities.

As a degree of calmness returns, more explanation and education about the illness should take place. The initial dose of medication can be cut down, but care has to be taken not to reduce too quickly and thus allow symptoms to get out of control again. Manic patients are good at pleading their case for lower doses: they are articulate, have little insight into the chaos they cause and do not feel unwell. Sometimes a compromise may be necessary to avoid the patient rejecting medication altogether, but the team must do all it can to avoid the symptoms flaring up. The team also has to be alert to a sudden swing into depression.

The patient with borderline personality disorder

A good CRT should be able to treat most people with a borderline personality disorder within the community. Where effective teams have been operating, inpatient staff comment on the disappearance of these patients from the ward. Often the point of first contact with patients with borderline personality disorder is in the A&E department following a self-harm episode; patients are quite likely to say that they will self-harm again if not admitted. Management is, therefore, mostly similar to that described in the section on the suicidal patient. However, the continual threat of self-harm is worrying for inexperienced staff. The first task is to take a long history, going into details about the triggers of this episode and about previous episodes of self-harm and their outcomes. This detailed history becomes a treatment in itself: a relationship develops, inconsistencies often appear and clues about how the episode can be managed emerge. Often the patient is seeking, even demanding, hospital admission. Usually such people have had many admissions, usually with uproar while in hospital, and little resolved at the end of it. Pointing this out to the patient opens the way to trying alternative strategies. Sometimes it is useful to pose the question, 'And how will being in hospital help solve that?' If the trigger to the present episode is interpersonal problems (as it often is), then the CRT staff point out that the problem lies in the community and that is where attention needs to be focused. If a relationship has irretrievably broken down, then the team comes up with strategies for dealing with this and rebuilding the patient's life. The sheer amount of talking usually results in the patient accepting home treatment.

There are some patients with borderline personality disorder who will maintain their demand for admission and continue to threaten disturbed behaviour unless it is granted. Here judgement is required; on the one hand, if experienced team members think the person is bluffing they may call this bluff; on the other hand, they may decide that the risk is too great and yield to what seems to be blackmail. The team should follow up what happens on the ward, since valuable clues may emerge that can be used in the next encounter with the patient.

For patients with borderline personality disorder who stay with the CRT, medication will usually be needed for the acute phase. Care must be taken to avoid drugs that are fatal in overdose, and the CRT should administer the medication so that the means of overdosing is not to hand. What has worked in the past may be a helpful guide. Many patients will say nothing has ever worked but still want medication. Antipsychotic drugs have anxiolytic and sedating properties. The selective serotonin-reuptake inhibitors (SSRIs) are occasionally effective antidepressants but take time to work. Benzodiazepines probably need to be given but if at all possible confined to only the first week or so; sleeping tablets will probably be needed for a similar period.

It is best not to keep these patients for too long: the phrase 'more is worse' is often true when managing them. The more time and effort devoted to them, the more their demands may escalate, and when the team cannot meet them they use this fact as a reason to self-harm or act out in some other way. Refer the patient on as soon as the crisis settles. Longer-term, consistent therapeutic relationships are likely to offer the best prospects of gradual improvement, with brief CRT contacts only at times of crisis.

First-episode psychosis

The first episode of psychosis is always a crisis for the family as well as for the patient and needs handling with much gentleness and sensitivity. Upon assessment, a nondescript diagnosis such as acute psychotic episode should be offered, with an explanation that resolution of symptoms within a short time is the likeliest outcome. The team needs to offer hope. The recommended medication in the initial phase is a low dosage of one of the new antipsychotic drugs, such as risperidone 1–2 mg per day. Patients experiencing a first episode generally respond to lower doses than may be necessary in established psychosis, and they are particularly vulnerable to side effects, so initiating higher doses than necessary creates a risk of adverse effects that may lead the patient to reject medication. Medication to ensure sleep will often be necessary, and benzodiazepines such as lorazepam often have a role. Sedation and control of anxiety and agitation should be achieved in the short term by using these and not by prescribing high doses of antipsychotic drugs.

If there is an early intervention service for patients with first-episode psychosis, referral needs to be made as soon as possible, and they will generally begin working alongside the CRT, engaging with the patient and social network from the earliest stages of management of the crisis. If there is no such service, the team continues to support the patient and relatives until the crisis is resolved. Counselling is critical and if access to psychological services is readily available they should be involved. It is important to avoid hospitalising people with first-episode psychosis if at all possible, something most likely to be achieved by close collaboration between the CRT and early intervention service. The experience of the symptoms is traumatic enough; being admitted to a psychiatric inpatient unit – especially one with disturbed patients – is a further traumatic experience and represents a turning point in people's self-image and, potentially, in their identity.

The contribution of psychological therapies

The emphasis in this chapter so far has been on using medication, practical social interventions and work with the whole social system to alleviate symptoms. However, the other potentially efficacious approach to many symptoms is, of course, psychological treatment such as cognitive therapy. A variety of professionals may deliver such interventions, but clinical psychologists continue very much to be the lead providers. A brief survey carried out to inform the writing of this chapter located fewer than 20 clinical psychologists currently practising within CRTs in England. Their presence in the teams appears to be increasing steadily, however, with most appointments being for part-time, sessional input. In the survey, the opinions of some of these psychologists were sought via their own professional network, which gives them a forum for peer support and discussion and meets regularly at different venues throughout the country. They were asked about their perceptions of their role and about the interventions that they employ within CRTs. This has informed the following account of how they work within CRTs.

Psychologists' training in formulation can allow them to support the team in making a more holistic assessment of the patient's difficulties, and consequently reduce excessive reliance on medication as the mainstay of treatment plans. The brief periods for which patients remain with CRTs can make it difficult for psychologists to plan a therapy 'package' in the usual way, hence their interventions often need to be pared down to fit into a handful of sessions with a patient.

The principal roles for psychologists in this setting are as follows.

Assessment and signposting for further treatment as appropriate. If it is thought that longer-term psychological interventions are needed, the CRT psychologist is unlikely to begin any treatment, as this cannot be followed through to completion, for example where sexual abuse has been identified. They can take part in initial assessment with other team members, and this is often valuable in determining whether the patient will be amenable to psychological interventions in the 'immediate' phase of the crisis.

Formulating the patient's difficulties and seeking to understand them in psychological and social terms. This leads on from assessment and continues throughout the treatment period. The aim is to promote understanding and self-awareness in the patient, and facilitate engagement and adherence.

Supporting their colleagues within the team. The psychologists who were surveyed saw this as important, and they described a variety of ways of providing this support. These included:

- one-to-one supervision sessions with individual staff, either as a named regular supervisor or on an ad hoc basis, as requested by colleagues
- providing training for colleagues in psychological approaches
- acting as a resource for research and audit activity
- generally broadening the thinking of the team in terms of using psychological interpretations for patients' difficulties, and promoting 'reflection' rather than 'reaction'.

Providing psychological therapies. Several brief therapies have the potential to be effectively employed in periods of crisis, including solution-focused therapy, brief cognitive–behavioural therapy, motivational interviewing, psychoeducation and relapse-prevention work. Longer forms of intervention are generally avoided. This work is by necessity focused, highly structured and fast paced, so that as much as possible can be fitted into the short time allowed.

Psychologists can work with most types of presentation, although some seem to have individual preferences and skills or are expected within their services to work with particular subgroups. Their work with acutely psychotic patients seems to be generally limited, however, and they tend to wait for acute symptoms to abate somewhat before attempting to engage. The CRT setting also gives them an opportunity to do some systemic work with families, which can often be more long term than the brief interventions identified above. One drawback with working in CRTs for the psychologists themselves is the possibility of becoming less skilled at longer-term work with patients, and family work is one way of 'keeping up to speed' in this respect. Working in other settings for one or two sessions a week is another way of preventing loss of skills.

The presence of psychologists in CRTs can bring tangible benefits for the wider services. Provision of psychological assessment and signposting does away with the need for people to wait, often for several months, to be assessed by a psychologist in an outpatient service, or within a CMHT. This can ensure that only people with the greatest need for long-term psychological treatment get referred on, avoiding a 'silting up' of other services.

The challenges identified as inherent in the CRT role centred on the psychologists having to try to maintain their own professional identity while being available to colleagues and 'pitching in'. Maintaining a balance between availability as part of the team and preserving a specific role may be difficult.

Clinical experience suggests that the use of some brief psychological interventions may be valuable in the management of crisis presentations, even though research evidence remains limited. Therefore, there is a role within the service for practitioners who can deliver these interventions safely and effectively. Psychologists are obvious candidates for this role, but there is also considerable scope for other professionals to be trained to deliver brief psychological treatments, either in conjunction with or instead of their usual roles. This is an area in which more research would be very helpful, since it would tell us which brief psychological interventions are effective within the framework of CRTs; which groups of patients are able to make use of them; and who can deliver them effectively.

Key points

- Management of symptoms in CRTs follows general guidelines for good practice, but some specific considerations are the need to begin achieving symptomatic control and control of agitation early, the adjunctive use of benzodiazepines and the need to monitor adherence and the early effects of taking medication very closely.
- Twice-daily visits are valuable initially for patients exhibiting significant behavioural disturbance, allowing not only close supervision of medication adherence but also close monitoring, reassurance for carers and early development of therapeutic relationships.
- Practical interventions and those focused on social networks are also of great importance in alleviating symptoms.
- Brief psychological interventions are in use in some CRTs where psychologists are employed, but more evidence is needed about which ones work, who can deliver them effectively, and which patients are likely to benefit.

11

Practical psychosocial interventions

Jonathan P. Bindman and Martin Flowers

All crises encountered by crisis resolution teams (CRTs) arise in a social context. In most, problems in the social environment have a direct role in precipitating the crisis, and even in those where the connections between psychopathology and environment are not obvious, therapeutic work must still be delivered in a way that is appropriate to the social context. This chapter describes practical interventions to address the psychosocial problems that trigger, exacerbate and arise from crises. It begins by considering how assessment must lead to an understanding of a person's social environment. The specific areas in which CRTs find themselves attempting to intervene with individuals are then considered in more detail (work with families and social networks is discussed in Chapter 12).

Who should provide psychosocial interventions?

Psychosocial interventions have traditionally been divided between the various professional disciplines involved in mental health: housing problems are seen as the province of the social worker; difficulties with cleaning, shopping and cooking are assessed by occupational therapists, and perhaps addressed by support workers; while nurses and doctors attempt to demarcate 'clinical' from 'social' problems. A CRT is unlikely to be able to maintain these traditional boundaries to the same extent as generic community mental health teams. The acute nature of the work and the necessity for each shift to be able to take on and deal with a full range of problems requires that all members of the team, even doctors (who are often the most resistant to multidisciplinary working), should develop a range of skills and be willing to make the attempt to step out of narrow professional roles in order to solve a problem. For this reason, in what follows we generally assume that the interventions suggested should be considered by all team members.

Crisis Resolution and Home Treatment in Mental Health, ed. Sonia Johnson, Justin Needle, Jonathan P. Bindman and Graham Thornicroft. Published by Cambridge University Press. © Cambridge University Press 2008.

However, the problem with entirely generic working is that certain professional skills (e.g. those of psychologists) may be undervalued or opportunities for learning missed. Ideally, teams lucky enough to have staff with a full range of professional skills should be able to make use of this resource by asking staff with expertise in certain areas for advice or encouraging them to teach, but the approach of simply referring, say, all housing issues to social workers or self-care problems to occupational therapists should be avoided. Handover meetings, which in most teams happen twice daily, provide the forum for interprofessional debate and inform care planning. Handovers need to be chaired and managed effectively in order to generate discussion within the multidisciplinary team and harness the different points of view (Chapters 25 and 26).

Assessing the social context

The amount of detail that can be obtained at an assessment will naturally vary with the urgency of the assessment, the availability of informants and the ability of the service user to provide information, but basic details about the social context and the way it relates to the presenting complaint will usually be obtainable even at the briefest of assessments (Chapter 8). It is always worth trying to get as much information as possible at the time the initial referral is received, before the assessment takes place. This helps to understand the full context of the crisis and decide who should be present at the assessment. The ability to respond to problems such as housing difficulties immediately can resolve crises that might otherwise quickly become intractable. Assessment information not perceived as immediately necessary is commonly left for the next shift to fill in, but later shifts may not feel the same sense of 'ownership' of the assessment as the one that takes the person on, and the initial gaps may be left unfilled indefinitely. The first visit to a person's home and the first contact with an informant, whether these happen at the initial assessment or later, will always reveal valuable additional information.

The standard method of psychiatric history taking gives considerable weight to psychopathology but rather less to social context. Staff providing home treatment will soon realise that, while it is certainly important to be as clear as possible about the nature of the psychopathology, detailed information about some of the social issues considered below will usually turn out to be equally valuable.

Housing and looking after the home

Assessment

Housing problems are perhaps the commonest social precipitants of contact with CRTs. Distress at unsuitable housing can drive people to contact mental health services, and people with long-term mental health problems often cope poorly with their housing or cause concern to neighbours. Hospital admission is commonly seen as the only readily available solution when housing problems, even long-standing ones, come to a head. A basic assessment, of the type carried out in a casualty department under time pressure, should elicit information about the type of accommodation, who else lives there, whether the rent is paid (and by whom) and whether the property is habitable (having heating, lighting, cooking and washing facilities). It may also become apparent at an early stage that a housing problem, such as rent arrears, problems with neighbours or the threat of eviction, is the principal precipitant of the crisis. However, it is when an initial assessment takes place at home, or at the first home visit, that the CRT has the great advantage over hospital-based services of being able to conduct a full assessment of the living situation.

Some of the questions which can be answered at a home assessment are listed in Box 11.1. In addition to these questions, conducting an assessment in the home environment is likely to allow most aspects of the history to be understood in more depth. For example, a person presenting with the features of depression can be assessed with reference to ability to care for the home, and the common problem of assessing whether complaints of noise or persecution from neighbours are psychotic in nature may be easier if assessors can hear for themselves how thin the walls are.

Interventions

Assessment often reveals housing problems that are long standing and not amenable to quick solutions. Local authority housing transfers, even when already clearly indicated and appropriately applied for, tend to take many months or years to complete, and the system may be too inflexible to allow acceleration of the process in order to resolve a crisis. The CRT must take a view at an early stage about the value of attempting to intervene; where the groundwork has already been done by the service user's regular care coordinator, the CRT may waste time if it attempts to interfere. Though offering practical help with housing issues is sometimes a useful way of engaging the service user (Chapter 13), it is important not to make a promise to facilitate a housing transfer if experience suggests that the CRT has little power to help. Short-term interventions are more likely to be effective, and some examples of these are given in Box 11.2.

A balance must be struck between helping people to help themselves and taking responsibility for actually resolving problems. Though the former approach is often preferred on the grounds that it does not encourage inappropriate dependence and disempower the service user, it is important to be realistic about what people in crisis can be expected to achieve. Sometimes the most helpful approach

Box 11.1. Questions for consideration at home assessments

Financial arrangements

- Who owns the property?
- Who is responsible for maintaining and securing the property if there are problems?
- Is rent or a mortgage payable? If so, are there arrears or has the person defaulted?
- How are utilities paid for and are there arrears or proceedings, or have essentials been cut off?
- Is there evidence of unpaid bills, unopened letters or threats to cut off utilities?

Physical security

- Is the property locked? (If the assessment is not being held in the property, who has the keys and how can it be accessed if the person is taken home?)
- Can doors and windows be secured?
- Is there evidence that the property has been left unsecured, or of unauthorised entry?

Basic facilities

- Do lights, heating, water work? If not, why not?
- Is there furniture for sleeping, sitting?
- Are there facilities for washing, and for washing and drying clothes?
- Is there a working and hygienic toilet?
- Is there a refrigerator or place for storing food? Is there edible food in it?
- Is there evidence of recent use of all essential facilities (e.g. for food preparation, laundry)?

Evidence of symptoms

- Is there damage to the property (e.g. interference with wiring, broken TV, boarded windows) that may have a pathological explanation?
- Is there written material, literature or graffiti suggestive of paranoid preoccupations?
- Is there evidence of severe neglect, squalor, uncleared rubbish?
- Is there a lack of personal possessions consistent with chronic mental illness or heavy drug use?
- Is there an excess of possessions, suggesting hoarding or inappropriate purchasing?
- Is there visible evidence of drinking or drug taking?
- Is there evidence of recent self-harm? Is there excess medication to be removed?

Evidence of psychological strengths

- Is the home better maintained than the person's mental state would suggest, or is any lack of care superficial and recent?
- Is there evidence of meaningful activity, interests and care for the home?
- Is there evidence of social activity and support (e.g. personal photos, letters and cards, evidence of entertaining)?

Box 11.1. (Continued)

Risks

- Is there evidence of self-neglect and inability to obtain or prepare food?
- Are there risks related to excessive cold (or heat)?
- Is there evidence of fire damage (e.g. from candles, dropped cigarettes or smoking in bed)?
- Are any neighbours encountered at the visit and is there evidence of hostility to or from neighbours (e.g. vandalism, graffiti on the person's or neighbours' properties)?

Box 11.2. Short-term psychosocial interventions: some examples

- Threats of eviction can often be deferred through advocacy from the team.
- Rent or mortgage arrears can be dealt with by arranging agreed repayment plans.
- Problems arising from failure to claim benefits can be resolved and arrears claimed.
- Minor repairs can be arranged and services reconnected.
- Accommodation can be tidied up.
- Major repairs and cleaning tasks can be initiated via appropriate services.
- Temporary accommodation with friends and relatives may be 'brokered'.
- Temporary accommodation may be funded by health or social services.
- Changes in permanent accommodation, including moves from independent to supported housing, can be initiated if this has not already been done, though only if the need for this is clear and not a temporary consequence of the crisis.
- Social systems intervention with housing officers, neighbours or hostel staff can clarify misunderstandings or disputes, and also establish relapse-prevention plans for the future.

is for CRT members to roll up their sleeves and unblock a sink or toilet, clean the fridge and take out the rubbish – attempting to encourage the person to do the work straight away, or trying to engage other parts of the care system to do it, may be time consuming and ineffective. Such interventions are often regarded as appropriate for support workers, particularly if sustained work is needed. However, all CRT staff may be called upon to make a home habitable with some timely intervention and should ideally be reasonably competent with practical matters, able to change a light bulb or charge an electricity meter key without calling in expensive professionals. It is, however, as well to know one's limits – one of the authors has on occasion experienced embarrassing failures to fix door locks or washing machines and other appliances, and has been forced to acknowledge that there are times when more appropriate professionals must be called in.

Special housing problems

A CRT is unlikely to be able to work with roofless individuals and will usually prefer to involve specialist services rather than attempt to treat people straight from the streets by finding them emergency accommodation. However, they are likely to find themselves involved with various types of people with insecure housing arrangements, including:

- refugees awaiting leave to remain in the country, or who have been refused leave but have not been deported
- immigrants with no legal status or established rights to statutory support
- people in temporary accommodation awaiting permanent housing
- people in temporary accommodation with disputed rights to permanent housing
- people in staffed accommodation that does not meet their needs
- people with a history of street homelessness in transitional settings
- former prisoners or drug users in resettlement settings.

Sometimes the solutions to such problems are legal, for example establishing the obligations of the local authority and advocating for the service user or providing reports on their vulnerability. Often, however, they require a detailed knowledge of the local context, including specialist services and housing providers, and sources of support or information. Sometimes no permanent solution can be found; if, for example, a refugee has been denied leave to remain in the country and exhausted rights to appeal, but no attempt is made to deport them (as is sometimes the case), then they remain in a legal limbo without clear rights or any prospect of obtaining them. They may exist in a fragile network of supports – perhaps involving churches, mosques or charity, sleeping on the floors of friends or compatriots, or illegal working – and may be vulnerable to exploitation. Though the CRT cannot provide definitive solutions, it can try to alleviate a desperate situation with food, money, advocacy and psychological support, or attempt to bolster a fragile network by making links with charities and formal refugee-support networks.

Though a majority of the patients of CRTs, in more deprived areas at least, tend to live in social housing, a number of interesting challenges can arise when working with people who own their homes. For example, CRTs may need to take an advocacy role and assist people in dealing with mortgage lenders, or help people to protect their own financial interests during a crisis. For example, we dissuaded a service user from selling her property at a very low price to a neighbour while unwell. Family members may also at times appear to be taking advantage of vulnerable service users who own property, and careful judgement is needed regarding people's capacity to manage their own affairs and the justification for interference by professionals. Healthcare provider organisations or their social service partners will have relevant policies on protecting vulnerable adults from exploitation and will be able to access legal advice in complex cases.

Money

Assessment

Lack of money is often the precipitant of a deterioration in mental state. The stress of unpaid bills, not having food in the fridge or being unable to afford the bus fare to visit friends can distract and disorganise. The individual's behaviour changes and protective factors, such as taking medication, get forgotten. A CRT needs to be able to deal quickly with this situation and should have a 'slush fund' for emergency needs.

A basic assessment should establish the service user's sources of income and the presence of any debts. The benefits system is complex and, fearful of fraud, places deliberate obstacles in the way of long-term claimants by requiring them to complete forms and attend interviews on a regular basis. It is, therefore, very common to find that people in crisis have failed to jump the required hurdles, and benefits have been cut off, leading to accumulating arrears in utility bills or rent. A full history of benefits previously and currently received, the contact details of the relevant offices and the exact amounts of any arrears or debts will need to be obtained. These may not be straightforward to ascertain simply from the history (someone who is too unwell to pay bills or who has given up opening letters is unlikely to know exactly what is owed), so a home visit provides an opportunity to go through letters and bills with the person.

Intervention

All CRT staff (not just social workers) will need to become adept at making contact with the benefits system, reestablishing entitlement to benefits and claiming arrears by obtaining medical certificates (backdated as necessary) and helping the service user fill in forms. Obtaining housing benefit arrears is particularly important, since if this has been cut off there will be rent arrears, which may be very large and lead to a threat of eviction. Housing transfers may be blocked until the arrears have been paid.

If service users are employed but have been missing work, the CRT may have a valuable role in providing medical certificates, securing a job under threat because of unexplained absence and negotiating a return to work. The CRT must, however, warn people of the possible adverse consequences of revealing contact with psychiatric services to an employer and it may be preferable to support people to negotiate sick leave and a return to work directly with the employer. In England, a doctor is permitted to complete the sick certificate for the employer ('Med 3') using a non-medical term like 'stress' or 'nervous disorder' if they feel it may be prejudicial to the service user to use a specific diagnosis. The doctor should then use another form ('Med 6') to notify the benefits system that additional information is available on request. Since it is not necessary to give a diagnosis, doctors should think carefully before using terms like 'psychosis' or 'schizophrenia', which may have unpredictable consequences for a person's employment.

Sometimes a service user's financial affairs will be more than usually complicated, perhaps because they have never claimed entitlements, have built up very large arrears which cannot be claimed, or because they have obtained large amounts of credit from multiple sources and have huge debts which cannot be repaid. People may be advised to go to a Citizens Advice Bureau or to another source of expert advice on benefits and debt management. However, CRT staff will usually develop some experience in negotiating repayment plans with credit card or catalogue companies, and in returning unwanted goods purchased during manic episodes (though one of the authors had great difficulty in returning a car purchased at a very high price by a service user without a driving license and could not save her from a loss of several thousand pounds). Among the more challenging problems are people who have substantial savings (and are, therefore, not entitled to benefits) but refuse to spend them on essentials, and those who refuse to claim benefits or cooperate with attempts to resolve problems (such as the patient with delusions who, believing himself in the pay of MI5, refused to sign claim forms). The local trust may employ a benefits adviser who can help in complex cases.

Food and self-care

Assessment

The psychiatric assessment includes questions about appetite and weight, loss of both being associated with a range of disorders, and problems with self-care will be apparent at the initial contact. Home assessment may reveal much more about people's ability to care for themselves and the underlying reasons for any deficits. As mentioned in Box 11.1, the team should ask the person for permission to check food cupboards and the refrigerator, and about cooking skills and the use of external sources of food.

Intervention

It is important that teams have the equipment to weigh patients (one of the few objective measurements a mental health team can make), and that they do so early in the period of treatment. An attempt should be made to determine from the history and examination whether the person is substantially above or below their usual weight (and whether this is within a healthy range), and then to monitor over the course of the intervention whether their weight is moving in the desired direction.

With many service users, an early intervention will be a visit to the shops to buy food, or the team may purchase and deliver basics or takeaway meals. Such meals are popular with staff, and often with service users, as they are quick to buy and involve no preparation, but they are also relatively expensive and may not be culturally appropriate or healthy (the combination of high-dose antipsychotic drugs and takeaway meals can lead to rapid weight gain). While it is reasonable for a busy team to adopt the quickest approach to ensuring that the person is nourished, it is important to make an early assessment of the person's own ability to shop and prepare healthy meals, and to support them in doing so as soon as possible. Families, where available, may be a good source of food in a crisis.

Work, meaningful occupation, education and daytime activities

Assessment

Assessment will always involve establishing whether the service user has work or other regular occupation, and how the crisis has affected their ability to carry out their usual activity. As described above, this may lead to short-term interventions related to sick certification and benefits. Whenever possible, a detailed educational and employment history should be taken, though this may be impractical in an acute situation. Even in a rapid assessment, it is usually worth asking the question 'How do you spend your time?' This should be followed by a few questions about the structure of the person's typical day (not least because it will help the team to plan visits for times when they are at home). It is important to probe standard answers like 'I'm at college'; this may mean a demanding full-time course, or an hour a week. Some exploration of the extent to which the person actually attends activities or is able to function in them is also important, or the assessor may be misled about the extent of disability.

A substantial proportion of service users encountered in crisis will turn out to have long-standing problems of unemployment or under-employment. As with all chronic problems uncovered during acute assessments, a view needs to be taken about what can realistically be achieved during an episode of acute care, and time may be saved by establishing at the outset what previous attempts have been made by the person or by services to find appropriate day care, education, or routes into work.

Intervention

Sickness certification for employees who are missing work because of the crisis is considered above. Though it will probably be helpful to support people in crisis to have time off work, this needs careful consideration. Some people, whether with depression or psychoses, may find work helpful even when unwell and should not always be encouraged to take time off (particularly if this may lead to the loss of a job). However, some hypomanic patients need to be actively discouraged from going to work when it is apparent that their own view of their abilities is at odds with everyone else's and they may put their job at risk.

The team needs to feel confident about negotiating with workplaces or educational institutions (with service users' permission), for example a CRT talked to a patient's manager about the patient's severe depression. When under stress, this patient, because of fear of relapse, often took time off without permission or explanation. The manager had a very high regard for the person's work but was frustrated by his erratic attendance. A dialogue was established that helped the employee feel more able to talk with his boss about his problems at work and manage his stress more effectively.

Though CRTs may not be best placed to deal with issues of long-term unemployment, it is useful to be aware of local projects and services aimed at helping people into work. There may be occasions when the CRT can reintroduce someone to a project with which they have lost contact, or make an initial referral if the person seems ready for it.

Relationships

Understanding the patient's relationship with family and carers, broadly defined, will be crucial to understanding the crisis and intervening effectively, and this is covered in more detail in Chapter 12. No chapter on psychosocial interventions would be complete, however, without some consideration of the central role of social and sexual relationships in precipitating and resolving crises. Assessing the nature of the social network and the roles of its key members, working out with the patient the appropriate level of communication with them, and then obtaining information from them is part of even the briefest assessment and is usually an ongoing process throughout the period of crisis care. Some particular problems arise from the nature of home-based treatment. The first is that relatives and carers who are present in the home may assume the right to be present at all assessments and contacts, or indeed may be unable to keep out of earshot even if they want to. If no opportunity arises naturally, staff need to feel able to ask for an opportunity to talk to the person alone, to check whether they have concerns that they cannot express in front of others. Second, staff may observe aspects of relationships that give rise to concerns. They may feel that carers are over-involved and encourage emotional dependency or, conversely, are cold, angry or hostile. Though relatively few staff will have formal training in the assessment of expressed emotion, most will be familiar with the concepts and may, therefore, be disposed to judge certain interactions between patient and carer as predisposing to psychotic relapse. It is important that such judgements are discussed in multidisciplinary meetings or supervision on a regular basis.

The opinions of staff about what kinds of interaction within families are 'appropriate' often turn out to be highly determined by the staff members' own family backgrounds or cultures. Multidisciplinary discussion may reveal that one person's 'over-involvement' is another's appropriate concern for a relative, or that one person's 'critical comment' is another's appropriate attempt to set boundaries on disturbed behaviour. Regular airing of views in team settings should reduce the tendency to judge and to set narrow boundaries on 'normality'. Similar issues can arise when CRTs are exposed to gay relationships, which, despite their widespread acceptance and the introduction of civil partnerships that establish the rights of gay partners to be carers, are still regarded judgementally by staff from some backgrounds (Chapter 17). Services are likely to have policies on non-discrimination that explicitly require them to treat such relationships with respect, but these are most likely to be effective if there is a culture of open discussion between staff about the way in which personal values affect their work.

Even where relationships are a long way from the norm – such as the situation we have encountered a few times in which relationships have an emotional component but also involve the selling of drugs or sex – the threshold for intervention should usually be high, not least because there are seldom practical ways of intervening in such relationships. There are, of course, some circumstances in which judgements have to be made, and if relationships appear to staff to be seriously physically or mentally abusive, then multidisciplinary discussion may lead to a decision to intervene. Advice should also be sought from specialists in the protection of adults, since the skills and legal knowledge required to manage such relatively rare issues are unlikely to be present within the CRT. In practice, the most readily available intervention is likely to be admission to hospital or, if available, a crisis house (Chapter 23), though there is little point in this if it cannot change the circumstances that will face the patient on discharge.

When intervening with a service user's social system, the team will often identify the needs of others, for example young people caring for parents. It is not uncommon for the main identified problem to become something quite different from the initial reason for referral, and the team needs to react accordingly, using its own network and social system to provide the best care for the people involved.

Communication

Communication problems, such as a language barrier or elective mutism, may be obvious at first assessment. These are common difficulties in mental state assessment generally and will not be dealt with in detail here. Home-based treatment may, however, present particular difficulties. For example, an interpreter can usually be arranged (either in person or via telephone) for an initial assessment, but it is less practical to arrange interpreting for twice-daily visits over an extended period. The CRT may either be faced with visiting someone with whom little or no communication is possible, thereby reducing the visit to medication delivery and practical support only, or be forced to rely on family members to interpret, with the associated problems which this brings of breaching confidentiality and risking biased or distorted interpretations. Telephone interpreting is sometimes useful but again may be less feasible on a regular basis than for an initial or hospital-based assessment. Sometimes a team member may speak the relevant language, though the shift system may make it impractical to rely on a single member of the team to do all of the visits, and in areas where dozens or even hundreds of languages are spoken this is often not an option.

A problem that must also be addressed at assessment is how to communicate with service users about visits in order to ensure that they are there, to get access to premises, to warn of delays or to rearrange times. Phone numbers, including mobiles, must be obtained and it is well worth taking the time to get alternative numbers, and to establish the person's views on relaying messages via relatives or even neighbours about visits that need rearranging. Teams should ideally have the option of lending mobile phones, since this will be cost effective if even a few failed visits can be avoided. Unfortunately, attempts to give patients goods perceived as desirable often face bureaucratic barriers ('What if they all want one, or won't give it back?'), but if the person has a mobile phone that is not charged, needs reconnecting or call time to be purchased, a bit of effort in getting it working is usually rewarded. Text messages are often an effective means of communication, especially with younger patients.

Service users with children

The presence of children at home may be a strong reason either to avoid hospital admission, since children may be distressed or put at risk by alternative care arrangements, or to avoid home treatment, if children are at risk from the patient. Deciding what to do is often complex and the team needs to have systems in place to ensure that difficult decisions can be supported by senior staff. Trusts will usually have a policy on child protection that requires that all concerns about risks to children are discussed with staff with special expertise who can advise on referral to social services, though the effect that this most threatening and potentially stigmatising of interventions may have on the relationship with the service user should not be under-estimated. Some service users and their children will already be subject to formal child protection procedures when taken on; others may be placed under them at the CRT's instigation. In either case, the relationship between the team and the service user tends to be compromised, the latter fearing, understandably, that their interactions with their children are under a microscope and that they could lose them. The team must attempt to emphasise the supportive and caring aspect of child protection procedures, and may use such procedures to access practical support (such as child care), but the threatening aspects of the process, and the fact that CRT staff may be obliged to disclose their observations to social care staff, need to be frankly acknowledged.

In most cases, patients who receive home treatment will be supported in continuing to care for their children, often with the help of other family members. Assessment must then include establishing the children's age-appropriate care needs and the extent to which the patient is able to meet them. The children's routines (meal, school and bed times) should be assessed with the parent and if these have been disrupted by the crisis, they should be supported in reinstating them. The CRT may broker support for the children by arranging for them to stay with relatives. It may seek short-term nursery places or child care in order to support the patient, and the CRT may be able to provide a range of other support, including ensuring that maximum benefit entitlements are received, accessing charitable funding and suggesting activities for toddlers (and older children during holidays) that will benefit the parent's mental state.

Transport and 'getting about'

Assessments may reveal problems with mobility or transport that have an important effect on people's quality of life. People who cannot get out of the home, whether for physical or psychological reasons, will be unable to access most healthcare services, as well as many aspects of 'normal' life such as socialising and employment. While anxiety or agoraphobia alone will not generally bring people into contact with a CRT, if it is a significant comorbidity, then a period of home treatment may provide an opportunity for some structured work using a cognitive–behavioural framework to increase the person's ability to leave the home. From a practical point of view, it may help the team if service users are able to visit the team base on some occasions rather than always being visited at home, and simple obstacles to travel, such as insufficient money or lack of knowledge or confidence about transport options, may be easily addressed.

Key points

- Mental health crises always involve a social aspect, but CRTs are often strongly influenced by the medical model of mental illness and may, therefore, see their principal role as being the delivery of medication.
- The importance of psychosocial interventions at the point of crisis cannot be over-stated and the time and willingness needed to implement them must be available. The ability to understand all the mechanics of the crisis can help to resolve it quickly and to stop it spiralling into a more destructive force.
- The role of the CRT is implicit in its title. To resolve crises, all CRT members need to value and continue to develop skills in a full range of psychosocial interventions.

12

Working with families and social networks

Christopher Bridgett and Harm Gijsman

In this chapter, we will use the term 'social network' to describe those people and groups with whom an individual has significant social contact. We will first examine the nature and importance of social networks, and will then go on to provide an account of what crisis resolution and home treatment teams (CRTs) can do to maximise the benefits to patients of support from key social relationships, both within the family and across their wider social networks.

The nature and importance of social networks

While for some the most important social relationships are within the family, for others they include a peer group, friends and acquaintances, neighbours or work colleagues. For most people there is a mix of all of these, varying perhaps with place of residence and state of health, and over time. Human beings are innately social in their behaviour, but it is important to remember that social relationships are not always supportive. For the mental health service user, relationships with and between informal and formal carers, and the relationships within the service between professionals and between the component teams, can have special importance (Chapter 7).

Bridgett and Polak (2003a) defined a social network as 'a series of overlapping social systems: sets of human relationships that vary in size, formality, function and permanence'. At the less-intimate end of the social spectrum, there is an unclear boundary, with a more general social cohesiveness referred to as the *social capital* of a community.

One of the possible disadvantages of admission to hospital for acute psychiatric care is a breakdown in the usual social life of the patient: once admitted, family and friends need to overcome practical, geographical and psychological

Crisis Resolution and Home Treatment in Mental Health, ed. Sonia Johnson, Justin Needle, Jonathan P. Bindman and Graham Thornicroft. Published by Cambridge University Press. © Cambridge University Press 2008.

barriers before visiting, and the patient can face similar barriers in visiting them – if they are allowed to leave the ward at all. Simply by providing an alternative to admission, acute home treatment can act to maintain existing social relationships.

However, the mission of home treatment needs to go beyond that. The *Mental Health Policy Implementation Guide* (Department of Health, 2001) explicitly states that an aim of CRTs is 'to provide interventions aimed at maintaining and *improving* the social network of a patient' (our italics). This recognises the importance of social context in establishing and maintaining mental health. When acute difficulties arise, both individual and social factors mould the form a crisis takes and the coping strategies implemented by the patient and his/her network.

When a psychiatric illness seems acute, and especially when the need for inpatient care is suggested, difficulties in key social relationships should be central to assessment and intervention. Hospitalisation is itself always a social intervention, providing a way of coping for both individuals and their overall social networks, including the mental health service itself. Crisis theory argues, however, that if admission can be avoided, and a different way of coping promoted outside hospital, then the crisis becomes an important opportunity for both the individual and the social network to learn more adaptive and healthy problem-solving strategies. This may partly explain the evidence that families do not generally experience a greater burden during acute treatment at home compared with during acute inpatient care (Joy *et al.*, 2006).

Confidentiality and significant others

As soon as professional caregivers begin to consider the predicament of the individual in relation to the family and the wider social network, the need to take account of rights to confidentiality becomes an important issue. Indeed, the need to respect confidentiality can become so difficult and contentious for the inexperienced team member that comprehensive psychosocial assessment and intervention are not accomplished, to the disadvantage of both the service user and significant others. A narrowly focused 'medical model', with a clinical emphasis on individual mental state, diagnosis and medication, is within a professional 'comfort zone', while working with social relationships can be unfamiliar and hazardous territory for clinicians more used to a hospital-based practice. For crisis resolution and home treatment, such work is, however, essential and it is useful to realise that confidentiality is not always a clear-cut issue and often depends on what and who is involved, and how things are done.

There are at least three types of information affected by confidentiality considerations:

- the information that a person is a patient of the service, is causing concern to others, or is being referred to the service
- personal information about the patient provided by others, and other third-party information
- personal information provided by the patient about themselves, and other information they provide.

How all of the above needs to be treated can vary with circumstances. For the individual patient, it is unusual for it to be acceptable to tell everything to everyone, but, equally, it is unlikely that there will be a blanket refusal to say anything to anyone. It is important to establish how confidentiality is understood, and to take account of any rules that a patient has set. Service users with unhappy past experiences may impose blanket injunctions against involving others, unless it is explained that agreements can be made about what is discussed with whom, and what is not. It can be useful to use an 'increasing dose' approach, where information exchange is modest to begin with and is only extended as all concerned become confident in the process, having seen how things have developed and the effect on the individuals concerned.

When taking an initial referral from a third party it is important to be clear whether information is being given with the informed consent of the person who is the subject of the referral. At this stage, however, it is the referrer who is potentially the service user, and their agreement to their account being shared with the person being referred is a relevant consideration. Next, depending on the circumstances of the referral, it may be useful and acceptable to take the opportunity to obtain further details from others involved, if this additional background information facilitates a safer, timelier and more comprehensive assessment. The first interview with the patient should be an opportunity to assess their capacity to deal with the account given by others and, therefore, to consent to further sharing of information as part of the assessment process. Capacity to make decisions about sharing information will sometimes be affected by illness and, depending on the issues involved, it may be evident that a duty to care for the patient, and to ensure also the safety of others, needs to take precedence over any claim of a right to confidentiality.

Provided the family and other social network members are already aware that their relative is in contact with the CRT, collecting information from them may be possible without specific consent from the service user, although care should be taken when the informant does not wish to be identified, or if the information is given on the understanding that it is to be kept secret. Likewise, staff may be able to give the family and significant others important general information about available services and procedures without specific consent. There may be circumstances in which it is necessary to provide information to a third party, even against the expressed wishes of a patient (Szmukler and Bloch, 1997). These include:

- when capacity to consent is affected by mental state
- when there are concerns about safety
- when there is no available alternative, and it is necessary
- when it is required to achieve evidently reasonable care and support
- when it allows care to be provided in the least restrictive setting.

Since more than one of these features may be applicable in any given situation, determining the appropriate course of action will often involve a delicate balance, especially given the need to achieve and maintain a trusting relationship between the patient and the CRT. Staff should also document carefully the reasons for any decision to disclose personal information without the service user's consent.

Assessment

As detailed in Chapter 8, while assessment for home treatment involves standard procedures such as gathering information regarding social circumstances, third-person accounts and risk assessment, there are important differences in emphasis. History taking and examining the patient's mental state is still a central feature of assessment (Chapter 9), but a further key component should be gathering information from a variety of sources about their social circumstances and networks, taking sufficient time to ensure this assessment is comprehensive and carrying out a substantial part of it where the patient usually lives. Indeed, since social context has such a powerful effect on individual behaviour, no assessment can be said to be complete until all relevant social factors have been accounted for and a home visit has been made. Some of the practical interventions to which such assessment can lead are described in Chapter 11. In this chapter, we focus on how the experience and behaviour of the individual can be understood in dynamic terms, by considering relationships with all significant others.

Care provided by a CRT involves informed teamwork and a collaborative approach involving other parts of the service (Chapter 6). Especially in the case of patients known to the service, understanding a referral within a 'whole system' framework includes taking account of the care arrangements and therapeutic relationships to date and highlights the importance of the team working with others within the service to resolve the crisis (Case study 12.1). Clear and detailed recording of social systems assessments facilitates a subsequent socially focused treatment approach.

CASE STUDY 12.1. HOSTEL RESIDENT

Presenting situation

A 39-year-old single unemployed woman with unstable chronic schizophrenia was referred for admission by her community mental health team care coordinator when her mental state deteriorated at the hostel where she had lived for six months; previously, she lived with her family. Her father died at home three months ago after a long illness. Recent paranoid agitation has led to angry disturbances, especially at night, and particularly towards male members of staff. Discussion over the telephone reveals non-compliance with medication over four weeks. She also stopped regularly attending the day centre where she has had most of her social contact for several years, but she remained in regular contact with her frail mother and her sister, who live nearby. Further assessment at the hostel on the morning of the referral revealed that she had shown no congruent emotional reaction to the death of her father, but recent changes in the management of the hostel have apparently upset her. There was now a danger of her losing her place if the disturbances continue, as the new manager thinks she is inappropriately placed. A social systems meeting involving all concerned was planned for the same afternoon.

Initiating a social systems meeting

The initial telephone calls suggested that the main social system involved was located at the hostel where the woman lived, and a meeting there with the patient, the hostel staff and the care coordinator would be necessary as soon as possible to achieve an initial resolution of the referral crisis. As the death of her father seemed important, her family lived nearby and she appeared to have a positive relationship with them, inviting them to the meeting was also judged important.

The meeting

Later on during the day of referral, two team members met with the patient, her sister, the care coordinator, her hostel key worker and the hostel manager at the hostel. Prior to the meeting, it was agreed that the patient's disturbed behaviour may have been directly related to non-compliance but, as she had apparently been compliant on first moving to the hostel, something more recent had clearly occurred to change her behaviour. There had been changes in the hostel management, but the death of her father appeared to be more important.

At the meeting, the patient initially refused to speak. The key worker described the recent incidents at night, which involved accusations against male staff invading her privacy (they were attempting to persuade her to take her medication) and, prior to that, her unwillingness to take more responsibility for the tidiness of her room (the manager explained that her recent habit of hoarding newspapers constituted a fire hazard).

When her sister then gave an account of their father's final illness, which had precipitated the patient's move into the hostel, the patient started to cry, angrily shouting at her sister about having to move out of their home and then being prevented from attending her father's funeral. Her sister explained how difficult it had been for the family caring for both her and her dying father at the same time, and how they had worried that she would cause a scene at the funeral.

The manager reminded everyone that the hostel felt it could not cope with her if she continued refusing to take her medication, and argued that she needed hospital admission. The sister then asked if, instead of admission, the CRT could for the time being help her and their mother take the patient home, on condition that she started taking her medication again. When the team agreed to this, the patient also agreed and, in tears, crossed the room to hug her sister. A further meeting at the family home was arranged for that evening, and it was agreed that the hostel room would be kept available for her.

An initial problem-orientated summary prepared at this stage (Figure 12.1) can usefully highlight the issues identified, suggest a plan for the team to follow and specify the people involved and how they can be contacted. If the summary identifies the *referral crisis* – the precise practical difficulty in coping that admission aims to solve – and the *social system crises* and related factors leading up to the referral, then the team's work can focus on crisis resolution. It can also be helpful for the team to display the social network relationships diagrammatically (Figure 12.2).

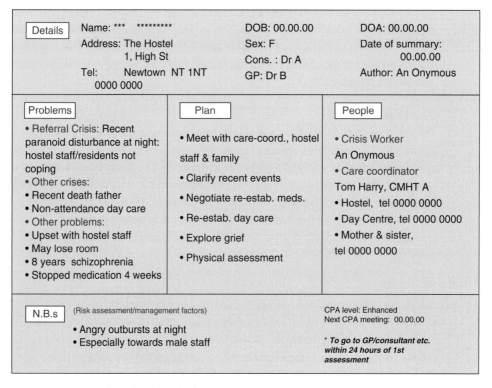

Figure 12.1 Summary for a hostel resident.

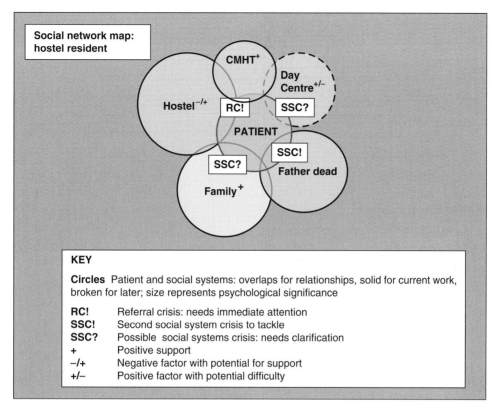

Figure 12.2 Social network map for a hostel resident.

General principles of intervention

Frequent visits by a team of well-trained nurses and other professionals to the patient in their own home – taking the service to the usual social environment of the patient, rather than vice versa – is perhaps the most important general intervention. Next, it is vital for the team to remember that a crisis can provide an important opportunity for families and other social groups both to understand themselves better and to change. Otherwise, the general principles recommended by McFarlane *et al.* (2003) for working with families, described below, can be usefully adapted for crisis resolution and home treatment.

Ensure coordination

Failures in coping, leading to requests for inpatient treatment, often require the CRT to pull together elements of care already available, enabling others then to work collaboratively with the team to reestablish the patient's ability to cope. For existing service users known to a community mental health team, the continuing work of the patient's care coordinator from that team is supplemented during the crisis by the more intense work of the CRT.

Adopt a social focus

The continuing importance of paying attention to the social as well as the clinical needs of the patient cannot be over-emphasised. Taking insufficient account of such needs may lead in the acute phase to an undue emphasis on, for example, medication, while after a few days the team's familiarity with the situation may obscure an opportunity to broaden the scope of intervention. Listening to and taking into account the concerns of the family and members of the wider social network help to make significant others equal partners in treatment planning and delivery.

Encourage communication

Key to enabling a return to adaptive coping is the skill of the team in ensuring that early and adequate opportunities are established for open discussion by all concerned about the origins of the crisis and how it needs to be managed. Conflicts need to be exposed and, if possible, accommodated, especially if they seem to be preventing resolution of the crisis. The opportunity to inform is important: misconceptions need to be identified and corrected. Taking into account the views of significant others can often be helpful in ensuring compliance with medication. When loss, following bereavement or retirement for example, is an issue, it may be important to suggest a renegotiation of family roles and functions. A flexible approach, involving both one-to-one and group discussion, is usually required.

Enable coping

Assessing the strengths and limitations of a family or social network allows additional support to be arranged where necessary, and it is important to explain clearly how extra help, including admission to hospital, may be enlisted. Teaching problem-solving strategies (see below), expanding a social network, anticipating future hazards and agreeing a crisis plan on discharge can play an important role in preventing future difficulties.

Specific interventions

Social systems meetings

Social systems meetings are a specific type of social systems intervention (discussed in more detail by Bridgett and Polak (2003b)) within an overall social systems approach (Bridgett, 2006a): the latter, derived from general systems theory, is applicable to all of the work done by a mental health service, not only by CRTs. Moreover, the theory – that the whole is more than the sum of its parts – helps to describe how a CRT works successfully within the whole 'service system' (Chapter 7), and especially as one of a range of interlocking alternatives to acute intensive psychiatric care (Bridgett, 2006b).

Given that complex interrelationships are an inevitable feature of social systems, it can be argued that all mental health interventions will have knock-on, or social systems, effects at some point or other. In crisis resolution and home treatment, the opportunity to implement social systems interventions by means of social systems meetings varies considerably. Experience suggests, however, that such meetings greatly improve the effectiveness of the approach, as does specifically designing an intervention to achieve a social systems effect.

After accepting a referral, the CRT should routinely collect certain key items of information by telephone from referrers and other key informants,[1] namely:

- which social systems are involved?
- which social systems crisis is it practical to tackle first?
- who to invite to the first social systems meeting?

A social systems meeting is an opportunity both for gathering further information and for 'natural group' work or therapy. Therefore, for the benefit of everyone at the first meeting, it should be possible to clarify the issues that have led to the referral and discuss how they can best be dealt with initially, while leaving further work for later. The meeting's venue is not always important, but a 'natural' rather than a formal setting helps to put people at their ease. It is recommended that two members of staff facilitate each meeting, with one perhaps being more active than the other. Discussion time should be allowed both before and after the meeting, and an account written up for future reference.

There are several factors to take into account in order to ensure a successful meeting. The choice of whom to invite and obtaining the patient's consent to this are clearly important. The approach should be collaborative, with the participants being encouraged to find their own solutions to the identified problems and put forward their own suggestions about possible solutions (Rosen, 1997). Holding an initial meeting early on in the assessment and treatment process can be especially effective in identifying the interpersonal problems that may have triggered or exacerbated the crisis (Fish, 1971), and a great deal of important work can be achieved in one meeting alone. Facilitation by active listening and promotion of understanding and communication is required. Caplan's (1964) principles of *adaptive coping* – confrontation with reality, expression of feelings and acceptance of help – may be important for all participants, not only the person referred.

---

[1] A minimum of three telephone calls is recommended (Chapter 8).

Psychoeducation

A crisis can be an important opportunity for learning, when arousal and increased receptiveness in both the individual and the family may enable rapid assimilation of several types of important and useful information. Psychoeducation – teaching a family and significant others about mental health and illness – is an effective general component of the treatment of schizophrenia, bipolar disorder, major depression and other disorders (McFarlane *et al.*, 2003) and is clearly specifically relevant to crisis resolution and to the social systems meetings described above. The topics of particular relevance are summarised in Box 12.1.

Box 12.1. Important topics in psychoeducation

A number of topics should be considered in psychoeducation:

- *causes*: stress and vulnerability, 'expressed emotion', alcohol and recreational drug use
- *symptoms and signs*: understanding and dealing with these, both positive and negative, clarifying what may and may not be caused by illness
- *diagnosis*: importance in psychiatry, compared with medicine generally
- *social and cultural factors*: taking account of these, both within the family and beyond; enabling early recovery by avoiding entrenched pessimism and acceptance of illness (Chapter 15)
- *treatments*: psychological and medical (Chapter 10), adherence (Chapter 13), coercion (Chapter 18)
- *prevention*: the relevance of adequate and appropriate social relationships, understanding how to access and use services, risk management, use of crisis plans.

When provided as a formal course, typically in an institutional setting, psychoeducation runs the risk of only reaching the well motivated. Crisis resolution and home treatment allows for psychoeducation to be provided for all referrals and offers the added advantage of contextual teaching and learning. The approach can be informal and piecemeal: we recommend that all members of the team should have training in psychoeducation and be encouraged to use it in their day-to-day work.

Communication training

In a crisis, adaptive coping by a social group is particularly dependent on adequate communication. When a crisis causes problems with coping, suboptimal communication within the group, and between the group and others, may be an important issue for the CRT to address. There is also evidence that certain family members of some patients with schizophrenia show minor but important communication deficits, such as vagueness, a tendency to make irrelevant remarks and a failure to complete statements in conversation.

Members of an acute CRT can usefully be trained to recognise and deal with the following issues (Falloon *et al.*, 1981):

- difficulties associated with non-verbal aspects of communication, such as voice tone, eye contact, facial expression and body posture
- problems caused by being too vague or general, rather than clear and specific
- when there is a tendency to speak for others rather than for oneself (i.e. people may say 'you must' when 'I would like' would be preferable)
- when there is a tendency to misinterpret 'cannot' as 'do not want' (e.g. when the family of someone with negative symptoms of schizophrenia construe the limitations resulting from these symptoms as laziness or uncooperativeness).

Problem solving

Problem-solving treatment (Mynors-Wallis, 2001) is a brief, structured cognitive–behavioural intervention that focuses on the here and now and enables the identification and solution of psychosocial problems significantly related to mental illness (Chapter 11).[2] It is a collaborative approach that has immediate relevance to the work of a CRT, especially when facilitating a social systems meeting (see above).

The therapist needs a neutral, enquiring attitude and should aim to follow, through guided self-help, the steps described in Box 12.2. Problem-solving treatment can be used flexibly by a team over several days but clearly needs good communication between the team members involved in order to maximise its effectiveness.

Family therapy

Formal family therapy is, unfortunately, not usually part of acute home treatment, being clinic based and subject to specialised assessment and often a waiting list. However, the interventions outlined above are clearly related to such formal treatment, especially systemic family therapy, and if the CRT has regular supervision by an appropriately trained clinical psychologist, important links between the team and a family therapy service can be established through case discussion. If sessional time can be provided to the team by such a psychologist, joint assessment visits to the home can be useful for in-service team training. With such help, the team can develop its skills in managing schizophrenia by reducing the effects of expressed emotion, and in the management of depression by the encouragement of positive reinforcement. Through appropriate discussions during crisis resolution, the team can also usefully enable selected families subsequently to engage in formal therapy.

---

[2] Its usefulness in family therapy for patients with schizophrenia is described by Falloon *et al.* (1984).

> ### Box 12.2. Steps involved in problem-solving treatment
>
> 1. *Identify the problem.* Clarification is crucial, especially when there is a range of views.
> 2. *List potential solutions.* Several solutions – perhaps five or six – should be asked for. To encourage 'brainstorming' by all present, all suggested solutions should be initially regarded as acceptable, even if at first sight they seem difficult to implement
> 3. *Discuss the 'pros and cons'.* Each possible solution should be discussed in turn, and a list of the 'pros and cons' of each assembled, with the therapist contributing as necessary.
> 4. *Choose the best solution.* Once everyone has had the chance to offer an opinion, a decision should be made. For some this is a difficult step to take without help.
> 5. *Implement the plan.* A balance between rushing and procrastination is advisable. A concrete plan is needed, perhaps broken down into manageable substeps that attend to crucial details.
> 6. *Review efforts.* Every success, no matter how modest, should be given recognition. Reasons for failure should be analysed and goals redrawn in the light of experience so that they are realistically achievable.

Key points

- Acute home treatment provides the opportunity for attention to the social factors that contribute to crises and for brief interventions that can change coping strategies for patient, family and wider social network.
- The challenge for CRTs is to ensure that the opportunity for working with relevant and important social relationships is not overlooked.
- For successful crisis resolution at home, the focus on the individual must always be widened to take into account the social systems involved.
- Working through a crisis gives an opportunity to see these significant links more clearly than at any other time, and allows the CRT to ensure that future care by others continues to recognise the significance of social context in maintaining the well-being of the individual.

REFERENCES

Bridgett, C. (2006a). The social systems approach. In *Crisis Resolution and Home Treatment: A Practical Guide*, ed. P. McGlynn. London: Sainsbury Centre for Mental Health, pp. 41–52.

Bridgett, C. (2006b). *Alternatives to Acute Admission: Crisis Resolution and Home Treatment.* London: Royal College of Psychiatrists. http://www.psychiatrycpd.org/learningmodules/alternativestoacuteadmissio.aspx.

Bridgett, C. and Polak, P. (2003a). Social systems intervention and crisis resolution. Part 1: assessment. *Advances in Psychiatric Treatment*, **9**, 424–31.

Bridgett, C. and Polak, P. (2003b). Social systems intervention and crisis resolution. Part 2: intervention. *Advances in Psychiatric Treatment*, **9**, 432–8.

Caplan, G. (1964). *Preventative Psychiatry*. London: Tavistock.

Department of Health (2001). *Mental Health Policy Implementation Guide: Crisis Resolution/ Home Treatment Teams*. London: Department of Health.

Falloon, I. R. H., Boyd, J. L., McGill, C. W., Strang, J. S. and Moss, H. B. (1981). Family management training in the community care of schizophrenia. In *New Developments in Interventions with Families of Schizophrenics*, ed. M. J. Goldstein. San Francisco: Jossey-Bass, pp. 61–77.

Falloon, I. R. H., Boyd, J. L. and Macgill, C. W. (1984). *Family Care of Schizophrenia*. New York: Guilford Press.

Fish, L. (1971). Using social-systems techniques on a crisis unit. *Hospital and Community Psychiatry*, **47**, 1–19.

Joy, C. B., Adams, C. E. and Rice, K. (2006). Crisis intervention for people with severe mental illnesses. *Cochrane Database of Systematic Reviews*, Issue 4, CD001087. Oxford: Update Software.

McFarlane, W. R., Dixon, L., Lukens, E. and Lucksted, A. (2003). Family psychoeducation and schizophrenia: a review of the literature. *Journal of Marital and Family Therapy*, **29**, 223–45.

Mynors-Wallis, L. (2001). Problem-solving treatment in general psychiatric practice. *Advances in Psychiatric Treatment*, **7**, 417–25.

Rosen, A. (1997). Crisis management in the community. *Medical Journal of Australia*, **167**, 633–8.

Szmukler, G. I. and Bloch, S. (1997). Family involvement in the care of people with psychoses. An ethical argument. *British Journal of Psychiatry*, **171**, 401–5.

13

Strategies for promoting engagement and treatment adherence

Mary Jane Tacchi and Jan Scott

Engagement is essential for the success of any mental health intervention. Intensive home treatment, when offered as a real alternative to hospital admission, represents a unique opportunity to provide acute treatment in a setting chosen by the patient. The safe and effective delivery of such treatment relies upon the patient's (and usually also the carer's) ability and willingness to accept and engage with the service provided, and to adhere to an agreed treatment plan. The potential promise of offering home-based rather than hospital care is that the experience of greater choice, more active participation in decision making and more acceptable treatment may increase engagement with services and active help seeking in the long term. This chapter will explore the general principles of engagement and describe the use of a health beliefs model to enhance this process and treatment adherence in day-to-day practice. Finally, the particular issues that arise in trying to engage and treat patients in their own homes will be considered.

Engagement

Literature from research on assertive outreach has focused upon the concept of engagement, and the principles outlined can be applied to most patient–clinician interactions in mental health services. Hall *et al.* (2001) developed an observer-rated measure of engagement that incorporated six dimensions of engagement:
- appointment keeping
- patient–therapist interaction
- communication

Crisis Resolution and Home Treatment in Mental Health, ed. Sonia Johnson, Justin Needle, Jonathan P. Bindman and Graham Thornicroft. Published by Cambridge University Press. © Cambridge University Press 2008.

- openness
- collaboration with treatment
- medication adherence.[1]

It is useful to think of engagement in this multidimensional way rather than as an 'all-or-nothing' concept. Engagement can be seen as a spectrum of behaviours and the number of components a person exhibits may change over time.

The *Keys to Engagement* report (Sainsbury Centre for Mental Health, 1998) describes various factors that can adversely affect engagement, and this and a subsequent report argued that strategies for engaging patients effectively are fundamental to the assertive outreach model (Sainsbury Centre for Mental Health, 2003; see Box 13.1). The importance of the needs and priorities of the patient, rather than a predetermined, clinician-led agenda, was emphasised. Thus getting involved with daily activities or sorting out practical problems can be a highly effective means for initial engagement in this setting.

Priebe *et al.* (2005) interviewed patients from an assertive outreach service who identified their three most important reasons for disengagement from the service as:

- a desire to be independent
- a poor therapeutic relationship
- a feeling of loss of control owing to medication effects.

The positive factors identified by patients as most salient in promoting engagement were:

- the time and commitment of staff
- social support
- a partnership model of the therapeutic relationship
- clinical engagement without an exclusive focus on medication.

The principles of engagement outlined for assertive outreach also apply to intensive home treatment and can be modified for use when briefer interventions are being provided without the benefit of long-term acquaintance with the patient. The themes that emerge are:

- the importance of listening to the patient and taking the time to find out about their perspective, rather than simply assuming it
- fostering a collaborative approach
- negotiating common goals.

The therapeutic alliance is the vehicle through which engagement proceeds. This is equally, if not more, important in intensive home treatment as in any other service setting.

---

[1] The paper uses the term 'medication compliance' but we feel that 'adherence' is a better representation of the outcome desired as it encompasses the notion of collaboration and mutual understanding, rather than a patient being compelled to take medication because the clinician says so.

> **Box 13.1. The *Keys to Engagement* Report**
>
> *Factors adversely affecting engagement* include:
> - past negative experiences of mental health services, particularly involuntary admissions
> - a lack of belief that services can help the individual
> - the perceived inappropriateness of services, in particular the perception that they are too focused on immediate symptomatic outcomes or medical treatment alone
> - factors directly related to illness, such as the presence of psychotic symptoms or hopelessness
> - negative staff attitudes
> - cultural and class barriers.
>
> *Effective patient engagement involves staff:*
> - developing a trusting relationship (or therapeutic alliance; see text)
> - working with patients on their own territory
> - spending time with patients
> - being highly flexible and creative in their approach.
>
> *Source*: From Sainsbury Centre for Mental Health, 1998, 2003.

The therapeutic alliance

The importance of the therapeutic alliance, and its impact upon outcome, has been described in detail in the psychotherapy literature. A recent review of studies using structured measures to study the therapeutic relationship in the treatment of severe mental disorders showed it to be a reliable predictor of patient outcome in mainstream psychiatric care (McCabe and Priebe, 2004). Various models have been proposed for conceptualising this association, many with the importance of an equal partnership between clinician and patient and of negotiation and collaborative decision making at their core (e.g. Charles *et al.*, 1977; Tarrier and Barrowclough, 2003).

DiMatteo (1979) is among the authors who have explored in greater detail the factors that are relevant to promoting positive doctor–patient interactions, prominent among which are warmth, positive regard, lack of tension and non-verbal expressiveness (Box 13.2).

McCabe *et al.* (2002) investigated how doctors engaged with patients with psychotic disorders. They showed that patients actively attempted to talk about the content of their psychotic symptoms but that doctors were reluctant to engage with their concerns if they were perceived as delusional in origin. The paper generated much discussion in the literature about the training of doctors,

> **Box 13.2. Features of the doctor–patient relationship relevant to promoting positive interaction**
>
> *Essential features* include:
> - warmth
> - positive regard
> - lack of tension
> - non-verbal expressiveness.
>
> *Other relevant issues* are:
> - communication style
> - how much the patient feels listened to
> - patient participation in decision making
> - the extent to which the doctor answers the patient's concerns and allows discussion
> - collaboration
> - mutual understanding
> - the extent to which each party takes the other's point of view into account
> - qualities of empathy and respect
> - the availability of enough time in the consultation.
>
> *Source*: From DiMatteo, 1979.

but one of the key points emphasised by the authors was that addressing patient concerns will lead to a more satisfactory outcome from the consultation for both parties.

Establishing the patient's model

The literature identifies a number of factors associated with non-adherence and poor engagement among individuals with severe mental disorders (Box 13.3; reviewed by Tacchi and Scott, 2005). Some of these can be addressed at an initial assessment, but detailed exploration of all of them is not necessarily helpful at this stage, even when trying to assess whether intensive home treatment is an option.

In order to develop engagement and to assess the likelihood of being able to implement intensive home treatment on an individual level, we advocate the use of a *health beliefs model*, involving exploration of the patient's beliefs and attitudes. We have found that a modified version of the *cognitive representation of illness model* (Leventhal *et al.*, 1992) can be employed to understand the patient's model of illness. Information from an exploration of the patient's 'cognitive representation' can then be used as a vehicle for establishing a therapeutic

---

Box 13.3. Factors associated with non-adherence and poor engagement in people with severe mental disorders

Demographic, illness and treatment factors associated with poor adherence:
- living alone
- comorbid substance misuse
- long duration of illness
- past history of medication non-adherence
- cognitive impairment
- lack of insight
- the subjective experience of side effects of medication
- complicated medication regimens.

Individual and relationship factors associated with non-adherence:
- high expressed emotion in the family
- lack of illness awareness
- an internal locus of control (i.e. the tendency to believe that events are always under one's own control)
- poor therapeutic alliance
- negative expectations or attitudes towards treatment
- the knowledge and beliefs of significant others
- fear of (rather than actual experience of) side effects from medication
- negative beliefs about taking medication.

---

alliance and thus promoting engagement and adherence to treatment (Tacchi and Scott, 2005). The cognitive representation of illness model describes how individuals organise information about what is happening to them when they experience physical or psychological symptoms, and how they react to this. The cognitive representation suggests that when an individual has a concrete experience of symptoms they attach an idiosyncratic or abstract meaning to what is happening that is usually organised around five key themes (Scott and Tacchi, 2002; Box 13.4). The content of the thoughts will differ between individuals, but clinicians can gain an understanding of the patient's perception of their problems by exploring these themes.

By exploring these five key themes, it is possible to gain an understanding of what knowledge or theories the patient has about their condition and to discuss any misunderstandings. The purpose is for the clinician to gain a clear understanding of the patient's model and of what the patient thinks is happening. This allows the clinician to make a judgement as to whether the patient's and the clinician's model are likely to be compatible, and what interventions will be most

Box 13.4. Key themes around which individuals' representations about what is happening are organised

Identity of problem. What does the individual think it is? Do they view it as a mental disorder?

Cause. What ideas do they entertain about what has caused their problem(s)?

Timeline. How long do they think it will last? Do they think it is transient, may persist or may be recurrent?

Consequences. How do they think it will affect them? Do they think there may be any serious consequences of not having treatment?

Cure. Does the individual think the problem can be cured or controlled? How has the individual attempted to cope with the symptoms and how do they appraise the effectiveness of their coping strategies?

Source: From Scott and Tacchi, 2002.

appropriate and acceptable to the client and their significant others, including whether intensive home treatment is the appropriate way of delivering care. The clinician uses the patient's model as a starting point for reinforcing accurate information and perceptions. The clinician and the patient can then explore what coping strategies the patient has been using, and together they can appraise how effective these have been in improving symptoms and quality of life. Any effective self-initiated strategies can be incorporated into the treatment plan alongside more typical service interventions, and by encouraging the patient to continue using both types of strategy, the message is reinforced that the treatment is a partnership, drawing on the resources of all those involved. The final step is to integrate the patient's model with the clinician's model, the aim being to develop a shared formulation of the patient's problems. This allows development and reinforcement of a rationale for involvement with mental health services and the production of a set of treatment goals that is rooted in these discussions. Because the goals have been developed collaboratively, they are usually more acceptable to the patient, who is, therefore, more likely to adhere to the proposed management plan.

The first meeting in a period of intensive home treatment is, therefore, crucial, and enough time needs to be allocated for the assessments and negotiations that we have described. While it is very desirable for some degree of engagement to be established at the first meeting, a shared understanding of the problems and jointly agreed management plan may evolve over the first few days of treatment.

Engagement in home-based treatment: specific considerations

Working with clients at home raises some considerations relevant to engagement that may not be addressed in other settings.

Structure

The first negotiation with the patient concerns the organisation of visits, for example how many people will be visiting and how often, and the acceptability of this to the patient. Convenient timing of the visits is essential, as is the resolution of any issues the patient may have with regard, for example, to the gender of clinicians. Cultural traditions within the home must be respected and the frequency of visits negotiated to take into account the patient's wishes, clinical and social needs, and the safety of patients, carers and clinicians.

Carers

Carer involvement is central to intensive home treatment, and this involvement usually begins right at the start of the work of the crisis resolution team (CRT) in a crisis. Issues of confidentiality must obviously be respected, but carer involvement is nonetheless a key to successful home treatment. Permission is usually sought from the patient for the clinician to have separate discussions with the carer during the course of the assessment, though joint meetings that include the patient are also important when the treatment plan is negotiated. The presence of children in the home is noted, and their safety and needs assessed, so that any other agencies can be contacted if necessary. Sometimes, both patient and clinician are willing to proceed with home treatment, but carer exhaustion or difficulty in providing consistent support can be an indication that admission to hospital or respite care is appropriate. There are cases in which home circumstances are not conducive to recovery, especially in the presence of high expressed emotion, difficult or abusive relationships or overcrowding, or where the patient is socially isolated; in such situations, alternatives to home treatment should be sought. Carers must feel that the provision of intensive home treatment is a positive and planned decision, not a means of avoiding admission at all costs.

It is important to establish with carers who is responsible for ensuring the safety of the patient (or others) in a given situation. It is often appropriate to enlist carers' help in monitoring symptoms and providing information about the home situation at follow-up assessments. However, clinicians must make it clear that they are responsible for ensuring patients' safety, and that carers are not being used to provide one-to-one continuous observation and monitoring. It is important that the carer is not left feeling that the burden of responsibility lies with them, or that they are being used to cover any deficiencies in the level of input available from the treatment team.

Risk

Engaging patients who are receiving intensive home treatment is the most important task to be accomplished in order to ensure their safety (see also Chapter 9). The process of constantly evaluating and reevaluating risk and planning how to keep patients and carers safe is much easier when relationships between patients and professionals are open and collaborative. The provision of a 24-hour helpline is only useful for patients who are able to use it, and intend to use it when necessary, otherwise it becomes a token provision that allows the clinician to feel more comfortable. Assessment of the patient's safety is essential, and it should be evaluated at every contact. Assessment of risk to staff from the patient, their carers or their environment is also a crucial part of deciding whether home-based treatment can proceed.

Containment

With intensive home treatment, there is not the physical security (or the sense of it) that is available in a hospital setting. Containment is provided by the clinician's behaviour and input, the engagement of users and carers and the shared knowledge and agreement that if the situation changes the intervention can change. Feedback from patients and carers has shown that the knowledge that help is available 24 hours a day via a telephone call, and that additional visits can readily be mobilized, allows users and carers to feel secure and confident about proceeding with home treatment.

Time

It is in the nature of intensive home treatment that patients are presenting in a crisis. While the need to establish a therapeutic alliance and undertake a risk assessment is urgent, it cannot be hurried. Spending time during the first visit establishing the patient's model of what is happening, comparing this with the model possessed by key significant others, and integrating their story with the clinical assessment is essential if engagement is to be promoted and a valid and reliable risk assessment undertaken. As stated above, engagement cannot necessarily be fully established at first contact, but it should also be borne in mind that this process often proceeds faster than in other treatment settings because of the intensity and duration of intensive home treatment visits and of the greater ease with which a collaborative relationship can be established in an informal community setting than in an institutional one.

Interactions and continuity of care

Intensive home treatment is provided 24 hours per day by a team of clinicians working shifts. While patients or carers may relate better to some team members than others, it is important to try to provide a coherent and predictable programme of treatment that the service users are able to understand and accept. Consistency of clinical staff should be ensured whenever possible, though it is inevitable that engagement will not occur exclusively with a particular member of the CRT. Realistically, therefore, a relationship has to be developed with the team as a whole. To facilitate this, the team must function as a whole, showing continuity and consistency in its approach and philosophy of care and maintaining excellent levels of communication, both within the team and with patients and carers. This can be achieved through:

- the rigorous use of daily handover meetings
- a system for communicating about urgent issues
- utilisation of information technology to maximise efficiency
- regular sharing of information and views
- repeated opportunities for re-stating of the team philosophy.

The most important aspect to engaging an individual and their significant others in intensive home treatment is to help them to understand that the critical component is the continuity of *treatment* and the treatment model, not necessarily the individual personnel, though where especially strong and empathic relationships are established with particular members of staff, this can also be a valuable tool in the treatment process.

Especially where engagement and adherence to medication are relatively difficult to achieve, the adherence therapy model (previously known as compliance therapy) may be a useful tool (Kemp *et al.*, 1998). Adherence therapy uses a health beliefs model to develop the therapeutic alliance so that clinician and patient can work collaboratively to reach common goals. In a formal course of adherence therapy, this initial process usually takes place over six sessions (lasting four to six hours overall). It can, however, be adapted for use in crisis work by shortening the initial stages and then consolidating and reviewing the five areas of the health beliefs model on further contact. As the visits from such a service will be more regular (often twice daily in the first instance) than with other psychiatric contact, the process of the adherence therapy is completed in a relatively short time. For patients who are more difficult to engage, such as those referred to assertive outreach services (see Chapter 7), the model is very useful in that it allows the patient's views and goals to be explored in a full and open way, and to be incorporated in the treatment plan. Negotiation takes place as to the timing, location and frequency of visits, and sometimes the intensity of contact has to be reduced as this is overwhelming to the patient and becomes counterproductive. The intervention is adapted to the patient's lifestyle, not vice versa.

Conclusions

Effective engagement is an essential part of providing successful intensive home treatment and is a complex, multifaceted process. The key dimensions are appointment keeping, the interactions between client and clinician, style of communication and collaboration with and adherence to treatment. The therapeutic alliance can be viewed as the vehicle through which engagement proceeds and is enhanced by listening, spending adequate time in discussion, finding out what the patient's agenda is and collaborating and negotiating with him or her from the outset. We have described a model that involves exploring clients' views and understanding in five key areas. This understanding is then used to develop the therapeutic alliance, a shared formulation and goals, and a treatment plan that is acceptable to both patient and clinician.

If patients and their significant others feel listened to and that their model and goals are being used as key determinants of the management plan, they are more likely to engage with intensive home treatment and more likely to adhere to the overall treatment package and accept medication. The converse is also true: a significant difference between the views of clinicians and patients and a failure to agree the goals of interventions are likely to militate against home treatment. However, the overview given in this chapter may offer some avenues to explore that will allow clinicians to avoid these difficulties or repair any ruptures in the therapeutic alliance. Once home treatment has been established, problems of the kind we have discussed in maintaining engagement in a therapeutic alliance can usually be identified and overcome, if not avoided altogether. If a decision is made against home treatment, this is more often because of risk or of potential burden for significant others. The patient's level of suicidal intent or severity of their symptoms, combined with inadequate insight or illness awareness, may impede their initial engagement with the process. Alternatively, social isolation or an inadequate level of social support – owing to the carers themselves being under stress, too distressed or unable to engage with the home treatment – may also mean that such an approach is counterproductive. Over time, many intensive home treatment teams develop a high level of skill in managing severe mental disorders in the community. It is clear that successful teams have a well-developed and comprehensive approach to service user engagement that makes it highly likely that patients and their families will not only accept but also actively choose this approach to their care and treatment. For patients whose mental health needs are long term, the aim is to maintain the sense of an effective therapeutic alliance with the team as a whole, allowing patients to be re-engaged in a similar way at each episode (Chapter 16). Patients who previously required recurrent admissions, sometimes on a compulsory basis, can instead receive care repeatedly in a community setting. Ideally this may result over time in a greater willingness to seek help early in a crisis and engage in active relapse-prevention strategies.

Key points

- Engagement is a multidimensional phenomenon comprising at least six key components: appointment keeping, client–therapist interaction, communication, openness, collaboration with treatment and medication adherence.
- The *cognitive representation of illness* model is a health beliefs model that identifies five core themes in a patient's beliefs about a disorder: identity, cause, timeline, consequences and controllability.
- This model can be used to develop a shared understanding between patient and clinician of the patient's problems that can enhance the therapeutic alliance and consequently improve the patient's adherence to the treatment plan.
- Successful home-based treatment teams attend to engagement, negotiation of the structure of the intervention, the role and involvement of carers, safety and containment, communication and responsibility issues.

REFERENCES

Charles, C., Gafni, A. and Whelan, T. (1977). Shared decision making in the medical encounter: What does it mean? *Social Science and Medicine*, **44**, 681–92.

DiMatteo, M. (1979). A social-psychological analysis of physician–patient rapport: Toward a science of the art of medicine. *Journal of Social Issues*, **35**, 12–33.

Hall, M., Meaden, A., Smith, J. *et al.* (2001). Brief report: the development and psychometric properties of an observer-rated measure of engagement with mental health services. *Journal of Mental Health*, **10**, 457–65.

Kemp, R., Kirov, G., Everitt, B., Hayward, P. and David, A. (1998). Randomised controlled trial of compliance therapy: 18 month follow-up. *British Journal of Psychiatry*, **172**, 413–19.

Levanthal, H., Diefenbach, M. and Levanthal, E. (1992). Illness cognition: using common sense to understand treatment adherence and affect–cognition interactions. *Cognitive Therapy and Research*, **6**, 143–63.

McCabe, R. and Priebe, S. (2004). The therapeutic relationship in the treatment of severe mental illness. *International Journal of Social Psychiatry*, **50**, 115–28.

McCabe, R., Heath, C., Burns, T. and Priebe, S. (2002). Engagement of patients with psychosis in the consultation: conversation analytic study. *British Medical Journal*, **325**, 1148–51.

Priebe, S., Watts, J., Chase, M. *et al.* (2005). Processes of disengagement and engagement in assertive outreach patients: qualitative study. *British Journal of Psychiatry*, **187**, 438–43.

Sainsbury Centre for Mental Health (1998). *Keys to Engagement: Review of Care for People with Severe Mental Illness who are Hard to Engage with Services.* London: Sainsbury Centre for Mental Health.

Sainsbury Centre for Mental Health (2003). *Mental Health Topics: Assertive Outreach.* London: Sainsbury Centre for Mental Health.

Scott, J. and Tacchi, M. J. (2002). A pilot study of concordance therapy for individuals with bipolar disorder who are non-adherent with lithium prophylaxis. *Bipolar Disorders*, **4**, 286–93.

Tacchi, M. J. and Scott, J. (2005). *Improving Adherence in Schizophrenia and Bipolar Disorders.* London: John Wiley.

Tarrier, N. and Barrowclough, C. (2003). Professional attitudes to psychiatric patients: A time for change and an end to medical paternalism. *Epidemiologia e Psichiatria Sociale*, **12**, 238–41.

14

Mixed blessings: service user experience of crisis teams

Alison Faulkner and Helen Blackwell

An argument often made for crisis resolution teams (CRTs) is that they are likely to be more acceptable to service users and to carers than hospital admission. The unpopularity of inpatient wards makes this a very important possibility, but as yet the literature on CRTs contains little exploration of the extent to which they fit with the views of service users about what helps them in crises. In this chapter, two people who have used CRTs as well as other forms of acute care discuss how far they fit with what we know so far about service user views and give their own accounts of using these services and of their potential advantages and pitfalls.

Introduction

Service users have been calling for alternatives to hospital admission in a crisis for many years. Indeed, it has been one of the key campaigning issues for the user/survivor movement in the UK. A review of over 40 reports and studies about service user views of services, prepared for the Audit Commission's (1994) report *Finding a Place*, revealed consistently strong support for community-based crisis services offering a 24-hour response and aiming to prevent hospital admission. One of the demands in the *Charter of Needs and Demands* (Survivors Speak Out, 1987) agreed at one of the first ever service user conferences – the Edale conference held in 1987 – was for the 'provision of refuge, planned and under the control of survivors of psychiatry'.

What people say that they want in a crisis – someone to talk to, sanctuary, support from someone and help with escalating practical problems – is often at odds with what is on offer: a busy ward, 24-hour television and regular routines of queuing for medication and meals. The Mental Health Foundation (1997) carried out a survey of service user views about a range of treatments and

Crisis Resolution and Home Treatment in Mental Health, ed. Sonia Johnson, Justin Needle, Jonathan P. Bindman and Graham Thornicroft. Published by Cambridge University Press. © Cambridge University Press 2008.

therapies in 1997. The overwhelming response to the question, 'What do you feel you want in times of crisis or distress?' was 'Someone to talk to'.

Admission to hospital has never been a popular outcome for people in a crisis, although it is sometimes unavoidable. Over the years, survey after survey has revealed poor physical conditions, understaffing, a lack of therapeutic activities and an increasingly high level of need amongst inpatients, particularly in inner-city hospitals (e.g. Levenson *et al.*, 2003; Sainsbury Centre for Mental Health, 1998, 2005). There is a sense of resignation about the state of our acute wards, and little evidence that very much is changing.

People's stories – often dismissed as anecdotal by those interested in evidence-based practice – paint a more personal picture of the situation. They relate how it feels to be a patient on those wards, and what effect being locked up for 24 hours a day without anything to do, an unchanging routine of meals, drinks and medication and little meaningful contact with staff might have on people. With the best will in the world, it would be hard to conceive of these conditions as creating a supportive or therapeutic environment. Coupled with the tendency to provide no information to patients about changes in meetings, appointments and ward rounds, these are conditions guaranteed to lead to high levels of frustration amongst all but the most drugged or compliant of patients.

Research carried out as part of the Mental Health Foundation's Strategies for Living Programme helps us to understand the experience better. This programme supported a series of user-led research projects (Nicholls *et al.*, 2003). One of these projects explored people's experiences of acute hospital wards and found that staff and patients rarely engaged in a relationship based on therapeutic interactions. The main role adopted by staff was 'to prescribe medication and to ensure that rules were adhered to'. The people interviewed said that they were more likely to speak to each other about their difficulties, although they still wanted to be able to talk to staff about the personal causes of their mental distress. Hospital routines were seen as more important for staff than addressing patients' needs. The few staff singled out for praise showed 'human qualities . . . the respect and dignity we expect from each other . . .'.

Responses to crises

The two main alternatives to hospital for people in a crisis are crisis houses and CRTs. The latter are now part of government policy in the UK and the main subject of this book, whereas the former have developed in response to locally identified needs, often of service users and/or the voluntary sector. The two models may be different in terms of the setting in which care is delivered but may embody similar approaches to crisis response. Campbell (1996) commented:

'What we would like to see, as part of community care, are places of refuge, of asylum in the original sense. They would be small, they would be local, they would take problems you experience on your own terms and they would omit much of the paraphernalia that is intrinsic to the psychiatric system.'

Crisis houses

The option often favoured by service users has tended to be the crisis house, a residential alternative to hospital offering a different kind of response to people in crisis. Over the years, a number of these have been established across the UK, developing differently in different areas, but often in response to service user/ survivor campaigning action. One of the first, if not *the* first, was a user-run crisis house in Wokingham. Current services include a survivor-led crisis service in Leeds, a recently funded new user-led service with Barnet Voice in North London, and the sanctuary/crisis house that Wokingham and West Berkshire Mental Health Association continues to provide. As Chapter 23 of this book describes, a number of other services operate in the UK, some provided by the statutory services, others by the voluntary sector or jointly by the two sectors.

The Mental Health Foundation and the Sainsbury Centre for Mental Health funded and evaluated eight crisis services a few years ago, and their report *Being There in a Crisis* (2002) found high levels of satisfaction with the residential crisis houses, with most service users feeling that the crisis house had met their needs. The following features were picked out for particular praise:

- the physical and emotional environment
- staff/quality of care
- the holistic/social approach to crisis
- recovery approach/use of complementary therapies (*in one house only*).

When asked if they could get similar help from any other service, the service users made favourable comparisons with hospital inpatient services. The following quotation in *Being There in a Crisis* illustrates this:

... it is completely different compared to the hospital. I was in hospital for seven months, the staff sit and read newspapers and dish out medication, you are not allowed out. It really does not compare, you get your own life back, people help to pick up the pieces.

I went into hospital voluntarily but they only try drugs and you just sit around smoking. There is no interaction, apart from you see the psychiatrist maybe once per week.

A survivor-led evaluation of the Leeds Survivor-Led Crisis Service (L. Allison *et al.*, unpublished) found some strikingly similar views: 'My whole life exploded and I tried to kill myself ... when I started coming here I haven't looked back' and 'Available, accessible, nice people, quick, responsive and welcoming ... the house itself seemed to glow.'

The experience of one of the authors (AF) of a crisis house in London reflects the findings of these evaluations: 'I received a far more humane and personal response to my crisis, with less disruption to my life, and within pleasant surroundings. I was able to think about what had been going on in my life and talk it through with members of staff, and to retain contact with my friends much more easily than when in hospital.'

The experience of crisis houses can help us to identify some of the key factors that help to support people through a crisis. These evaluations show us that service users value a holistic response – something that goes beyond or outside the medical model – with time to talk and work through the crisis, in an environment that is safe and pleasant and suggests that they are valued as individuals. The question is whether these elements can be found in a CRT based on home treatment.

Crisis resolution/home treatment teams

The government's chosen form of crisis response is the CRT. The *Mental Health Policy Implementation Guide* (Department of Health, 2001) stated that CRTs should have the following characteristics (see also Chapter 6):

- a multidisciplinary team
- availability to respond 24 hours a day, 7 days a week
- staff in frequent contact with service users, often seeing them at least once on each shift
- provision of intensive contact over a short period of time
- staff remain involved until the problem is resolved.

The team local for AF says that it offers:

- an alternative to hospital admission for people aged 16+ who are experiencing acute episodes of mental health difficulties
- rapid assessment
- intensive home-based intervention in the early stages of a crisis
- individualised care plans drawn up in conjunction with you and your carer
- help with resolving your crisis and to help you discover ways of preventing future crises
- monitoring medication in the early stages of a crisis.

There has been some evidence over the years that families, both service users and carers, are more satisfied with home treatment than with hospital treatment (Chapter 5); it may provide both with some useful support. An Internet search revealed a number of relevant websites and articles. One of these is a brief feedback survey of service user views of the Leicester CRT. This is notable because while the survey reports high levels of satisfaction with the team, as do many other surveys of CRTs, it also identifies a minority of service users who would have preferred to be in hospital and, significantly, a majority (over 80%) who would have liked to have the option of going to a crisis house. Other reports point to higher satisfaction levels, as measured on various scales, and a reduction in hospital admissions (Chapters 4 and 5). For example, in Easington, County Durham, an evaluation of a recently introduced CRT indicated very high levels of service user satisfaction and a 70% fall in acute hospital admissions (National Institute for Mental Health in England, 2006).

Crisis teams: service user experiences

The following section relates the personal experiences of the authors with crisis teams.

Alison Faulkner

In two different London boroughs, I have had two very different experiences of CRTs. In the first borough, the team was very new and I had no idea who they were when they walked in on the assessment I was having with a doctor at the hospital's emergency reception centre. They did not introduce themselves very well but were able to offer me a bed in the local crisis house, which seemed to me to be a good option. There were, however, difficulties with liaison between the team and the house. Evidently, the team had the right to admit up to three people to the eight-bedded crisis house, and continued to be responsible for those in their charge. This did not work very well for me because I had been to the house before and in my distressed state I found it difficult to work out how things were happening in a different way from my previous stay.

Unfortunately, there was a bad outcome on this occasion. While staying in the crisis house, I took a serious overdose, which was easy to do in the relatively free environment of the house. On reflection, I believe that I should have been admitted to hospital rather than the crisis house, although I would not necessarily hold the team entirely accountable for this.

Two members of the team came to pick me up from the accident and emergency department after the overdose and return me to the crisis house. One of them said to me: 'If you know so much about mental health, why did you do that?' I felt really upset by this and subsequently did not feel able to talk to them easily (which raises another issue about how those of us who are 'involved' in the mental health system – whether locally or nationally – are treated when in distress).

After I had returned home, problems with this first team continued. For example, I turned up at the hospital for an appointment – a journey of two bus rides – to find that there was no one there for the meeting. I was never given any information about the team and was not properly informed when I ceased to be on their books.

In the second borough, things were very different. Perhaps the team had been in existence for a bit longer, and their procedures were, therefore, more well developed. The team comes to the hospital or to the accident and emergency department to assess the potential user and then decides if their support will be helpful. I have felt well supported on the two or three occasions when I have needed their support. People more or less turn up when they say they will, and they treat me more like a human being – with respect and an appreciation of me as an individual with my own life to lead. As with all teams, wards and services, there are good, bad and indifferent members of the team and people you hope will not be visiting you, but on the whole it has been a positive experience.

The important things to me about a team supporting me at home are that they are able to see your whole situation and (preferably) not turn up simply to ask if you are eating, sleeping and taking your medication. There is generally more time to talk to someone, which is something you rarely get in hospital. You can receive support at home after a short hospital admission, something that in my experience never used to happen at all. Practical help is valuable, such as taking you shopping when you return home from hospital, or helping to sort out some of the chaos at home – although personally I find it hard to ask for these things. It is helpful to have some continuity – to see the same one or two people on each visit so that you do not have to repeat your story. However, this may not always be possible. In a similar way, the thoroughness of the handover and the communication between team members are important in providing continuity of care.

As for the issue of team members coming into one's own home, I think this is a mixed blessing. Some people find this intrusive. I have a nice flat and generally present myself reasonably well, which sometimes means that people think I am in a better mental state than I feel, and this does not always work well for me. In general, though, I have found team members to be polite and not overly intrusive on their visits. I suspect that the very fact of seeing you in your own home almost obliges team members to see the broader social context, and thus acts to de-medicalise the crisis to some extent.

Clearly, one of the key aims of CRTs is to reduce hospital admissions, but it seems to me that there is a significant difference between just aiming for a reduction in numbers and trying to provide service users with genuine alternatives and real choices. One of the potential dangers of this is that the aim of avoiding hospital admission may become paramount and lead people to misread a crisis and fail to admit someone when, in fact, admission might be what is needed. I think that this did happen to me on the first occasion described above, although the duty doctor also agreed to the CRT's plan.

The features of CRTs that I have found helpful are:

- time to talk
- practical help
- a holistic approach
- responsiveness to fears/risks
- information about the team
- clarity about discharge arrangements
- good communications with other healthcare professionals, such as the community mental health team, general practitioners and psychiatrists
- staying at home – at times.

Unhelpful features and approaches have included:

- replication of hospital approach
- judgemental comments about your home/person
- unreliability about turning up for visits or meetings
- lack of clarity regarding what the team can do, the limits to the help they can offer, and so on
- avoiding hospital admission is more important than responding to individual crises
- avoiding questions about risk and harm
- coercion to comply
- staying at home – at times.

Overall, I believe that the key to this is in being able to offer a different ethos in the way a crisis is dealt with, whether in a crisis house or by a CRT. There needs to be an element of choice for people and a realistic assessment of the risks, undertaken jointly, for such services to be both effective and responsive to individual needs. Some people do not feel safe at home and others feel strongly that home is a safer and better place to be. We need to see CRTs as one part of a whole service. I still strongly believe that we need to revise and reform the acute wards and their role in the service if we are ever going to treat people in acute mental distress as if they are human beings. And I would like the option of a crisis house as a source of sanctuary and support.

Helen Blackwell

While in hospital four years ago, my health deteriorated and I took a life-threatening overdose. My psychiatrist declared that I was no safer in hospital than out. Since then I have remained out of hospital but have been supported by the CRT on four occasions, for periods varying from two to six weeks. The level of risk I have presented to myself on these occasions has often been extremely high, but I – and the team supporting me – have judged that I would be safer, and recover more quickly, if supported at home.

I do not know if my local CRT uses a stated approach or model. However, in my experience many elements of the recovery approach are integral to their work. Here I will highlight three aspects of the recovery approach: first, users having a greater degree of choice and control than in traditional services; second, viewing service users as members of their own community, with a variety of strengths and roles; and third, adopting a positive approach to risk taking.

Choice and control

In using the CRT I have felt that I have had a greater degree of control of the process than if I were in hospital. This has been evident in small but significant ways, for example, being asked whether I would prefer to be visited by worker A on the morning shift or worker B on the evening shift. The team have insisted that they would work round my existing commitments, rather than the other way round. This has helped me to see my mental health difficulties – even during a crisis – as one aspect of a much wider picture. I have continued to function as a worker, family member and friend – though with support in thinking through how to minimise stresses and ensure my needs were met.

Strengths and resources

By staying at home during a crisis, I am able to draw on a much wider range of support than hospital – or mental health services in general – can provide. I can continue to attend my regular psychotherapy sessions, draw on the support of friends, book a massage and be with my dog! The CRT has asked how they can support me in this, which has included walking my dog with me and dropping me off at the swimming pool after visiting me at home.

It initially came as a surprise to me that a member of the CRT would spend a considerable amount of time helping me to develop strategies for managing my professional work during a crisis. This was an enormous help for a number of reasons. I felt that she did not see me just as a 'patient', but as someone who could perform valued work at the same time as managing a personal crisis. It respected my preferred individual coping strategy: using a combination of rest, support and a 'cycle of achievement' to combat depression. It also recognized the basic realities of my life – that as a self-employed worker it is sometimes a fine balance whether to take time off work, with potential anxieties about money, or continue work and be paid. These are considerations that are individual to me, but the model operated by the CRT allows workers to respond to my individual needs.

The CRT in my locality has gone further than many in using local community resources. If they feel a client needs to get away from their home environment but does not need hospital admission, they may offer up to three nights in a local hotel. This has attracted mixed reactions from local service users: for some, the idea of an empty hotel room, even with visits from the CRT, is a nightmare; for others, it is a welcome offer of respite and 'time out'.

Positive risk taking

I see an effective CRT approach as an example of positive risk taking. The CRT worker who took the lead in my care helped me to identify specific risks, early warning signs, strategies, supports and safety nets. I was assured by the whole team that they were there to be contacted, day or night, and constantly reassured that they *wanted* me to contact them. This contributed to a sense of emotional safety, as did the warmth of staff and the fact that they remembered, and communicated to each other, details about my needs.

Crisis teams in context

However, my experience is that there are limitations both in the model and operation of CRTs. The support I have described above has only been possible when the team has been adequately staffed. If it was under-resourced, this has been evident in phone calls not returned, messages not passed on and visits cancelled. At these times, the frustration of the CRT members, who cannot offer the quality of service they want to, has been evident. For me as a client, it has meant the loss of the sense of safety that the team provides.

The second potential difficulty is that of recruiting a team with consistently high skill levels. While some of the things I value are down to the way the service is structured, other things depend on the skills of individual team members. I have found that I choose to talk about more complex or personal issues to team members who are both sensitive and skilled in helping me to express feelings and solve problems. I do not talk at that depth with team members who just ask the 'sleeping, eating, medication' questions. A team will only be effective if it has more of the former and fewer of the latter!

Finally, I do not think that the home treatment model is sufficient as a standalone service (even in conjunction with acute wards). There are times when I do need time away from home with support. Two years ago, I spent four days at Maytree, a sanctuary for people feeling suicidal. At that point, I needed the safety of people around me 24 hours a day, knowing someone could sit with me and listen for as long as I needed. It was a safe environment, planned to be peaceful, uncluttered and calm. There are times when home, with its memories, demands and easy access to methods of self-harm, is not the right place to start recovery. More recently a local crisis house has been established that is staffed and managed entirely by service users. I have stayed in the house on two occasions. It also offers a calm and warm welcome, time to talk, rest, paint and enjoy complementary therapies. It is amazing how far one can travel emotionally during a three- or four-day stay in a crisis house, if the approach is designed to help guests actively make sense of their crisis. The combination of home treatment and access to a crisis house has been key to my recovery, but both need to be adequately resourced.

Key points

- Service users have been calling for alternatives to hospital admission in a crisis for many years.
- Alternative ways of managing a crisis involve a holistic response to people, a non-medical approach and the opportunity to talk to someone about what is happening.
- The CRT needs to be seen as part of a whole system, within which the acute wards still need to be revised, modernised and refocused on crisis management.
- There is still a place for the crisis house, a residential non-medical place of sanctuary where people can stay for a short respite away from home.

REFERENCES

Audit Commission (1994). *Finding a Place. A Review of Mental Health Services for Adults.* London: HMSO.

Campbell, P. (1996). What users want from mental health crisis services. *Mental Health Review*, **1**, 19–21.

Department of Health (2001). *Mental Health Policy Implementation Guide.* London: Department of Health.

Levenson, R., Greatley, A. and Robinson, J. (2003). *London's State of Mind: King's Fund Mental Health Inquiry 2003.* London: King's Fund.

Mental Health Foundation (1997). *Knowing Our Own Minds.* London: Mental Health Foundation.

Mental Health Foundation and the Sainsbury Centre for Mental Health (2002). *Being There in a Crisis: A Report of the Learning from Eight Mental Health Services.* London: Mental Health Foundation.

National Institute for Mental Health in England (2006). *10 High Impact Changes for Mental Health Services.* London: Care Services Improvement Partnership.

Nicholls, V., Wright, S., Waters, R. and Wells, S. (2003). *Surviving User-led Research: Reflections on Supporting User-led Research Projects.* London: Mental Health Foundation.

Sainsbury Centre for Mental Health (1998). *Acute Problems: A Survey of the Quality of Care in Acute Psychiatric Wards.* London: Sainsbury Centre for Mental Health.

Sainsbury Centre for Mental Health (2005). *Acute Care 2004: A National Survey of Adult Psychiatric Wards in England.* London: Sainsbury Centre for Mental Health.

Survivors Speak Out (1987). *Charter of Needs and Demands.* Edale, UK: Survivors Speak Out.

15

Early discharge and joint working between crisis teams and hospital services

Fiona Nolan and Sylvia Tang

In this chapter, we will examine some ways in which crisis resolution teams (CRTs) liaise and work with other acute care services, especially in facilitating early discharge from hospital. Ways of establishing strong and effective working relationships between hospital and crisis services will be described. Finally, different approaches to facilitating early discharge will be explored in three case studies.

The relationship between crisis and acute services

Much of the focus in the literature discussing CRTs tends to be on providing an alternative at the point of hospital admission. However, another important role, particularly where one of the main goals of introducing them is to reduce bed use and divert resources into community-based mental healthcare, is their potential for becoming involved following admission in order to allow early discharge from hospital. As yet, very little research has focused specifically on the effectiveness of strategies for reducing hospital stay.

Early discharge is perhaps the activity for which strong relationships between CRTs and ward teams are most important, but this relationship is also important when CRTs offer intensive home treatment to patients who present significant risks: rapid access to inpatient beds is needed if escalating risk and lack of treatment response make management at home unsustainable. An effective relationship with inpatient teams is important to allow CRTs to engage in positive risk taking with this group. For CRTs to sustain an effective gatekeeping role, they also need to have good relationships with inpatient teams and with the staff who assess patients presenting in the casualty department with acute mental health

Crisis Resolution and Home Treatment in Mental Health, ed. Sonia Johnson, Justin Needle, Jonathan P. Bindman and Graham Thornicroft. Published by Cambridge University Press. © Cambridge University Press 2008.

problems. These staff are often called mental health liaison teams. Therefore, CRTs should not be isolated groups, working to their own distinct agenda, but should ideally be an integrated component of a local acute mental healthcare system (Chapter 7), in which shared aims and clearly defined care pathways facilitate continuity of care throughout the service.

In some areas, specific models have been developed to promote joint working between CRTs and hospital services. As this chapter will discuss, these have involved rotating or sharing staff and joint assessment work with inpatient staff, liaison teams and day hospital services (Chapter 22). If we think of acute care services as lying on a spectrum, at one end would be completely separate CRTs, inpatient wards and liaison, day care and community care teams, at the other an integrated acute care service with staff moving fluidly between each component as required, one point of entry/assessment to the service and each element of the service involved in care and discharge planning. Currently, most parts of the UK probably operate a model that lies somewhere towards the 'separate services' end of the spectrum.

Early discharge within an effective acute care system

In order to have an impact on length of stay for people who have been admitted, CRTs need to remain involved after admission so as to identify the point when the initial obstacles to successful home treatment have to some extent resolved and continuing treatment at home may be feasible. In order for early discharge to be used effectively and safely, it is essential that CRTs and inpatient services enjoy a good working relationship, and that ward staff fully understand the process of early discharge and the role of the team in shortening admissions. One possible misconception of the CRT's role is that it picks up the patient at the point of discharge, when the crisis has fully resolved. If a CRT operated in this way, it would not be providing an alternative to hospital care, but rather it would be prolonging the period of acute care unnecessarily. Prompt provision of continuing care and support in the community following discharge for a patient who is no longer experiencing a crisis should generally be the role of the team that will care for the patient long term (e.g. a community mental health team (CMHT)), not of the CRT.

While the threshold for management of risk within the CRT is high, there will always be cases where inpatient treatment cannot be avoided, whether for the duration of a crisis or only in the initial stages until the threat to self or others has reduced to a level that can be safely managed at home (Chapter 8). In some cases, an aspect of the home situation, such as a carer's need for respite, may have necessitated an admission, and discharge can only occur when this has been addressed. Regular communication between CRTs and ward staff is essential. In this way, the patient's progress can be followed and both teams can agree on the point at which discharge to the team should occur. The level of communication can vary but should occur at least weekly, with the CRT visiting the ward in order to discuss each patient's progress and suitability for home treatment. Weekly ward rounds may be a convenient time for this to be discussed, although within a more cohesive system of acute care, communication should occur more frequently and within less formal settings (in addition to planned meetings), allowing better and swifter communication about the appropriateness of early discharge. Rotation of staff between services also enhances liaison between the teams.

Early discharge will be promoted by having the same senior psychiatrist retain overall responsibility for care throughout the crisis period, whether the patient is being treated at home or in hospital. This element is common to all of the service models we describe below. The ways in which consultant psychiatrists work across services and the extent to which they work closely with CRTs varies considerably. Models include:

- senior psychiatrists dedicated to CRT work only, which maximises such expert input to the team but may be less successful in terms of continuity of care
- psychiatrists dedicated to acute care, including inpatient and CRT care
- psychiatrists working with CRTs and with CMHTs
- psychiatrists working across all the components of a sector service, taking responsibility for patients receiving inpatient, CRT and continuing community care.

Psychiatrists dedicated only to CRTs maximise their availability and influence within these teams, but from the perspective of early discharge, there are considerable advantages to structures where the same psychiatrist is responsible for both inpatient and CRT patients. This senior psychiatrist should generally have at least weekly dedicated sessions with the team, which not only facilitates appropriate early discharges from hospital but also supports the team in acting as gatekeeper to hospital beds. In the case of patients who have not had previous contact with mental health services, or who are not under the Care Programme Approach[1] at the time of crisis, the CRT psychiatrist consults on care during their period of treatment by the team.

Box 15.1 summarises the essential elements of a successful early discharge system.

---

[1] The Care Programme Approach was introduced by the UK Government in 1991 and provides a framework for assessment of needs and care planning.

> **Box 15.1. Essential components of a successful early discharge service**
>
> - Clear systems for regular and frequent face-to-face contact between CRT and inpatient team.
> - CRT and inpatient team understand clearly the other's remit and ways of working.
> - Effective systems for transferring information between teams, including, if possible, easy access to shared electronic records and/or summaries of risk and history in electronic form.
> - Multidisciplinary meetings at which clear joint care plans are agreed, involving inpatient and CRT staff, as well as other key staff involved with patients, such as CMHT care coordinators and carers.
> - Experience of joint working between the teams, including conducting joint assessments with patients and carers.

Determining whether early discharge is appropriate

One general requirement for early discharge is that patients should be willing to work with the team and should prefer to, or at least be willing to, continue receiving treatment outside hospital. Where carers are involved, they should be willing to accept the patient back home at the point when early discharge is being considered. Patients need access to accommodation that, even if temporary, must be stable for the duration of treatment. Where a CRT has access to community crisis beds in a hostel or flat (Chapter 23), the immediate concerns regarding accommodation are addressed and treatment can take place outside hospital. The risk factors that indicated hospital admission in the first instance (Chapters 8 and 9) should have resolved to a point where home treatment can safely be considered. At the same time, CRT support following discharge is only appropriate if there is still a need for intensive home treatment, for example because of persisting positive symptoms or elevated mood, or because there is an immediate need for a family to receive substantial support and education if they are to sustain their role as carers. Case study 15.1 illustrates the process of negotiating and planning early discharge by describing an example of a patient's journey through the acute system.

Care planning may involve an initial period of leave from the hospital rather than complete discharge, and in England and Wales, Section 17 of the Mental Health Act, which allows a time-limited period of home leave for compulsorily detained patients, may be used. Carers should be involved as much as possible throughout, including attending professional meetings.

Features that facilitate successful early discharge are:

- patient has reasonable insight into need for treatment
- patient would definitely prefer to be at home
- stable accommodation is available, even if temporary
- carers feel able to receive patient back home
- patient agrees with the short-term care plan and is willing and able to adhere to treatment.

CASE STUDY 15.1. A PATIENT'S JOURNEY THROUGH THE ACUTE CARE SYSTEM

Mary is 30-year-old woman of white UK origin who was admitted to an acute mental health inpatient ward after presenting to the casualty department of the local general hospital. She had been ritualistically self-harming and exhibited thought disorder, rapid speech, increased speed of thoughts and delusions involving religious ideas about being sacrificed. She was observed to be responding to auditory hallucinations of God communicating with her. It was noted that she may have misused substances prior to admission. She was known to mental health services and already had an allocated care coordinator in the CMHT.

The severity of her self-harm and the strength of her belief that she should continue this meant that the conclusion from a joint assessment by the CRT and the liaison team was that she should be admitted to hospital. Initially she agreed to admission as a voluntary patient, but she tried to sabotage the treatment of her self-inflicted injuries and attempted further self-harm on the ward, resulting in compulsory detention under Section 2 of the Mental Health Act.

After 10 days support on the ward and treatment with antipsychotic medication, there was a substantial improvement in her mental state, with lessening of her psychotic symptoms, cessation of her self-harm attempts and the recovery of some insight. She expressed a keen desire to be discharged home although she continued to hear sporadic voices and her mood seemed to be becoming increasingly low as her insight increased. Her parents and her sister, with whom she lived, supported her wish to go home. A multidisciplinary meeting was held on the ward, attended by CRT staff, Mary's primary nurse on the ward, her consultant psychiatrist, who was responsible for her care in the CMHT as well as on the ward, and her CMHT care coordinator, who had already had two meetings with her since admission and several telephone discussions with the family. An agreement was reached at this point that early discharge was appropriate, initially on a trial basis. In the first instance, it was agreed she should have a week's trial leave from the ward, after which the effectiveness of home treatment and the appropriateness of final discharge would be considered.

She agreed to work with the CRT, which initially visited her at her family home twice a day. She was reluctant to take another type of medication even though her consultant felt that an antidepressant would be of benefit. It became evident that there were tensions within the family, some of a long-standing nature and others resulting from the recent situation. Several family meetings took place involving different combinations of relatives: interventions provided included psychoeducation for family members who had been unaware of the details of Mary's illness and meetings focused on trying to resolve some immediate family conflicts. Mary's depressed mood gave rise to continuing concerns about suicide risk, so her mental state was closely monitored and her daytime activities carefully planned. She began to re-engage with a local day centre where she had been attending for a number of classes and activities until the recent deterioration in her mental state: CRT staff accompanied her on the first of her visits there and met with the day centre staff to ensure they were aware of current plans and risks.

After a few days at home, Mary agreed to try taking an antidepressant. As well as her frequent contacts with the CRT, she had weekly sessions with the community psychiatric nurse who was her regular care coordinator in her CMHT. These sessions were dedicated to considering Mary's future activities and plans, and psychoeducation regarding the recent relapse. They also used the sessions to develop a relapse-prevention plan, specifying early warning signs and action to be taken in response to these to prevent a further full-blown relapse. The CRT and Mary's mother contributed to this relapse-prevention plan. After just over three weeks of intensive home treatment, the CRT was able to disengage, gradually reduce the number of visits and hand care back to the care coordinator and the CMHT.

Potential pitfalls of using early discharge

It is possible that patients who receive shortened periods of inpatient care might be at risk of early relapse and readmission. Other possible negative outcomes include increased risk behaviours, greater burden on carers and less complete recovery than in hospital. As mentioned above, there is a dearth of evidence around this aspect of home treatment, and we do not know whether readmission is any more likely following early discharge than after a hospital stay of conventional length (i.e. until the crisis has completely resolved), nor is there evidence regarding differences in other clinical and social outcomes. However, early discharge was a component in the CRTs evaluated in the Islington Crisis Studies (Chapter 5): these CRTs overall appeared to result in outcomes similar to or better than conventional care, but the contribution made to this by early discharge cannot be ascertained.

Approaches to integrating the acute care system: three case studies

The approach outlined above is compatible with a variety of organisational relationships between the CRT and the other components of the local service system. However, as previously discussed, it is likely to work more effectively when there is a high level of integration and continuity of care between different components of the acute care system. In this final section, we will use three case studies to illustrate different approaches to ensuring continuity of care across this system. In the first two (Case studies 15.2 and 15.3), one of the main distinctive elements is that a single manager is responsible for more than one element of the local acute care system. In the final example (Case study 15.4), in contrast, the focus has been more on close integration of the services within a small mental health sector, with the senior psychiatrist having a key role in ensuring continuity of care.

CASE STUDY 15.2. THE WEST NORFOLK ACUTE CARE SERVICE

The service in West Norfolk was initially set up in 2003 as a telephone crisis service. A fully operational home treatment service was established in 2004. The local acute care system now has four integrated components:

- an inpatient ward with 30 beds
- a home treatment service
- an acute day-care service
- the liaison team service in the accident and emergency department.

In addition, there is a free telephone helpline that operates at all times and, like the liaison service, is staffed by people from across the acute care service.

The acute services have one overall manager and staff are moved freely from one service to another depending on how busy each is at any given time. The service's catchment area includes both a rural and an urban population, totalling 160 000, with some inpatient beds also provided for a neighbouring Primary Care Trust with a population of 40 000. The total staff complement is 72; most are mental health nurses or support workers.

The service works closely with the 'continuing support team' (community team) and active outreach team and provides additional support through one of its treatment components when this is requested by either of these teams, without performing additional assessments. The community services are thus trusted to judge whether a patient requires treatment within the acute care service.

Approved social workers, who have specific responsibilities in relation to compulsory admissions under the Mental Health Act, work within the community team and provide emergency duty services in the community and within the liaison service. They liaise closely with the acute care service and use all the options available within this system during Mental Health Act assessments.

The community team care coordinator and consultant psychiatrist retain their overall responsibility for care while a patient is being treated by the acute services.

In this way, a high level of integration has been achieved within the local acute care system. Following this, there has been a reduction in the number of inpatient beds in the service's catchment area, from 75 in 2003 to 30 in 2006, with corresponding reductions in admissions (47 to 27 per month), length of stay (27 to 19 days) and occupied bed days (1262 to 573 per month). There has also been a 50% reduction in the overall use of the Mental Health Act over the same period.

CASE STUDY 15.3. THE CITY AND HACKNEY HOME TREATMENT SERVICE (EAST LONDON)

In this inner London service, the main focus has been on achieving close integration between the liaison service in the casualty department and the CRT. An acute service, incorporating both home treatment and a liaison service to the casualty department, was established in 2001. There are now also plans to incorporate an acute day service element, with the existing day hospital changing its role to brief periods of crisis treatment. These three overall services have a single manager. The inpatient unit functions and is managed separately, although there is close liaison between the home treatment team and ward staff, with approximately one-third of their referrals coming from the wards for early discharge.

This acute service serves an inner-city catchment area population of 210 000, with high levels of social deprivation. The home treatment team is divided into two sector teams, one dedicated to the northern part of the London Borough of Hackney, the other to the southern part, which incorporates the City of London. The total staff complement across both sectors is 31 and comprises sixteen nurses, five support workers, four social workers, two occupational therapists and four psychiatrists. The team also currently staffs the liaison service and will staff the planned acute day-care service, although this will necessitate additional recruitment.

One important element of this service is that it does not act as gatekeeper to inpatient beds. It may perform this role in the future, but the fact that, up to now, patients could be admitted without the knowledge of the CRT is thought to have reduced the team's impact on admissions and bed use over the four years it has been operating.

CASE STUDY 15.4. CAMDEN AND ISLINGTON MENTAL HEALTH AND SOCIAL CARE TRUST (NORTH LONDON)

The London Boroughs of Camden and Islington span another deprived inner London area and have been the subject of two major evaluative studies, described in Chapter 5. The main aim in this mental health trust has been to integrate services at the level of small geographical sectors rather than across the acute care system as a whole. Each sector has a population of around 35 000, and one consultant psychiatrist retains responsibility for patients whether they are currently on the ward, under the care of the CRT or receiving continuing care from the CMHT. The first of four CRTs was set up in this inner-city trust in 1999 and the last in 2003. All elements of the acute care service system operate separately in terms of management, staffing and referral procedures. However, the four teams have developed different procedures for early discharge and prioritise it to different degrees. The team serving the North Islington area has developed a particularly strong focus on early discharge. Among the factors influencing this are the good relationships that have grown between the team and inpatient wards, inpatient staff developing a good knowledge of how the CRT works and what its role is, and the enthusiasm of sector consultants. This team has also had an effective gatekeeping role since it was established in 2000. The CRT aims to follow up actively in hospital patients who are not initially judged suitable for home treatment, and to attend ward round reviews with the aim of facilitating early discharge at the earliest opportunity.

There is no transfer of staff between services, although there are plans for the liaison team service to perform some of the CRT's roles in assessing patients on wards for early discharge and in assessing the suitability of patients presenting to the accident and emergency department for home treatment as an alternative to hospital. The CRT complement is 17 full-time equivalent staff, comprising ten nurses, three social workers, two support workers and one junior psychiatrist, with three sessions dedicated to the team by the senior sector psychiatrists.

Key points

- Reliance on inpatient beds can probably be reduced not only by diverting patients from admission but also by promoting early discharge from hospital, although there is a lack of research in this area.
- Very effective liaison between CRTs and ward teams is required for significant numbers of early discharges to be achieved.
- CRTs are best viewed as one element within a local acute care system. Pathways between different elements of this system and the maintenance of continuity of care need to be considered carefully if the system as a whole is to function effectively.
- Patients may be suitable for an early discharge at a stage when the symptoms and psychosocial difficulties underlying the crisis still persist to a degree, but the immediate impediments to home treatment, such as high risks or uncooperativeness with care, have diminished.
- An acute care system may function more effectively where there is integration between its elements, for example between inpatient teams and the CRT, and/or between the CRT and the liaison team in the casualty department. Models that increase integration in this way have been developed though not yet subjected to robust evaluations.

16

Working with repeat users of crisis resolution services

Martin Flowers and Jonathan P. Bindman

Some users of the mental health services experience repeated admissions to hospital, sometimes over many years, and their complex needs mean that a high level of support may be required. In any area served by a crisis resolution team (CRT), there are likely to be some local service users who present in crisis frequently, often out of hours when other mental health services are not available. Consequently, they are likely to be seen many times by the CRT. While this may sometimes reflect gaps in other, more suitable long-term provision (such as assertive outreach teams, or services for people with borderline personality disorder that are sufficiently containing), this is also a group who may benefit considerably from CRT care. Working with the same service users through repeated crises allows the team to develop and refine an effective response to their individual needs, and if the crises are managed well, there is scope for the development of a therapeutic alliance with service users and carers of a strength that is likely to be hard to achieve in a single episode of crisis care. In some cases, it is only after the CRT and service user have worked together in several crises that they develop effective strategies for reducing the frequency of crises or alternative methods of dealing with them.

In this chapter, a case study is used to highlight important aspects of how CRTs can work with repeat service users and how they can engage social systems in crisis management. The management of repeat crises requires collaborative working with other services involved in the client's care, so that effective plans can be developed for containment of crises and transfer back to the regular team.

When working with repeat attenders, the CRT can develop crisis plans that allow the lessons learnt from one crisis to inform the next. These crisis plans will ideally include information on 'relapse signatures' – the patterns evident in repeated crises that enable the team to predict their course and intervene effectively. The CRT

Crisis Resolution and Home Treatment in Mental Health, ed. Sonia Johnson, Justin Needle, Jonathan P. Bindman and Graham Thornicroft. Published by Cambridge University Press. © Cambridge University Press 2008.

will also have the opportunity to work with other services to develop long-term plans that allow crises to be anticipated.

Content of crisis plans

A crisis plan (for all patients, but particularly for those with repeated crises) should:

- provide consistent and clear plans for communication, both between the client and services, and between different services
- outline a coordinated and shared approach by all services that may encounter the client in crisis
- enable reliable and consistent responses to the individual's requests
- aim to prevent hospitalisation as a default response to crises
- avoid having too many people involved, and facilitate cooperation and frequent liaison between all those involved
- help to provide a secure environment that enables and facilitates the development of independence.

The crisis plan needs to be reviewed, both during the period of the crisis and at its end, to ensure that the plan is effective and that lessons are learned from each crisis that can be used in the next. Adequate time is needed for team discussion and shared reflection.

Crisis plans, crisis cards, advance directives and joint crisis plans

The crisis plans typically developed by UK services at present consist of a list of actions to be taken in a crisis. This list is usually drawn up by clinicians, sometimes with limited involvement of the service user. The format of these crisis plans may be driven by standard local documentation or computerised information systems, such as those used to support the Care Programme Approach, the framework which all services in England and Wales are required by law to use for assessing needs and planning care. Such systems tend to require that case managers include a crisis plan in the care plan of all service users, but this does not generally have to be very detailed or well worked out, or to follow a fixed format. Some more developed models of crisis planning, which may helpfully be incorporated in the work of CRTs, will now be described briefly.

Crisis cards – written statements designed to be carried by service users to provide immediate information on preferences in crisis situations – were first developed over 20 years ago by service user organisations. They were intended to ensure that service users' own preferences for treatment in crisis would be known and taken into account at a point when they might be unable to express their choices directly.

A crisis card is a form of advance statement or advance directive. In general, advance directives are declarations made by service users, anticipating a future situation in which the capacity to make decisions might be lost. They are intended to influence the practice of professionals towards treatment plans that are acceptable to the service user. This, therefore, provides a way in which clinicians can be helped to determine what is in a service user's best interests. Because mental health laws in the UK do not specifically require that the clinician consider the client's best interests, in the medicolegal sense, the preferences expressed in the advance statement can be over-ridden by the treating clinician. However, it is increasingly recognised that advance statements are an important way for patients to exercise some dignity and control over their treatment, and that clinicians should respect them unless they can explicitly justify over-riding them.

A more recent development in crisis planning is the 'joint crisis plan'. This is also a form of advance statement but differs from a crisis card in two respects. First, the joint crisis plan is formulated by the service user in collaboration with the care team, the aim being to resolve any conflicts between service user preferences and the care team's views as the plan is being drawn up, rather than leaving them to cause difficulties when a crisis arises. Second, a neutral facilitator works with the service user and care team on development of the plan. Thus, in terms of both clinician and facilitator time, the resources required are greater than when service users are simply asked to prepare a statement for a crisis card. A randomised controlled trial in the UK (Henderson *et al.*, 2004) found that joint crisis plans halved the use of detention under the Mental Health Act (1983): 27% of a group of 80 people without such plans were compulsorily admitted during the study period compared with 13% of 80 people who had them.

Given the pressure under which many CRTs work, it is understandable if they often keep crisis plans as brief as possible. However, when service users present repeatedly in crisis, developing a more sophisticated and detailed joint crisis plan, which takes into account the service user's own view of the crisis and the clinicians' views about what courses of action are most helpful, is likely to be a good investment of resources. Joint crisis planning is a model that may become increasingly useful as CRT practice develops.

Relapse prevention

A further approach that may be particularly useful in responding to repeat service users is relapse-prevention work, in which triggers to relapses of mental illness and early warning signs are identified and strategies for preventing or attenuating the severity of such relapses developed (Birchwood *et al.*, 2000). The accounts of the service user, their social network and the clinicians who have come into contact with them during relapses are combined to produce a detailed description of the relapse signature and the characteristic pattern followed by a relapse, and a detailed plan for how all involved should respond at each stage of relapse. Typically, CRTs only see people at a relatively late stage of relapse, so that the involvement of others who have seen the service user at an early stage is also likely to be required, but CRTs will often have an important role in contributing to and, sometimes, initiating relapse-prevention work.

People with borderline personality disorder

The considerations already discussed apply as much to people with personality disorders as to those with other problems, but there are some additional issues with this group. People with borderline personality disorder who present frequently to casualty departments following self-harm, or to mental health services with suicidal ideation, may be repeatedly referred to CRTs. Given that many of them are frequently admitted to hospital during such crises, they meet the basic criteria for CRT involvement. However, as with other services they try to make use of, they are often rejected by CRTs or, if accepted, are regarded with some ambivalence regarding whether they are 'appropriate' recipients of the service. Services may even set out specifically to exclude them from CRT care. This is unfortunate, as there are many situations where a hospital admission may be appropriately avoided by CRT involvement (see also Chapter 10). As with other frequent CRT users, repeated contacts may allow for the development of a therapeutic relationship that speeds up assessment, contains the anxieties of the team and the client alike and allows brief but effective interventions. Recurrent contact with the CRT may also be used to develop better crisis plans for the individual, which may reduce the need for crisis care over the longer term.

One respect in which the needs of people with borderline personality disorder may differ from those of other groups of recurrent CRT users is that, because of the difficulty in forming appropriate attachments experienced by most people with this diagnosis, they may find it particularly difficult to relate to multiple members of the team, something which is usually required by the shift pattern of working. 'Splitting' may result, with the client attempting to develop a very close relationship with some members of the team while rejecting others as unhelpful. If the team tries to deal with this by allocating only a limited group of workers to the client, the problem may be exacerbated, with some staff perceiving the client as a 'special' patient and reacting with hostility to what is felt as a threat to team cohesiveness. The CRT must be alert to the development of a situation, fortunately not common, in which their involvement actually destabilises such clients and contributes to a pattern of recurrent crises.

The solution to such problems should be individual to the client, but it is important to consider how the client's distress can best be contained within a single, or very limited number of, therapeutic relationships. If the client already has a containing relationship with a particular consultant, care coordinator or psychotherapist, it may be best to avoid CRT involvement in favour of encouraging the earliest possible contact with the regular worker, even if this means that some clients need to be admitted to hospital overnight in crisis. If the client has no containing relationship, though CRTs may play useful roles in recurrent crises, the CRT should also be trying to support the development of suitable containing relationships with other parts of the service over the longer term.

A case study

The remainder of this chapter is devoted to a case study that demonstrates some clinical strategies which may allow CRTs to promote change in coping strategies and in patterns of service use among frequent users of mental health services.

Presentation

The first time the CRT received a referral for John was when he was referred for a hospital admission after once again having been taken to the accident and emergency department on a Section 136 of the Mental Health Act (this provides for the police to take to hospital someone they find in a public place and suspect of being mentally ill). He had been involved in a fight in a local bar, was angry and aggressive and was not taking medication that had been prescribed for him.

History

John was 57 years old and had had 22 admissions to hospital over a period of 27 years, with relapses of a schizophrenic illness. An only child, he was living with his mother in council accommodation. His father had died many years previously. John was unemployed and had not worked for 30 years.

Care plan

He had a care coordinator from the local community mental health team (CMHT) and had a good relationship with him when well. His written care plan stated that he needed to be admitted to hospital when the following relapse signature was present: 'stops taking medication, starts to drink heavily, begins to experience auditory hallucinations of a derogatory nature, becomes irritable and hostile, threatens to self-harm including OD of prescribed medication'.

Risks

Records indicated that he had committed several acts of violence towards others in the context of drinking in local bars and responding to auditory hallucinations. He had been brought to the local accident and emergency department by the police under Section 136 of the Mental Health Act on six such occasions.

Pattern of admissions prior to involvement of the crisis resolution team

His admissions to hospital were typically of three to four weeks in duration, during which time he would stop drinking heavily and re-start antipsychotic medication, which he was happy to do. When well, John was a gentle man who was very upset and embarrassed about his behaviour in crisis.

Involvement of the crisis resolution team

The CRT was able to treat John at home and break the existing pattern of admissions. A lengthy assessment at the point of crisis, with a social systems focus (Chapter 12), suggested that many of John's difficulties, his deteriorating mental health and his subsequent behavioural problems, stemmed from his worries about his mother, Helen, who was 86 years old and had been suffering from a chest infection. John was concerned that he was a burden on her and had contributed to her illness. He also began to express fears about how he would cope if and when she died. When the CRT spoke to Helen, she also expressed fears about what would become of John once she was unable to care for him.

A full review of John's psychiatric history revealed that many of his 22 hospital admissions had taken place over the previous 10 years, and on discussion with John and his mother it appeared that admissions were correlated with periods when she was not well. This had been alluded to in case notes, but the significance of this connection seemed to have been less apparent during hospital admissions than to the CRT, which had a high level of contact with Helen at home visits.

John's hospitalisation increased his fears and his anger, driving a wedge between him and the hospital staff. Once he had stabilised on the ward, the situation at home had usually eased as well and the fears of both John and Helen at the time of the crisis were not expressed when it came to planning John's follow-up care.

Repeated contact with the crisis resolution team

After an initial period of contact with the CRT, which successfully averted hospital admission, crises recurred on several occasions over the next four years, and John became a frequent user of the team, with which he became well engaged. The team was able to develop a crisis plan in partnership with his mother and the CMHT care coordinator.

The issues that needed to be addressed included beginning a dialogue between John and Helen about her physical health, and helping John to understand her needs when she was ill and how his behaviour affected her well-being. John needed to express to his mother his fears about the future and how these affected his mental health. These discussions helped them to understand the repeating patterns of his relapses and allowed them the safe space needed to plan for the future. This included some very difficult subjects, such as where John would reside after Helen died.

John's care coordinator was involved in some of these meetings and was active in developing plans at the time of crises and in ensuring they were seen through once John had been discharged by the CRT back to continuing CMHT care. Other members of the social system were involved over time, including the general practitioners of both John and Helen, and John's aunt, who was very involved with the family.

John's response to stressful situations was discussed and it became clear to everyone that he found it difficult or embarrassing to say when he was upset or worried. Furthermore, he did not want to 'be a nuisance or worry anybody'. Over time, work with the CRT and the care coordinator helped John to discover the paradox that, in his attempts to 'not be a worry', he used coping mechanisms, such as heavy drinking, which caused great distress to himself and his mother.

Strategies to promote change in his responses were discussed. An early plan was that he should contact the CMHT by telephone early in the development of a crisis. The initial effect of this plan was that he called the CMHT very frequently about a range of life problems, major and minor, was put through to different team members and received confusing and conflicting advice at times. He also called the CRT out of hours when not under their care, including on occasions when he was drunk or threatening self-harm. This caused them the not uncommon difficulty with people who move repeatedly from CMHT to CRT and back, of deciding whether his level of crisis made it more appropriate to respond or to direct him back to the CMHT. Shared relapse-prevention and crisis plans were developed at joint multidisciplinary meetings between the CMHT and CRT, and these helped both teams to give consistent advice and to assess the appropriate level of response. Gradually boundaries were established around the use of telephone contact, and he made more effective use of his care coordinator in heading off crises, only calling the CRT when in treatment with them.

It was only after involvement of the CRT over a number of periods of crisis that it was possible to address fully the painful question of what should happen to John, and to the tenancy of their shared home, when his mother died. Other important areas of work included development of a detailed understanding of his drinking behaviour, leading to a drinking partner becoming involved in supporting him and alerting the CMHT when his drinking increased sharply, and to an understanding of his erratic use of medication during the development of a crisis, which was helped by the use of a dosette box.

Over four years, the periods between crises lengthened, his night-time phone calls stopped almost completely, he worked far more closely with his care coordinator and was able to manage his difficulties effectively. A clear plan was established about what would happen when Helen eventually died, including where John would live. This was reassuring for the whole family and John's social system, and clarified the role of the CRT in his future care.

Key points

- For repeat service users, CRTs are well placed to achieve gradual change by a consistent approach through a series of crises. The crisis provides an opportunity for understanding underlying problems in social systems and developing strategies to prevent or attenuate future crises.
- The CRTs, CMHTs, service users and their social networks can work together to develop crisis plans, test them and refine them. Joint crisis plans and relapse prevention are particularly useful models for management of repeat users of CRTs.
- All CRTs are under pressure to treat and discharge quickly, but a substantial proportion of patients will be seen more than once, and effective relationships can be built over time.
- Recurrent crises do not generally reflect failure of either the CMHT or the CRT. Patterns of behaviour leading to crises that have developed over many years may take years of careful collaborative work to change.

REFERENCES

Birchwood, M., Spencer, E. and McGovern, D. (2000). Schizophrenia: early warning signs. *Advances in Psychiatric Treatment*, **6**, 93–101.

Henderson, C., Flood, C., Leese, M. *et al*. (2004). Effect of joint crisis plans on use of compulsory treatment in psychiatry: single blind randomised controlled trial. *British Medical Journal*, **329**, 136–40.

Mental Health Act (1983). London: HMSO.

17

Responding to diversity in home treatment

Danny Antebi, Waquas Waheed, Sonia Johnson
and Lisa Marrett

When patients are treated in their own homes rather than in an institutional setting, their social circumstances and identities are necessarily much more visible and salient. This offers very valuable opportunities to assess social determinants of the crises, to deliver interventions that are appropriate to clients' social and cultural needs and to engage the key members of their social networks in the management of their mental health problems. Considerable challenges accompany these opportunities. Home treatment clinicians cannot avoid having their own values and preconceptions challenged by the great range of ways of living and thinking that they will find among patients and their social networks, and adapting interventions so that they are appropriate to the full range of clients' values and social circumstances requires considerable imagination and sensitivity to diversity. In this chapter, we will explore the ways in which crisis resolution teams (CRTs) can try to respond effectively to clients' diverse needs. Our main focus will be on responding to ethnic, religious and cultural variations, but in the latter part of the chapter, we will also address gender-specific needs and home treatment for gay men and lesbians.

Ethnic diversity: background and current service provision

Migrants from Asia, Africa, eastern Europe and the Caribbean Islands permanently reside as ethnic minorities in many Western countries. Numbers both of asylum seekers and economic migrants have substantially increased, driven by wars and global political upheavals and by economic disparities. The UK Census (Office for National Statistics, 2001) indicated that the proportion of the population belonging to a non-White minority ethnic group increased by 53% between 1991 and 2001, from 3 million to 4.6 million (or 7.9% of the total UK population), and similar demographic changes have occurred in many European countries.

Crisis Resolution and Home Treatment in Mental Health, ed. Sonia Johnson, Justin Needle, Jonathan P. Bindman and Graham Thornicroft. Published by Cambridge University Press. © Cambridge University Press 2008.

Ethnic disparities in mental healthcare have been a significant focus of concern in recent UK policy (Department of Health, 2003). South Asian minority groups report significantly higher levels of psychological distress and lack of social support, particularly among immigrant women from Pakistan (Weich *et al.*, 2004). In younger women of Asian family origin, rates of deliberate self-harm (Cooper *et al.*, 2006) and completed suicide have been rising over the years. The suicide rate among young Asian women is reportedly twice the national average (Khan and Waheed, 2006).

Reasons documented for this higher prevalence are housing problems, lack of social support, unemployment, racism, low literacy levels, lack of English language skills and marital and family relationship problems (different traditional or religious expectations, including beliefs on marriage, divorce, widowhood and family honour) (Chew-Graham *et al.*, 2002). Another important factor is that symptoms of depression in South Asian patients seem to persist for longer periods and follow a chronic course. The main reason for this may be lack of treatment seeking, treatment provision and/or adherence in this group. This leads to poor resolution of symptoms and hence higher prevalence (Husain *et al.*, 1997).

Patients of African-Caribbean and Black African family origin have higher rates of compulsory treatment and more complex pathways into mental healthcare (Bhui and Bhugra, 2002). Compared with White patients, they are admitted at three times the rate to medium-secure units (Maden *et al.*, 1999) and eight times more to high-secure units (Leese *et al.*, 2006). Younger African-Caribbean men with psychosis report a lower level of satisfaction with services (Parkman *et al.*, 1997). Increased rates of psychosis have been reported among people from Black ethnic minorities in the UK and various other countries with White majorities, with social factors such as discrimination and social defeat prominent among the possible explanations (Selten and Cantor-Graae, 2005).

The complexity of the needs of the UK migrant population is increased by its fluidity, and demographic data quickly become out-dated with new influxes and indeed outward migrations. For example, Eastern Europeans now constitute a substantial part of the UK population, but research on their mental health needs is as yet unavailable. A group with particularly complex needs is asylum seekers and refugees, for whom the stresses associated with migration and experiences of social exclusion in the UK are often compounded by the effects of trauma and loss, resulting in high levels of unmet need among those in contact with mental health services (McColl and Johnson, 2006).

Current service provision

The capacity of current services to respond to diverse needs sensitively and without discrimination is often criticised as limited, perpetuating disparities in access to care and adverse experiences of service contact among minorities. Evidence of inequalities is seen throughout the care pathway, from issues around access and detention rates to recovery and social inclusion. Reasons for these differences are complex and various, and are well-rehearsed elsewhere, but they are likely to include both issues related to the mental health services, such as direct and indirect discrimination, inflexibility of response and lack of appropriate skills, and the more general effects of the social exclusion and racism encountered by minorities in many social contexts.

There is no lack of national legislation and guidance in this area: the Race Relations (Amendment) Act 2000, *Delivering Race Equality in Mental Health Care* (Department of Health, 2005), *Inside Outside* (Department of Health, 2003) and *Breaking the Circles of Fear* (Sainsbury Centre for Mental Health, 2002), to name the most significant. Despite the fact that discrimination has been evident for many years, some argue that to an extent it is a lack of political will, both nationally and locally, that has led to a failure to bring about significant changes in approach. Any efforts that have been made have as yet fallen significantly short of what is needed to bridge the gap.

The way forward

There is an urgent need to review the way mental health services are organised and delivered in order to make them sensitive and responsive to the needs of people from diverse backgrounds. However, the recent emergence of home treatment offers some potential solutions to these problems, with the opportunity for treatment to be delivered in a comparatively non-stigmatising way within familiar, non-threatening surroundings, such as patients' own homes. From an ethnic minority perspective, the issues described above have been among the main reasons for lack of trust in and under-utilisation of mental health services. It is important to address these pivotal issues in the planning and delivery of home treatment services from the very beginning, and to adopt components and strategies which help to ensure that they are culturally sensitive. In this way, the pitfalls encountered by other services may be avoided.

Making home treatment culturally sensitive

In this section, some of the processes that contribute to making home treatment culturally sensitive are discussed. Many of these are relevant to all mental health services, but some are especially salient for crisis resolution teams (CRTs). Some of these processes are illustrated in Case study 17.1.

CASE STUDY 17.1. CULTURALLY SENSITIVE HOME TREATMENT PRACTICES

A 30-year-old Somali woman has been referred by a general practitioner (GP). She has four children under seven years, the youngest being 10 months. She has been in the UK for 18 months and speaks no English; her only support appears to be her husband. She told her GP through her husband that she was having visions of blood and graves and could hear dead people talking to her. The GP has referred her as psychotic and had initiated antipsychotic medication.

At first contact, the CRT should:

- arrange an interpreter, ensuring they speak the correct language
- arrange the assessment separately from the children as far as is possible
- ensure the husband is able to be present for part of the interview
- clarify the patient's legal status
- clarify her religion and ensure gender of assessor is considered.

The CRT should talk to the health visitor/GP prior to assessment.

Assessment should cover the following issues:

- be mindful of the husband as family spokesperson (it can be easy to offend) but bear in mind that it may also be valuable for her to speak to staff without him being present
- clarify how she wishes to be referred to and how her name should be recorded
- gain information about why and how she left Somalia
- gain information about her experience in the UK
- ask about khat[1] use: social or solitary use, does she chew all day?
- any history of mental illness in Somalia and her experience of that (e.g. hospitalisations)
- role of her extended family.

Outcome.   The assessors feel that this is the first occurrence of mental health problems. The woman is currently experiencing significant psychosocial stresses with a lack of social support and she has been expressing her distress and depression the only way she knows how and thought the assessors might understand. It is concluded that she is probably not psychotic. Of particular note is the fact that her mother and extended family were a prominent support during the first year of bringing up her other children. Loss of contact with them has exacerbated her social isolation.

Initial intervention will include the following:

- arrange increased support for the older children
- arrange contact with local Somali support groups
- review the appropriateness of current medication
- arrange some individual support for her to talk about her distress
- review on a daily basis initially.

---

[1] A shrub with mild stimulant properties that is chewed or taken as tea by many people with Somali, Ethiopian and Yemeni backgrounds. Its legal status varies from country to country and an association with psychosis is suspected.

Organisational structure and policy

Mental health providers in the UK are now obliged to address diversity in areas such as training, recruitment, service improvement and audit. Organisations have an obligation to work towards ensuring cultural competence in all processes and procedures. O'Hagan (2001) described cultural competence as

The ability to maximise sensitivity and minimise insensitivity in the service of culturally diverse communities, and its successful application will depend a great deal upon cultural awareness, attitudes and approach. The workers need not be, as is often assumed, highly knowledgeable about the cultures of the people they work with, but must approach culturally different people with openness and respect – a willingness to learn. Self awareness is *the* most important component in the knowledge base of culturally competent practice.

If this approach is to be effective, local teams must own the process of working towards cultural competence in the operational detail of organisational systems and service delivery, and the practice of individual staff must be based on the openness and respect that O'Hagan described and on awareness of the characteristics and needs of the population that their team serves.

Staff recruitment

The aim of recruiting a diverse workforce across all UK public services has not proved easy to achieve. There is provision within the UK Race Relations Act (Section 5 (2)d) for the recruitment of staff such as support workers from specific minorities who are highly represented in the local community, but it is questionable whether official encouragement to make use of this opportunity has had a significant impact. Both services and user groups struggle with dilemmas such as whether the team should reflect its client base or the population it serves? Rather than engaging in this debate, change is more likely to occur when teams focus on embedding an approach in which prejudices and assumptions are examined, both individually and on a team basis. Creating such a team culture will have a positive impact upon service delivery and relationships with service users and the community. This may well also have a positive long-term impact on recruitment. Awareness and mindfulness of diversity must drive recruitment, and this is likely to produce a workforce that, through reflective practice, is able to deliver home treatment to a diverse population. Nevertheless, how and where jobs are advertised should be considered, and guidance sought from local minority communities.

Staff training and attitudes

Responding to diversity is not the realm of the specialist, but the duty of all practitioners. The purpose of training should be to promote culturally competent practice through self-awareness. Such training contributes to the development of a working environment and practices that enable individuals to change attitudes and behaviour, especially where they have statutory powers conferred on them. Diversity training should not be seen as a separate, add-on topic; rather, the importance of diversity awareness should be emphasised in training generally. This does not mean that race and diversity must be covered within every course, but that trainers should consider the issues relevant to the subject covered, thereby 'mainstreaming' diversity into all training. The approach should, therefore, be one of bringing diversity into training rather than training in diversity.

Training alone can never achieve necessary organisational change. Line managers and team leaders need to be not only culturally competent themselves but also trained in addressing cultural competence with individual staff and within team cultures. Their training should also emphasise legislation and policy frameworks, including relevant employment legislation, methods for challenging discrimination, responsibilities under the Race Relations (Amendment) Act 2000, how to implement race equality schemes, service benchmarking and equality impact assessment training.

As a starting point for training, an introduction to the culture and traditions of local ethnic communities is important, particularly as the staff will be working with the patients and their families inside their homes. There is huge ethnic variation in the ways people live their lives, for example in greeting strangers and showing courtesy. Seemingly innocent acts may, through lack of knowledge, be seen as inappropriate and can adversely effect the therapeutic relationship. Specific training programmes have been created for health professionals for this purpose and have been found to be effective (Dogra, 2001). We live in an increasingly multicultural society and, therefore, assessment procedures must increasingly be appropriate for cross-cultural application. Staff need to be trained in carrying out assessments across cultures and to be aware of potential obstacles and techniques to overcome these (Bhui and Bhugra, 1997).

As well as having awareness of culture and traditions, it is helpful for staff to have some knowledge of the history of important local migrant groups, and of the main reasons why they have left their homelands and settled in the UK. It is crucial, however, that such awareness is accompanied by vigorous avoidance of making stereotypical assumptions about the values and lifestyles of service users based purely on nationality or ethnic group. Rather, staff need always to be aware of the great complexity of identities that occur, above all in metropolitan areas where a very wide range of groups live alongside one another. Ethnic group is a very blunt tool for understanding ways of living or thinking: the Black African category used in the UK Census encompasses a great continent with vast variations in culture, religion, language, economic situation and tradition. Within the Caribbean, different islands have very distinct histories and cultures. Even where people share countries of origin, nationality and religious affiliation, their social circumstances in the countries from which they come may have been very different: a polyglot university professor and a shepherd with limited literacy skills cannot be assumed to share a world view and way of life just because they come from the same place. In the UK, degrees of acculturation vary greatly, especially among second and subsequent generations of migrants, some of whom may have largely adopted the values and ways of living of the country in which they have grown up. People with mixed origins are also more and more highly represented in European populations. Social class, educational background, professional identity, sexuality and, in particular, religious affiliation may all be at least as salient as elements in many people's social identities as their ethnic backgrounds. Thus, while a broad awareness of the cultures and traditions to be found among local ethnic groups is a useful tool for staff in seeking to understand patients' social situations, they above all need an open, curious and unprejudiced approach to exploring and seeking to understand each individual's narrative and the complexities of their identities.

Approaching change

An early task when considering the cultural competence of the team is to gain a sense of its strengths and weaknesses. Tools for organisational analysis such as 'appreciative inquiry' (Bushe and Coetzer, 1995) and 'process mapping' (Damielo, 2006) help to generate an overview of the system and how it behaves in practice. This assessment must take into account the perspectives of all interested parties, including service users, carers and other agencies such as voluntary sector organisations that work with minority groups. It is not a 'consultation' but a sharing of agendas and priorities. Where in the care pathway does the service respond thoughtfully, and where inflexibly? Carefully mapping the care pathway in collaboration with other parties highlights not only areas of agreement about change but also points along the pathway where the aspirations of the service and of the patient may diverge. This can provide a focus for dialogue and the development of possible solutions. Points along the pathway that can be easily audited can also be identified.

First contact

A crucial factor in the development of therapeutic relationships between patients and staff is the quality of first contact between service users and statutory organisations. This is often the point in the engagement process when trust and confidence between service users and services are either won or lost. Current models of service delivery mean that early contact is often made by a CRT. Consequently, the manner in which such teams respond to a diverse population will be a significant factor in the longer-term outcome of intervention by services. Ideally, practitioners should prepare for the first contact carefully. They should remember that service users from minority ethnic backgrounds may be feeling particularly vulnerable. As well as suffering from mental health problems, they may be anxious about how they will be treated and whether they will be stereotyped in any way. Acknowledgment of and respect for such vulnerability will contribute to confidence building.

The preparation for first contact should involve consideration of language requirements, physical disabilities and the domestic situation, for example whether the client is a single mother with young children. It is important to understand the family structure as early as possible and identify the person likely to act as family spokesperson. Good preparation will ensure that the assessment occurs in the right place, at the right time and with the right people present, and that it addresses the right issues, including, for example, immediate social problems such as housing and uncertain immigration status and important aspects of personal histories, such as past persecution or torture.

Matching patients with therapists

Some patients will request a worker who shares their own perspective. For example, a Black patient may prefer a Black worker, a Christian patient may want someone who shares their religious views, or a female patient may request a female worker. These are always difficult decisions, and our current practices are inconsistent. Most people would be comfortable with a woman who has a history of sexual abuse requesting a female worker, whereas a White patient requesting a White worker immediately raises the spectre of a racist motive. Similarly, a member of staff who is gay may be put in a very difficult position through seeing an overtly homophobic patient. Decisions taken by teams in response to such situations are inevitably value-laden and as such leave huge scope for discrimination. It is, therefore, important that teams have in place a transparent and standardised process for responding to such requests. They may, in any case, often not be in a position to respond to a specific request because suitable staff are not available: this needs to be carefully and respectfully explained to patients, and it may be possible to find other solutions, such as involvement in the care plan of staff from appropriate voluntary sector organisations.

Language and interpreters

It can be difficult enough describing distressing experiences in a way that can be understood using one's first language, but many service users have to do this in a second language or through an interpreter. This leaves both patient and assessor at a disadvantage, and it is easy to envisage a misunderstanding about symptoms leading to diagnostic error. Distress may be described, for example, in terms of 'having visions' and it can be difficult in such cases to determine whether these are psychotic hallucinations.

The role of interpreters is a complex one (Phelan and Parkman, 1995). Clinicians may feel de-skilled and are often unsure how to accommodate a third party in an assessment and treatment process. Interpreters may have difficulty remaining neutral and may perceive themselves as advocates for the patient, whereas mental health staff may expect them to adopt a neutral position. Therefore, establishing a working relationship with the interpreter in which the expectations of each party are negotiated is an essential part of preparation. It is sometimes necessary for a family member to act as an interpreter because there is no other option, but this should be avoided unless there is no good alternative, as some objectivity may be lost. Care is needed in establishing that the interpreter does indeed speak the patient's first language: confusion not infrequently arises where a country has a variety of national languages, and sometimes it is necessary to ensure that the interpreter speaks not only the right language but the right dialect in order to be confident of full comprehension. Interpreters should have some knowledge of the environment from which the patient has come. Historical community conflicts can mean that two people from the same country may be highly suspicious of each other, for example recently following the war in Rwanda. Interpreters and staff of local voluntary organisations, as well as online sources such as news sites and the UK Foreign Office, can help staff to understand such complexities better – it is also helpful for staff to get into the habit of reading good-quality media reports about events in the areas of the world from which local asylum seeker groups come.

The Care Programme Approach and risk assessment

UK CRTs will always be working within the framework of the nationally mandated Care Programme Approach, which sets out requirements for assessment of needs and written formulation of care plans for secondary mental health service users. The recording of information is an essential part of this and should be culturally sensitive, for instance when asking for and recording people's names, which may not conform to a familiar format. Understanding family structures, belief systems and previous negative experiences of mental health services, either in the UK or in the country of origin, is essential in delivering a good care plan.

The use of risk assessment is sometimes seen as a negative, stigmatising and ultimately harmful process, particularly by ethnic minorities, and this is arguably a consequence of the way it has been used. It must, therefore, be employed in a way that does not discriminate. We all stereotype and make assumptions about others, and these will be reflected in our approach to patients. Stereotyping can be reduced by ensuring that the actuarial part of the risk assessment is accurate and factual. For example, 'stories' about a previous assault should be checked as far as is possible. Access to accurate conviction records is essential. Approaching risk assessment and management collaboratively throughout the Care Programme Approach process (i.e. with the service user and support network involved wherever possible) is more likely to promote a therapeutic engagement. This will lead to improved outcomes and ultimately a reduction in risk. Collaborative working will also promote a culturally sensitive approach, thereby reducing labelling and preconceptions.

Interventions provided

Where medication is part of the treatment plan, staff need to bear in mind that differences in explanatory models of mental health problems may lead people from some backgrounds to be particularly sceptical about medication and inclined not to adhere to it. Providing information in multiple languages is necessary, covering the purpose of the treatments, the likely delays in improvement of symptoms once medication is initiated, dose titration and likely side effects. With regard to non-pharmacological interventions, in the NHS there has historically been a lack of provision of psychological therapies for patients in general, and for those with a limited grasp of English in particular. Innovative approaches to delivering psychological interventions, such as via the telephone if local linguistic expertise is not available, should be explored.

Collaborative working with families

It is extremely important to work closely with families, as often they have more influence in the day-to-day life of people from certain ethnic minorities than is typical in the indigenous population. Their explanatory models of illness need to be explored in order to engage them with a collaborative care plan, and their levels of English literacy taken into account.

Collaborative working with the voluntary sector and communities

In terms of access, the voluntary sector can act as a route into services and should be viewed as an essential component of the care pathway. Patients may feel more comfortable in a non-statutory environment and may prefer to present themselves to and be supported by such agencies and by groups other than statutory health services. To achieve the best possible engagement, there needs to be a working relationship between statutory and voluntary sectors. That relationship will consist of formal agreements or practices, for example information sharing, and informal agreements, such as using their premises for assessment.

Special considerations

Specialist ethnic minority services

The fact that certain groups receive different levels of service has led to the emergence of some services directed at specific populations, such as the Antenna Outreach Service (McKenzie, 2003), and the debate about whether certain groups should have separate services continues (Bhui and Sashidharan, 2003). There are advantages and disadvantages to this approach but, given the large number of groups represented in the populations served by many services, establishing specific services for each main group is often not very practical. However, a degree of specialisation may be helpful in managing such diversity. In order to respond to and engage a diverse population, it is generally not necessary to establish specialist home treatment services; CRTs should instead approach this through reflective and flexible working practices. There may, however, be a need to consider innovative arrangements for access to services and assessment for particular groups: one way of developing this may be through access to a specialist 'cultural consultation' team, whose remit is to support other teams in culturally sensitive service development and in complex assessments where cultural factors appear important (Waheed *et al.*, 2003).

Refugees and asylum seekers

The legal position of asylum seekers and refugees may complicate and limit the range of interventions the CRT can deliver; for example, failed asylum seekers usually have limited access to benefits, housing and primary care. This group is particularly vulnerable to developing mental health problems, and services have a duty to respond to acute presentations of illness. Particular care should be taken about making assumptions concerning motive for presenting. Someone reporting suicidal ideation may do so in the contexts of despair or depression, or as a political gesture – any or all of these may be true. This is when relationships with community groups are invaluable: they may know the person and can help to promote understanding of the situation and development of a support package.

Audit and evaluation

Audit and evaluation address the gap between what has been shown to be effective and what is actually practised. The starting point is to be clear about the strategic and operational objectives of the team; for example, whether the team is an assessment service, a home treatment service or a gatekeeper to acute inpatient beds. Performance objectives should then be set and the team's practices evaluated against them (Box 17.1). Some of these, such as reduction in

> **Box 17.1. Examples of practices suitable for audit**
>
> - Provision of multilingual materials.
> - Rates of referral for Mental Health Act assessments for minority ethnic people compared with others.
> - Prevalence of service users requesting interpreters and their availability when required.
> - Pathways to care among service users. Are ethnic groups at higher risk of adverse pathways such as via the police or the courts? Do Asian women make use of primary care to gain access to services or are they referred via voluntary sector organisations?
> - Extent to which service use by ethnic minorities reflects the composition of the underlying population.
> - Comparison between satisfaction among ethnic minority and among White British service users.

use of inpatient beds, are likely to be set by NHS commissioners. The team may also want to set its own objectives, such as ease of referral, outcome of assessments or outcome of interventions. Process mapping will highlight points along the care pathway that are easily identifiable and measurable and, therefore, suitable for audit.

Other aspects of diversity

The focus so far in this chapter has mainly been on diversity in terms of ethnic groups. However, diversity obviously has many other facets, including religion, social class, gender and sexuality. Many of the principles discussed above can also be applied to other aspects of diversity, especially the importance of understanding patients' individual narratives without relying on stereotypes, and of a respectful, self-aware and open attitude to all service users. Some further considerations in working with particular groups follow.

Home treatment for women

Critics of psychiatry's approach to women have suggested that it tends to be based on out-dated gender role stereotypes and that women's social powerlessness is reinforced by explanations in terms of illness for distress that, in fact, results from the discrimination and adverse social circumstances that women often experience (e.g. Showalter, 1987). Home treatment has the potential to serve women better than traditional institutional care, as the social contexts of distress and the diversity of women's roles, experiences and mental health needs may be more visible and ways of delivering services can be flexible (Johnson and Buszewicz, 1996). The benefits of this model for women may be reflected in the finding that availability of CRTs appears to reduce admission rates for women more than for men (Glover *et al.*, 2006). In order to ensure that women do indeed benefit from the availability of CRTs, there are a number of questions that staff should consider regarding every patient.

Does treatment at home mean that current stresses and adverse experiences are perpetuated?

Hospital admission has many disadvantages but can sometimes offer respite from poor home circumstances and difficult and abusive relationships. Experiences such as domestic violence are important factors in women's mental health problems; consequently, resolution of a crisis may require a temporary or permanent refuge from home, either in hospital or in another setting such as a crisis house (Chapter 23) or women's refuge. Therefore, the assumption that remaining at home is always beneficial should be avoided.

What will happen to caring roles during the crisis?

Women are more likely than men to be carers for children or disabled or elderly relatives, and this may have an impact on their mental health. Women with severe mental illness are considerably more likely than their male counterparts to have children. When a crisis involving a woman who is her children's main carer results in hospital admission, some form of assessment of and response to the children's needs generally ensues, albeit not always one that is in the long-term interest of mother or children, as custody loss often occurs at this point. Home treatment offers better possibilities for parental and family relationships to be maintained during the crisis, but this also comes with some hazards. At worst, children may be at risk if there is inadequate assessment of the ability of a woman who is receiving home treatment to continue caring for her children during a crisis. Resolution of a crisis may also be impeded if women do not have any respite from onerous caring roles. With regard to children, CRTs need to develop strong relationships with children and family social services teams and to have protocols in place for prompt assessment and management of women with children, aiming to provide whatever short-term respite and support are needed for the long-term maintenance of caring roles and relationships. Another consideration for home treatment services is the burden that may be placed on women as carers for their patients during crises: carers are often enthusiastic about home treatment, but staff need nonetheless to remember that the risks and burdens they are expected to tolerate during a crisis can sometimes become excessive, especially if they care for someone who experiences recurrent crises (Chapter 16). Carers may themselves have physical and mental health needs that compromise their ability to cope with crises at home, and teams also need to remember that most women in the UK and other northern European countries now work and, therefore, cannot be assumed to be available throughout the day to support patients at home.

Are women's voices clearly heard during assessment and treatment planning?

The need to identify the 'family spokesperson', quite often a male member of the household, among some minority groups has been discussed above. However, it should also be remembered that in both minority and majority groups, household dynamics are sometimes disempowering for women; consequently, their husbands, partners, fathers and sons should not be allowed to speak for them without real efforts being made to establish the women's own views about their needs and experiences. Therefore, CRTs should generally ensure that whenever possible women have some opportunities to talk to staff without other family members being present.

Home treatment for men

In the UK, men now outnumber women on psychiatric wards, greatly so in forensic and secure facilities, and so they are now the sex for whom alternatives to admission are most relevant. However, some evidence is now accumulating that they are less likely to be diverted from admission through CRT care than women (Chapters 3 and 5). The reasons for this need to be better understood. Possibilities include a different diagnostic mix, higher rates of substance misuse, poorer social support, greater actual or perceived risk of violence, and less actual or perceived willingness to engage with services: some, though not all, of these factors are potentially remediable. If men tend more often than women to be assessed as unsuitable for home treatment, we need to establish how far this is based on real clinical and social differences and how far on stereotypes. Men have tended to have fewer advocates for their mental health needs than women, yet evidence of poorer outcomes in illnesses such as psychosis and of a greater tendency for care to be institutional rather than community-based suggests that more attention may be needed to their specific needs and relationships with services.

Gay men and lesbians

Relatively little research has been devoted to the mental health problems and needs of gay men and lesbians, but a recent study suggests increased rates of consultation with mental health professionals, self-harm and recreational drug use among both gay men and lesbians, as well as higher alcohol use among lesbians than heterosexual women (King *et al.*, 2003). Staff should, therefore, be particularly aware of these risks. Growing public acceptance of same-sex relationships and the introduction in many Western countries of legally recognised same-sex marriages and civil partnerships have potential to reduce health inequalities based on sexuality (King and Bartlett, 2006). However, we are not yet at a stage where all gay men and lesbians feel able to be fully open about their sexuality, and CRTs need to be even more focused than usual on privacy and confidentiality in this area. Being treated at home may make it harder for people to conceal their sexuality and significant relationships; consequently, if gay men and lesbians do not feel confident that these will be accepted and understood, they may sometimes be reluctant to engage with CRTs. In order to facilitate (though not force) disclosure of sexuality, CRT staff need to avoid making an automatic assumption that their patients are heterosexual, to convey a consistently open and accepting attitude to gay sexuality, and to make it clear that confidentiality will not be breached, for example where patients' relatives are unaware of their gay relationships. As with other aspects of diversity, avoidance of stereotypes is important: the range of lifestyles, values and sexual behaviours encountered among gay men and lesbians is as wide as among the heterosexual population.

Conclusions

Diversity is an approach and an attitude towards patients that balances their individual needs against those of a highly complex organisational system that will inevitably tend toward inflexibility. Responding to diversity is, however, not a specialism but an obligation for everyone, and the creation of specialists or specialist teams may allow generic services to abrogate responsibility. Working with the great range of groups currently living in the UK and other Western countries is challenging but can also be fascinating: few other jobs offer as rich an opportunity as mental health work to meet, develop relationships with and hear the life stories of people with a vast variety of experiences. Staff who are comfortable with and stimulated by such opportunities will come to regard them as a privilege.

Training and service delivery should emphasise self-awareness, reflection, transparency and respect. These features, rather than a focus on obscure cultural nuances, represent the most important components of culturally competent practice.

CRTs have a special responsibility since they are often the point of first contact and can set the scene for a positive therapeutic relationship between patient and services.

The golden rule is a time-honoured principle that tells us to treat others as we would wish to be treated. Its intentions were sound since it was designed to prevent us from doing harm to others. Yet, with the increasing complexity of society, we cannot simply assume that others need the same things and wish to be treated in the same way as we do, since in doing so we perpetuate the values and beliefs of the dominant culture. We, therefore, now need to go beyond the golden rule and adopt the maxim: treat others as *they* would wish to be treated. This 'platinum rule' respects and values diversity.

Key points

- Respecting, valuing and responding to a diverse population, in terms of characteristics including ethnic group, religion, gender and sexuality, should not be a specialist task but the obligation of all mental health staff.
- Home treatment makes variations in people's ways of life more visible; this offers opportunities to tailor interventions to people's social circumstances, values and networks, but it also challenges clinicians' prejudices and preconceptions.
- Accurate knowledge about cultural variation in values, beliefs and ways of life and about the histories of minorities is helpful, but the most valuable attributes for CRT staff in responding to diversity are unwillingness to stereotype, an awareness of the complexity of people's identities, and an open and respectful attitude to all service users.

REFERENCES

Bhui, K. and Bhugra, D. (1997). Cross-cultural competencies in the psychiatric assessment. *British Journal of Hospital Medicine*, **57**, 492–6.

Bhui, K. and Bhugra, D. (2002). Mental illness in Black and Asian minorities: pathways to care and outcomes. *Advances in Psychiatric Treatment*, **8**, 26–33.

Bhui, K. and Sashidharan, S. P. (2003). Should there be separate psychiatric services for ethnic minority groups? *British Journal of Psychiatry*, **182**, 10–12.

Bushe, G. R. and Coetzer, G. (1995). Appreciative inquiry as a team development intervention: a controlled experiment. *Journal of Applied Behavioral Science*, **31**, 13–30.

Chew-Graham, C., Bashir, C., Chantler, K., Burman, E. and Batsleer, J. (2002). South Asian women, psychological distress and self-harm: lessons for primary care trusts. *Health and Social Care in the Community*, **10**, 339–47.

Cooper, J., Husain, N., Webb, R. *et al.* (2006). Self-harm in the UK: differences between South Asians and Whites in rates, characteristics, provision of service and repetition. *Social Psychiatry and Psychiatric Epidemiology*, **41**, 782–8.

Damelio, R. (2006). *The Basics of Process Mapping*. New York: Quality Resources.

Department of Health (2003). *Inside Outside: Improving Mental Health Services for Black and Minority Ethnic Communities in England*. London: The Stationery Office.

Department of Health (2005). *Delivering Race Equality in Mental Health Care*. London: The Stationery Office.

Dogra, N. (2001). The development and evaluation of a programme to teach cultural diversity to medical undergraduate students. *Medical Education*, **35**, 232–41.

Glover, G., Arts, G. and Babu, K. S. (2006). Crisis resolution/home treatment teams and psychiatric admission rates in England. *British Journal of Psychiatry*, **189**, 441–5.

Husain, N., Creed, F. and Tomenson, B. (1997). Adverse social circumstances and depression in people of Pakistani origin in the UK. *British Journal of Psychiatry*, **171**, 434–8.

Johnson, S. and Buszewicz, M. (1996). Introduction. In *Planning Community Mental Health Services for Women: A Multiprofessional Handbook*, ed. K. Abel, M. Buszewicz, S. Davison, S. Johnson and E. Staples. London: Routledge, pp. 1–5.

Khan, F. and Waheed, W. (2006). Suicide and self harm in South Asian immigrants. *Psychiatry*, **5**, 283–5.

King, M. and Bartlett, A. (2006). What same sex civil partnerships mean for public health. *Journal of Epidemiology and Community Health*, **60**, 188–91.

King, M., McKeown, E., Warner, J. *et al.* (2003). Mental health and quality of life of gay men and lesbians in England and Wales. *British Journal of Psychiatry*, **183**, 552–8.

Leese, M., Thornicroft, G., Shaw, J. *et al.* (2006). Ethnic differences among patients in high-security psychiatric hospitals in England. *British Journal of Psychiatry*, **188**, 380–5.

Maden, A., Friendship, C., McClintock, T. and Rutter, S. (1999). Outcome of admission to a medium secure psychiatric unit. 2. Role of ethnic origin. *British Journal of Psychiatry*, **175**, 317–21.

McColl, H. and Johnson, S. (2006). Characteristics and needs of asylum seekers and refugees in contact with London community mental health teams. *Social Psychiatry and Psychiatric Epidemiology*, **41**, 789–95.

McKenzie, K. (2003). Services for African and African-Caribbeans: the Antenna Outreach Service. *Mental Health Review*, **8**, 16–21.

Office for National Statistics (2001). *Census 2001*. London: Office for National Statistics. www.statistics.gov.uk/census/.

O'Hagan, K. (2001). *Cultural Competence in the Caring Professions*. London: Jessica Kingsley.

Parkman, S., Davies, S., Leese, M., Phelan, M. and Thornicroft, G. (1997). Ethnic differences in satisfaction with mental health services among representative people with psychosis in south London: PRiSM study 4. *British Journal of Psychiatry*, **171**, 260–4.

Phelan, M. and Parkman, S. (1995). How to do it: work with an interpreter. *British Medical Journal*, **311**, 555–7.

Race Relations (Amendment) Act 2000. London: The Stationery Office. www.opsi.gov.uk/acts/acts2000/20000034.htm.

Sainsbury Centre for Mental Health (2002). *Breaking the Circles of Fear: A Review of the Relationship between Mental Health Services and African and Caribbean Communities*. London: Sainsbury Centre for Mental Health.

Selten, J.-P. and Cantor-Graae, E. (2005). Social defeat, a risk factor for schizophrenia? *British Journal of Psychiatry*, **187**, 101–2.

Showalter, E. (1987). *The Female Malady: Women, Madness and English Culture, 1830–1980*. London: Virago.

Waheed, W., Husain, N. and Creed, F. (2003). Psychiatric services for ethnic minority groups: a third way? *British Journal of Psychiatry*, **183**, 562–3.

Weich, S., Nazroo, J., Sproston, K. *et al.* (2004). Common mental disorders and ethnicity in England: the EMPIRIC study. *Psychological Medicine*, **34**, 1543–51.

18

Coercion and compulsion in crisis resolution teams

Jonathan P. Bindman

One of the aims of crisis resolution is to offer treatment in a less coercive manner than inpatient care, which always imposes the constraints of institutional living on patients, whether or not they are also subject to legal compulsion, physical restraint or forcible injections. While many people do indeed recognise and value the freedom to be treated in their own environment, treatment at home may also be applied coercively, and crisis resolution teams (CRTs) use a range of 'treatment pressures' in the course of their work, including, but not confined to, the use of legal compulsion. In some cases, the degree of intrusion into the patient's home environment and social network may be so great that they may find hospital treatment preferable. This chapter describes a simple hierarchical model of treatment pressures and illustrates how these may be applied in practice by CRTs, and the dilemmas that arise. The use of legal powers to compel acceptance of treatment in the community and some of the practical difficulties of using coercive powers in a community setting are also discussed.

Defining coercion

Szmukler and Applebaum (2001) have conceptualised a hierarchy of 'treatment pressures' (Figure 18.1). Only the highest levels of the hierarchy (threats and force) are conventionally recognised as coercive, but the lower levels of treatment pressure, commonly used in practice, raise some of the same ethical dilemmas as the higher ones, and all can be regarded as forms of coercion. The hierarchical model provides a useful way of classifying the complex interactions between CRTs and patients, and may help to decide what level of pressure is ethically justified.

Crisis Resolution and Home Treatment in Mental Health, ed. Sonia Johnson, Justin Needle, Jonathan P. Bindman and Graham Thornicroft. Published by Cambridge University Press. © Cambridge University Press 2008.

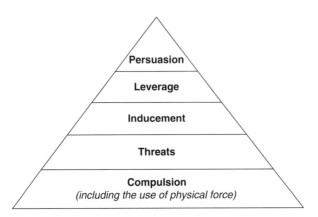

Figure 18.1 Hierarchy of treatment pressures (Szmukler and Applebaum, 2001).

Persuasion, leverage and inducement

The lowest level of treatment pressure is *persuasion*, in which the professional sets out the benefits for the client of a particular course of action and attempts to counter objections. The patient is free to reject advice.

The next level of pressure – *leverage* – assumes an interpersonal relationship between patient and professional that has an element of emotional dependence. This gives the professional power to pressure the patient by demonstrating approval of one course of action or disapproval of another.

Greater pressure may be exerted by *inducement*, in which acceptance of treatment is linked to material help, such as support in accessing charitable funds.

Threats and compulsion

The highest levels of pressure in the hierarchy are overtly coercive. A *threat* could be made to withdraw services on which the patient normally relies (which is more coercive than simply failing to offer inducements over and above normal services) or to detain them in hospital.

Finally, at the highest level of the hierarchy, patients may be *compelled* to take treatment against their will, by detention in hospital or, if necessary, by the use of physical force.

Ethical justifications for treatment pressures

Professionals may feel uncomfortable about the use of coercion and avoid careful examination of the coercive aspects of their work, despite acting coercively on a regular basis. They may prefer to avoid considering their own role in coercion by attributing the necessity for it to someone else: the person must be coerced because they will be 'sectioned' by the consultant, arrested by the police, assaulted by the neighbours or evicted by the council if they do not cooperate with the treatment plan.

The risk with this approach is that people who believe they are acting on behalf of others and do not examine their personal role in coercion are likely to act more coercively, and are more likely to go beyond an ethically justified level of coercion, than those who take responsibility for their coercive actions and carefully consider their ethical justification.

It is important, therefore, that CRT members all understand that coercion can be legitimate, ethical and justifiable, and there should be open discussion about which coercive acts are or are not acceptable.

The usual justifications for pressuring patients to accept treatment concern risks to the health or safety of the patient, or to the safety of others, though these risks are often rather poorly defined and rarely quantifiable. Deciding what level of pressure is commensurate with the risk is not straightforward but it may be helpful to try to apply an ethical framework commonly used to assist decision making in general medicine. This requires consideration of the person's capacity to take treatment decisions in their best interests. Capacity is usually defined as the ability to understand and retain information about the proposed treatment, and to weigh in the balance the consequences of alternative decisions about it. In the UK, the legislative framework for considering capacity has become much clearer with the implementation of the Mental Capacity Act 2005. Capacity needs to be considered in relation to a specific treatment decision, and people may lack capacity to take some decisions while retaining it for others. People with capacity can determine what treatment is in their own best interests, even where their views do not accord with those of clinicians, and minimal pressure, perhaps limited to persuasion, is all that can be justified in such cases. If capacity is lacking, the treatment that is in the person's best interest may need to be determined by clinicians, though taking into account, if possible, the past and present wishes of the patient and the views of significant others. The minimal level of pressure necessary to achieve the objectives of this treatment can then be exerted.

While the application of this framework is helpful in clarifying the decision to be taken, community teams are often faced with situations where a simple judgement of capacity is not easy to make. A person may, apparently through choice, live in squalor, or even on the streets. Does such an apparently irrational choice necessarily imply a lack of capacity, or must delusional reasoning be established? Even if capacity seems to be absent, what minimum standard of living is in the best interests of a patient who expresses no desire for material comforts?

Faced with such complex issues, it is tempting to resort to the traditional medical approach of assuming that best interests are best determined by a beneficent doctor. However, attempting to apply a capacity-based approach makes it clear that it is patients' reasoning about their situation that is the starting point for the decision, and makes it less likely that the values, anxieties or prejudices of others will prevail over patients' expressed views. Sharing difficult decisions with multidisciplinary teams, carers and advocates similarly reduces the risk of poor or hasty judgements.

Though the Mental Health Act 1983 allows compulsion on the grounds of risk to others, and mental health services are exposed to strong societal expectations that they should prevent violence by their patients, attempting to take an ethical approach to treatment pressure on these grounds presents considerable difficulties. There are very few circumstances in which citizens without mental disorder can be detained preventatively on the grounds of risk, and it is hard to justify taking a different approach to people with capacity. The challenge for community mental health services is to avoid being pressured into applying an ethical double standard, in which behaviour that would not justify significant sanction in the absence of mental disorder is used to justify loss of liberty, or in which levels of treatment pressure are not commensurate with the actual level of risk.

Coercion in practice

Actions that are coercive are often undertaken by CRTs. Most professionals believe that they apply the minimal level of coercion necessary, but there may be situations in which this is not, in fact, the case. A CRT is usually under pressure to arrive at a formulation of the patient's problem and make management decisions very rapidly. Indeed, the referrer may give the formulation and the solution to the CRT even before the person is assessed. For example, the CRT may be told that the person has had a relapse of psychosis as a consequence of discontinuing medication, and the role of the CRT is to ensure that medication is resumed. Other common scenarios include:

- a patient with chronic negative symptoms is not caring for him or herself adequately
- a patient's behaviour is alienating carers or neighbours and putting their accommodation at risk
- someone with a history of depression is at increasing risk of suicide
- misuse of drink or drugs is leading to a deterioration in mental state.

Psychotropic medication is usually assumed to be a key part of the solution to all of these problems, though a variety of other interventions suggest themselves in each case. The CRT is, therefore, likely to approach the person with a clear view about what action they should take. In addition to the pressure to come up with quick solutions, the need to unite a large number of staff around a treatment plan that can be handed over in a straightforward manner from shift to shift may tend to encourage the development of a firmly held collective view about what the patient should do. Unsurprisingly, such views often conflict with the patient's own view of the situation and the stage is set for coercive approaches. However, what is the minimum level of coercion appropriate to the situation?

Avoiding coercion

The first question must be whether coercion needed at all. It may be possible to avoid approaching the patient in the first place with a treatment plan that can only be delivered coercively. If the initial interview with the person can be approached without preconceptions or instructions from the referrer, in a spirit of genuine enquiry about the person's perception of the problem and the solution, then a consensus may be achieved at an early stage between patient and CRT, and the issue of coercion need not arise.

Insight

Achieving consensus on treatment with the patient is sometimes assumed to be a hopeless task because they 'lack insight', and the use of coercion is, therefore, deemed inevitable. This may be a simplistic view. Insight has been described as consisting of three components (Birchwood *et al.*, 1994), which are to some extent independent:

- the acceptance of a problem
- the ability to relabel symptoms, e.g. to recognise the association of hallucinations with illness
- the acceptance of treatment recommendations.

Though the assessor and the service user may not achieve consensus on all three aspects at once, it is also unusual for all components of insight to be entirely lacking (if they are, then the person is perhaps unlikely to accept home treatment in the first place). It is usually possible to reach agreement either that the person has a problem and is in need of help or that particular symptoms are illness related. Sometimes, even when these components cannot be agreed, the patient will accept treatment offered without the need for coercion.

Persuasion

If no consensus about treatment can be achieved, and it is decided that treatment pressure is justified, then persuasion is the appropriate starting point. As above, this involves explaining to the patient the benefits of the treatment plan, countering objections by reasoned argument, and giving authoritative advice. This can only work if the assessment has been sufficiently thorough. It is usually futile – and potentially very embarrassing – to set out to persuade someone of the necessity of taking medication on the basis that 'someone told me at handover that you are supposed to be starting your tablets again'. Effective persuasion will be based on a clear understanding of the person's problem, and on either convincing evidence of the effectiveness of medication generally for the kind of problem the person has or evidence of the previous benefits of treatment for that particular individual and an understanding of why they have discontinued it. Persuasion can be highly effective if people feel that their problem has been properly understood and a rational solution proposed, but in practice an argument all too often falls flat because the person feels that the professional is advocating a 'one size fits all' solution in ignorance of the person's own experience. The use of authority needs to be carefully considered and adapted to the individual service user. It is seldom possible to be completely confident that a particular treatment will work, particularly if it is being used for the first time, and some people respond well to an honest acknowledgement by the clinician of the level of uncertainty, since the risk of loss of trust if the treatment subsequently fails is reduced. However, some people will be made very anxious by obvious lack of confidence on the part of the clinician, and will be helped more by reassurance and professional optimism.

Leverage

Leverage is an extension of persuasion in which the patient's emotional relationship with the professional adds to the force of persuasion. Someone who is unconvinced by a rational argument may still accept treatment from a professional who is trusted and believed to be acting in a caring way. Most CRTs are faced with the problem that they are unlikely to have the sort of trusting relationship with a patient that is built up over time (though they may develop this with people who are seen repeatedly in crisis). The CRT members are sometimes skilled at developing such relationships quickly and bring either a high degree of empathy or 'natural authority' to their role that gives them effective leverage. The CRT may also use 'proxy' leverage, mentioning to the person that they know that their care coordinator, consultant or other trusted person is supporting the treatment plan (and, by implication, will be disappointed if it is not followed).

Inducements

Direct inducements, such as paying people to take medication, are not usually given (in the UK, at least), though they are not necessarily harder to justify ethically than any other sort of coercion. In practice, however, it is difficult for health services to access cash for this purpose, and there is also, perhaps, an anxiety about setting precedents that will be hard to maintain. That said, other sorts of inducement are often offered, such as small amounts of cash to buy food or other essentials, help with accessing benefits or practical help with the home. More substantial inducements include offers of help with obtaining housing transfers, interceding in legal problems such as helping to avoid prison, helping with asylum applications or avoiding deportation. Such offers need to be handled with great care as the CRT may not be in a position to deliver them.

One recognised issue with inducements has been referred to as the problem of setting a 'moral baseline' (Wertheimer, 1987). An inducement is a material benefit over and above what the person has a right to expect. Defining an inducement, therefore, involves defining baseline entitlements. For example, a level of benefits sufficient to live on is (in the UK) an entitlement, and professionals should assist people with mental illness to access this without linking help to acceptance of treatment. However, the disability living allowance is an additional benefit awarded on the basis that it will alleviate the consequences of disability. It might be legitimate to offer to assist someone in accessing this if they are engaging in treatment, but to withhold it if the money is likely to be used to worsen the disability (e.g. spending it on drink or drugs). Some professionals are happy to engage with such issues of moral judgement, while others might see their role as maximising benefits and prefer not to seek to use them as inducements.

Similar moral debates may arise over the use of 'petty cash'. It is usual for CRTs to be able to access small quantities of cash for service users who have no money to buy food or essentials (or for the team to buy food and deliver it). This may be used as an inducement – more readily provided for people who are perceived to be cooperative than those who are not – but it can also be argued that it should be provided purely on the basis of need, in which case it should not be withheld, regardless of the degree of cooperation.

Threats

The use of threats by CRTs is rather common, with many patients agreeing to accept treatment on the basis that they feel (or have been quite explicitly) threatened with compulsory admission to hospital if they fail to cooperate. Though professionals may feel some repugnance at issuing threats, and defend against this by attributing the threat to someone else (the consultant psychiatrist of the community team who will make the application for detention, perhaps), like all forms of coercion a threat may be ethical if justified in the way described above. But while it may be legitimate, working on the basis of this threat can be unsatisfactory because the sanction – compulsory admission – can be hard to apply in practice and is an 'all or nothing' response. A reluctant patient might agree to a treatment plan involving regular visits and acceptance of medication, but if they are then unavailable for some visits, or decline medication on some occasions but not others, then it may be hard to justify admission on the basis of partial cooperation. Yet, if any breach of the agreement is ignored, or dealt with by repeated warnings but no actual sanction, then the threat may lose its effectiveness. Furthermore, even if the CRT does decide that the threat must be acted on, this may fail, either because the approved social worker or nearest relative does not regard detention as justified or for practical reasons, such as lack of beds or difficulty getting the police or ambulance service involved.

Other threats to which CRT users are often exposed include eviction, loss of benefits or rent support, the threat of violence from neighbours and sanctions from partners or family. While it is tempting to present these as reasons why the person should cooperate with treatment, the CRT cannot make use of them as threats since it will usually have a moral obligation to protect the person from them, and even if the team feels that it is not ethically required, for example, to prevent an eviction, they are unlikely to be in control of the sanction.

Force and legal compulsion

In the UK at least, physical force is not used in the community by CRTs, though in some other countries forcible medication may be given in community settings with police assistance. Patients may, however, be forcibly treated in hospital during a crisis, and may be treated by the CRT while subject to legal compulsion. The commonest situation in which this arises is when patients who have been compulsorily detained in hospital are granted leave in the community (under Section 17 of the Mental Health Act 1983 in England and Wales) subject to conditions set by the detaining psychiatrist, which may include accepting visits or medication from the CRT. It is important that the CRT is involved in agreeing the conditions of such treatment. These should be written clearly and in detail, giving the frequency and location of visits and the exact doses of medication to be taken, so that there can be no doubt about what is expected of the patient and about when conditions have been breached. Breaches should result in recall to hospital for compulsory treatment, unless the CRT and the detaining psychiatrist agree that the breach is unimportant. In practice, there are a number of obstacles to this. If the conditions are not carefully written, there may be debate with the patient or within the team about the existence of a breach, and also differing views about its seriousness and the necessity for readmission. There may also be difficulties in communicating the breach to the hospital consultant, who may not share the CRT's view of the need for admission. It may be hard to get police assistance to readmit, or to secure a hospital bed. Some of these problems may be alleviated by having a psychiatrist in the CRT take responsibility for the legal order, though CRT psychiatrists may encounter problems in accessing beds for readmissions. In practice, therefore, threats that involve the sanction of forcible treatment in hospital may lack credibility and should be made with care.

Proposals are currently (as of 2006) before Parliament to strengthen the legal powers in England and Wales to treat with compulsion, through the introduction of a form of community treatment order. Such powers have been available to community teams, including CRTs, in Australia for over a decade (Mark Hinton, personal communication). Community treatment orders affect CRT practice in two ways. First, a patient subject to a community treatment order can readily be transported to hospital for assessment, with police assistance if necessary, if the CRT has concerns about risk. This can be effected much more easily than is currently the case in England, where removing someone from the community requires a Mental Health Act assessment, which is time consuming to organise and requires a high threshold of concern. Second, if a patient being managed by the CRT in crisis refuses treatment from the CRT, having previously been made subject to an order requiring treatment, they can be taken forcibly to hospital to receive medication, then returned to the CRT's care. If the Australian CRT is satisfied that it is both ethical and necessary to use the threat of force to ensure that such a patient takes treatment, then it has the power to act on this threat in a way that English CRTs do not. It remains to be seen whether the new powers proposed in England and Wales have a significant impact on CRT practice, or whether difficulties in obtaining police support or finding beds place a practical limit on the use of threats and force.

Key points

- Coercion is a routine part of CRT practice.
- Coercion may cause discomfort on the part of professionals, which can be alleviated by using a framework of ethics to justify a level of coercion commensurate with the benefits to the patient and the risks to others.
- Open discussion of these issues within the team will minimise the likelihood of the excessive use of coercion that can arise when professionals' concerns about risk are not adequately shared and contained.

ACKNOWLEDGEMENT

Thanks to Mark Hinton for discussion of CRT practice in Australia.

REFERENCES

Birchwood, M., Smith, J., Drury, V. *et al.* (1994). A self-report insight scale for psychosis: reliability, validity and sensitivity to change. *Acta Psychiatrica Scandinavic*, **89**, 62–7.

Mental Capacity Act 2005. London: The Stationery Office.

Mental Health Act 1983. London: The Stationery Office.

Szmukler, G. and Applebaum, P. (2001). Treatment pressures, coercion and compulsion. In *Textbook of Community Psychiatry*, ed. G. Thornicroft and G. Szmukler. Oxford: Oxford University Press, pp. 529–43.

Wertheimer, A. (1987). *Coercion*. Princeton, CT: Princeton University Press.

Section 4

Variations and enhancements

19

Integration of the crisis resolution function within community mental health teams

Alan Rosen, Paul Clenaghan, Feleena Emerton and Simon Richards

There is now a substantial body of evidence to support the inclusion of a 24-hour mobile community crisis response (Hoult *et al.*, 1984; Rosen, 1997; Johnson *et al.*, 2005) and case management based on a continuity of care principle (Rosen and Teesson, 2001) as components in all local psychiatric service systems. At the same time, there is considerable confusion and blurring in the literature between crisis and emergency psychiatric response services (e.g. American Psychiatric Association Task Force on Psychiatric Emergency Services, 2002), and between discrete crisis teams and combined crisis and case management teams (extended hours teams (EHTs)). While Thornicroft and Tansella (2002) endorsed both crisis and case management components as essential parts of a balanced hospital and community mental health service, Rosen (2002) has emphasised the importance of integrating all these components of a local service as much as possible. Thornicroft and Tansella (2004) proposed that combined generic community mental health teams (CMHTs) without differentiation into specialised components (e.g. crisis, early intervention, assertive case management) represent a stage of evolution of a service. Enhanced material resources will allow it to become a more differentiated service, including these components as linked but distinct elements. They argued that the evidence base is stronger for such specialised components than for generic teams. While there is evidence to support this in some cases, no proper test has ever been carried out of whether specialist crisis resolution teams (CRTs: also known as intensive home treatment teams, crisis assessment and treatment teams, access teams and psychiatric emergency teams) are preferable to combined crisis and case management teams (Glover *et al.*, 2006; see Chapter 5).

In this chapter, we will describe a model of combined crisis and case management services in its historic and functional service development context and will contrast this with other models.

Crisis Resolution and Home Treatment in Mental Health, ed. Sonia Johnson, Justin Needle, Jonathan P. Bindman and Graham Thornicroft. Published by Cambridge University Press. © Cambridge University Press 2008.

Definitions

The term 'extended hours team' describes a local CMHT that combines the two functions of crisis intervention and ongoing case management, ensuring continuity of care between these phases. Such teams are also called acute care community teams, in contrast to community teams that focus on rehabilitation/recovery functions, including offering an assertive community treatment (ACT) model.

Extended hours teams at Lower North Shore and Ryde Mental Health Services

In the Lower North Shore Mental Health Service of Sydney, Australia, a successful randomised controlled trial of a crisis team providing follow-up for one year as an alternative to hospital-centred acute care (Hoult *et al.*, 1984; Chapter 2) led to the establishment of a separate crisis team as a regular component of the community service in 1981. By 1983, the crisis team and the case management functions of the two CMHTs in the catchment area had been merged, and this system has been in place ever since. Each local CMHT operates its own crisis intake system and has its own subcatchment area of two municipalities during office hours, though sometimes drawing on assistance from its sister CMHT. At nights and weekends, each centre contributes one professional staff member to the crisis service, so at least one of the rostered crisis staff is likely to know (or have easy access to information about) any established or ex-client who presents for assessment. Similar merging of crisis and case management teams has occurred in other areas of Sydney.

The Lower North Shore EHT is closely linked to an early intervention in psychosis mobile team, while the neighbouring Ryde EHT oversees and regularly visits an acute community respite care household and an early intervention in psychosis household, each for up to four residents. Each service has access to these specialist services provided by its neighbour. These geographically distinct local services have been administratively amalgamated recently as the North Shore Ryde Mental Health Service. Lower North Shore EHT provides first-line mental health assessments to general hospital emergency departments (in the UK, usually referred to as accident and emergency departments) when their own psychiatric triage staff are not available. The EHT staff and all other community case managers are expected to visit their clients regularly when they are inpatients. Reciprocally, ward staff are expected to include a person's community case manager in all key meetings (e.g. with the family) and in all major decisions throughout the admission, not just before discharge. The wider context of these mental health teams includes growing integration of the full spectrum of community and acute inpatient services, including acute general hospital services, recovery/rehabilitation teams (including ACT), residential, vocational and social/leisure activity services, and general practitioner (GP) shared care programmes.

The tiered model of care that operates can be described as a continuum of involvement, moving from the provision of full case management, through episodic contact to full discharge to GP case management (see below). The last is indicated when the client is stable, has a supportive caring system and established accommodation, and is able to manage their own medication and seek emergency assistance. In an external study of mental health services on the Lower North Shore of Sydney, Slade (1995) concluded that, regarding EHTs,

> One of the key practical issues for developing community care teams . . . is the configuration of crisis teams. The extended hours team began as a separately staffed (and researched) crisis team (Hoult *et al.*, 1984), but over time was integrated with pre-existing community mental health teams. Separate crisis teams gave better short-term outcomes, because of the intensive, dedicated support. It was also a helpful configuration when setting the service up, because both teams were motivated to 'out-perform' the other. Longer term, however, it was found that better outcomes were associated with an integrated team, since episodes of illness were more rapidly detected by a staff member who is familiar with the person, and the continuity of service was helpful for clients in crisis – a client sees the same person (or a close colleague) at nights or weekends as they would at midday (during the week). Furthermore, the reduced rivalry [between service components] led to higher morale in the team.

Manchester integrated home treatment service and community mental health teams

Following the closure of a psychiatric institution in Manchester, England, in 1991, funds earmarked for a traditional day hospital were used to set up a home treatment service (HTS) in 1992. By 1995, it was evident that trying to operate such a service within the framework of a traditional service model was problematic: the CMHTs were often closed to referrals, there was a five-month wait to see a psychiatrist and it was difficult to access the HTS owing to its inability to transfer service users to appropriate follow-up services to free up some of its limited number of places. In 1996, an integrated new service combining a HTS and CMHT was piloted and in 1998 this model was extended to the remainder of the local trust with three integrated teams being established within existing resources. These are 24-hour, seven day a week services operating 365 days a year, with a single point of entry for all referrals and providing management for all severe and persistent disorders. The perceived strengths of this model are continuity and consistency of service for each client, eliminating the need to transfer care, and the ability of the team to increase or decrease levels of support rapidly to meet assessed needs. Since 2005, further developments have included an increasing focus on recovery and social integration, and incorporation in the Gateway Project, which involves formally linking inpatient services and community teams by pre-planning admissions and setting discharge goals prior to admission (Adrian Galloway, personal communication, 2006).

Organisational choice points

Choosing between crisis services and the emergency department

Crisis services are one component of a comprehensive mental health system and are as crucial to it as an emergency department is to the overall health system. However, the crisis model is not synonymous with or an extension of an emergency department model. Table 19.1 summarises differences between the roles of services that respond to mental health crises and the roles of emergency services, including the emergency department, although it cannot always be assumed that people will seek help in ways that are appropriate to these distinct roles.

Table 19.1. Distinguishing crisis and emergency responses

	Crisis	Emergency
Key characteristic	Intensely stressful turning point	Immediately life-threatening situation
Appropriate personnel to call	General practitioner, community mental health professional, local authority social services	Police, ambulance and paramedics, fire brigade, hospital casualty department
Appropriate response time	Timely (e.g. phone back within 15 minutes of call) and arrange crisis visit as soon as possible and strategically timed to include all participants and personal supports	Immediate (e.g. phone and expect immediate connection) or arrive and expect urgent action on 24-hour basis, subject to triage arrangements on the basis of assessed level of urgency and emergency resources available
Appropriate response type	Crisis assessment and support	Life preserving: secure physical safety
	Defusing stress and interpersonal strife	Defusing violence or potential violence
	Harness emotional arousal: use as opportunity for new solutions	Psychosocial first aid, or critical incident counselling
	Practical assistance with pressing problems of living	Urgent physical or psychiatric assessment and treatment
	Physical or psychiatric assessment and treatment when necessary	

Choosing between integrated crisis and case management teams or discrete teams

The key choice that this chapter is concerned with is between EHTs, which integrate case management and crisis responses, and CRTs. One of the key differences is that CRTs are usually completely separate teams within a mental health service, whereas the professionals in EHTs are drawn from local CMHTs on a rota basis to provide crisis response in and out of office hours (Table 19.2).

Teams that respond to mental health crises range from those performing crisis work exclusively, with time-limited follow-up, to those providing crisis interventions integrated with a continuity of care case management function. This spectrum is described in Box 19.1.

While service planners often debate whether to have specialist crisis teams separate from the case management services, or to integrate the two models, few evaluation studies distinguish between them (Chapters 4 and 5). In New South Wales, most areas started with discrete crisis intervention teams and discrete case management teams. These teams have in many areas integrated fully into one team, whereas in other services the crisis intervention team has extended its role to include case management, or the two teams have remained separate.

We, therefore, have three levels of integration.

Separate.   CRT only provides crisis intervention and a case management team based in a community mental health centre is separate (models A and B in Box 19.1).

Table 19.2. Contrast between separate crisis resolution teams and integrated extended hours treatment teams

	Crisis resolution team	Extended hours team
Service user type	No exclusion criteria for local residents with any psychiatric disturbance; service users have a wide ability range	No exclusion criteria for local residents with any psychiatric disturbance; service users have a wide ability range
Location of service	Often home centred at height of crisis; separate team	Centred at home and at community mental health centre; crisis service combined with the centre
Case management approaches	Open-ended caseload with high-intensity input for a short period only	Open-ended caseload with intensity of input limited by caseload
Type of service	Crisis responsive (to pressing concerns and symptoms); short-term crisis care and treatment	Crisis responsive and proactive to prevent crises; crisis care, and treatment and ongoing case management

Box 19.1. Crisis team spectrum

Minimum scope and integration	A	Crisis only: assessments and referral for continuing care by other services within 24 hours (e.g. emergency department model, but in the community)
	B	Crisis and team management until crisis is manageable; then referral
	C	Crisis and individual treatment delivered by one key clinician, complemented by a crisis team; then referral when crisis is manageable
	D	Crisis and individual treatment delivered by one key clinician, complemented by an integrated team; a treatment package is provided (with an end-point identified)
Maximum scope and integration	E	Crisis and individual treatment delivered by one key clinician, complemented by an integrated team; a treatment package is provided (with or without an end-point)

Partial integration. There are distinct crisis teams and case management services, but they work very closely together and the case manager leads on the management of the crisis (in collaboration with the crisis team) as well as on continuing case management (model C).

Full integration. Case management and CRTs merged as one team (models D and E).

Some clinicians prefer model C, on the grounds that in models D and E care is too generalist and none of the clinicians become specialists in delivering crisis care. Models A, B and C involve a crisis treatment package with an identified end-point, whereas models D and E are designed to involve a seamless transition from crisis phase to continuing care. Consequently, other clinicians argue that the latter models are preferable because they provide much more continuity of care. As the end of the crisis approaches, such models invite continuity rather than requiring that clients are referred on to a new clinician, who has to start the process of engagement again. Engagement, trust and other interpersonal gains made during the crisis can thus be built on.

In reviewing the two models within Sydney, there is some evidence that distinct specialist crisis teams extend the length of the period of crisis treatment. Camperdown and Marrickville (two areas in inner-city Sydney each with populations of approximately 100 000) use the partial integration model (C), and where ongoing community care is required it generally involves a transfer to another team. Hornsby and Lower North Shore (populations of 260 000 and 175 000, respectively, and also in metropolitan Sydney) have the full integration model (D and E). Evaluation reviews indicate that:

- 30% of the caseload of the specialist crisis team remained in treatment with the team after one month in teams based on model C, with crisis work accounting for 80% of service providers' time (Marrickville and Camperdown) – the vast majority of this group constituted people with psychosis
- less than 5% of people remained in 'crisis treatment' as delivered by an integrated team approach after one month in models D and E (Lower North Shore and Hornsby), with 45% of service contacts crisis related, and 50% of service providers' time expended on crisis work.

We hypothesize that the combined models D and E favour increased retention of clientele in follow-up. Furthermore, the combined model supports an earlier entry into individualised case management and it may be that earlier connection with a case manager provides better outcomes than a team approach in terms of continued engagement and individually tailored longer-term treatment planning. Whether the best results are achieved by having a separate crisis-orientated team or combined EHT case management and continuity of care teams may, however, depend more on local geography, demography and resources than on the inherent superiority of either model.

Basic structure of extended hours teams

Staff numbers and rotas

Urban EHTs are often multidisciplinary, with all professions sharing the extended hours roster, two at a time, backed at all times by a rostered junior and a senior psychiatrist, who may also be on call for home visits and the local general hospital. Staff are available on a call-out basis overnight; these arrangements are appreciated and generally respected by our service users and their families, and are very rarely abused. Night-time call-out rates, excluding calls to the emergency department, average five per month for urban teams covering populations of approximately 100 000 (Camperdown and Marrickville). Factors influencing this rate include service availability in the emergency department and the options available for assessment and treatment there. In the Hornsby area, for example, call-outs after 10.30 pm can occur on over 50% of nights owing to high demand in the emergency department and lower levels of staffing and skills there in assessing mental health problems.

An EHT needs to have at least eight members available each week to cover the rota for responding to crises. Mondays to Fridays between 9.00 am and 9.00 pm, two EHT members at a time are dedicated to doing a combination of intake and crisis work, while a further four to six do continuing case management work. Two team members then provide crisis care from 2 pm to 10.30 pm. One member of the team is available on call overnight. At weekends, two members do crisis work from 9.00 am to 9.00 pm and two others from 2.30 pm to 10.30 pm.

Interdisciplinary skill mix

The overall staffing of community teams that deliver crisis care is generally 50% mental health nurses, with allied health professionals (psychologists, occupational therapists) and social workers making up the other 50%. The role of medication dispensing in a combined crisis response and case management team is important but can be over-stated – it is one of the tools of the trade and, therefore, most teams operate with a minimum of 50% nursing staff. Recruitment should be based more on the skills required rather than on the profession:

- evidence-based psychosocial interventions
- problem-solving skills
- non-intrusive home visiting skills
- assessment skills (including suicide assessment)
- clinical skills
- family work skills
- understanding short-term and long-term treatment of a range of mental disorders
- expert understanding of psychosis
- good understanding of medications and their management (adherence strategies etc.).

Key qualities for crisis and case management work which are often undervalued include:

- low levels of hostility, criticism and over-involvement (i.e. low 'expressed emotion') tempered by sufficient involvement (Bentsen *et al.*, 1996)
- a desire to understand a person and their lived experience rather than to 'objectify and medicalise'
- a flexible working style and the ability to be comfortable with complexity and uncertainty, as solutions to problems of living and crises involving mental illness are often shades of grey, not clear-cut.

Organisation and operation of the Lower North Shore extended hours team, Sydney

All staff operate across the continuum of community care, including access and entry, crisis intervention, acute treatment, ongoing care and treatment, integrated hospital and community care, and discharge planning.

Staffing

The EHT at Lower North Shore includes nurses, an occupational therapist, psychologists and social workers. Staffing is rostered over a seven-day week, working day and evening shifts. All staff except medical staff are case managers.

A psychiatrist and a trainee psychiatrist are based with each EHT and are on an on-call roster out of office hours but also provide some sessions at the hospital and with the ACT/recovery team.

Workload

Caseloads for each EHT member are a mix of diagnostic groups, including psychotic disorders, mood (depressive, bipolar) and anxiety disorders, personality disorders, adjustment disorders and situational crisis problems (Table 19.3).

Frequency of contact with each client depends upon the severity of their illness or current crisis situation and may vary from twice daily contact in and out of hours during periods of being acutely unwell to contact every three to four weeks if the client is stable and managing well.

Caseloads for full-time staff members range between 30 and 40 clients. There are two main 'pressure valves' to allow regulation and adjustment of caseloads: the ACT team and the GP shared care transfer. If client contacts remain very frequent and their needs complex and time consuming after several weeks or months, the individual may be transferred to the ACT team. If client contact is required less than every four weeks and the person's condition stabilises, transfer to GP case management (the 'CLIPP' model; Meadows, 2003) may be negotiated. This entails work with the service user's family and GP with a detailed individual care plan, an explicit action plan for early warning signs and a GP shared care coordinator arranging annual psychiatric reviews and providing crisis access back into the service if and when necessary.

Table 19.3. Primary diagnostic groups for clients seen during 2005 by the Lower North Shore extended hours team, Sydney

Group[a]	Percentage
Mood (affective) disorders	29
Schizophrenia, schizotypal and delusional disorders	38
Anxiety, stress-related and adjustment disorders	9.6
Drug and alcohol use disorders	7.3
Specific personality disorders	2.8
Eating disorders	0.5
Mental retardation	0.5
Organic brain disorders	0.5
Mental health diagnosis not allocated or not applicable[b]	12.9

Notes:

[a] There is extensive additional comorbidity of most other categories with substance use and personality disorders.

[b] Includes not yet specified personality disorders.

Work phases

The phases of work within the EHT for each team member include time allocated for case work, office hours 'intake' (crisis) periods, out of hours (evenings and weekends) crisis work, continuity of care and administration work.

Crisis intake triage and bridging care

Crisis duties within office hours involve active clinicians working for two four-hour periods during office hours each week triaging all (not just crisis) calls for assistance with new referrals. Referrals may be made by individuals themselves, GPs, police, department of housing or other government agencies, friends or family, or concerned others. They are accepted by telephone or face to face on a 'walk-in' basis. Intake duties involve multitasking, from providing an access point for all mental health information to providing ongoing care for clients whose case manager is on leave. It is beyond the scope of this chapter to comment on the many issues relating to access to a mental health service when someone is not in crisis, but we recognise that the risk of performing a combined crisis and intake role is that the effectiveness of both could be diluted.

After hours crisis work

In the evenings and at weekends, crisis work involves providing additional support or assessment for known clients via telephone or home visits. New referrals are also received and are triaged via hospital switchboard, answer phone, mobile phone or the drug and alcohol triage service. Assessment and support is also provided by the EHT to clients of the early psychosis team, child and adolescent teams and older people's mental health services, which do not operate after hours.

Emergency department

Assessments in the emergency department at the local teaching general hospital are conducted seven days and nights per week between the hours of 8 am and 12.30 am (though occasionally until 2.00 am if necessary) by a mental health nurse consultant who specialises in such assessments, providing psychiatric triage, developing effective treatment pathways from the emergency department and building helpful relationships with that department's clinical specialties and other emergency services. When the emergency department's nurse consultant is not available, mental health assessments are conducted jointly by an EHT member and a psychiatric registrar, or by two EHT members (one from each community mental health centre during their hours of operation). The EHT member from the community mental health centre covering the catchment area of the present-ing client is then allocated whenever possible as the client's case manager, thus providing subsequent continuity of care. Some people assessed in the emergency department live outside the local catchment area (20%) and are, therefore, referred to their local mental health services following assessment.

Case management

This involves the allocation of the client to a case manager, usually through the intake process of the community mental health centre or by crisis workers. The case manager is then responsible for assessment and coordination of treatment, referral to other agencies that may assist the client (e.g. drug and alcohol services) and liaison with and education of the client's significant others.

Review phase

Following assessment and initial treatment, review of each client occurs at a daily team meeting then at regular review meetings. Current mental health status and functional capacity and stability are discussed. Decisions are made about whether further management should be through continuing case management as at present, referral to the intensive case management team for more intensive care or discharge of the client to their GP (often in conjunction with the general practice shared care coordinator based at the service) or to a private psychiatrist or therapist.

Range of interventions

The range of interventions provided to clients includes mental health assessments, usually performed initially by non-medical staff, followed by joint assessment involving psychiatrists, medication supervision and adherence training; short-term supportive counselling; cognitive–behaviour therapy; and functional capacity assessment. Family intervention is provided via referral to the family education evening support group or individually by the team members and the family work coordinator. Assistance can be sought from our own work enterprise and/or specialist employment rehabilitation agencies, rehabilitation and drug and alcohol services.

Administration

Administration duties include completing file documentation, including individual care plans and reviews; liaison letters to GPs; attendance at the daily clinical staff meeting; and completion of daily service contact statistics, quarterly nationally mandated outcome measures for each client, car logbooks and reporting of critical incidents.

Outcomes of extended hours teams

A suite of outcome measures is currently nationally mandated in Australian mental health services. These include the Health of the Nation Scales (Wing,

1989) and the Life Skills Profile (Rosen *et al.*, 1989). A third, self-report subjective measure is required, but the measure mandated varies from Australian state to state. Other ways of assessing EHTs and crisis services include their population penetration (i.e. the proportion of the population seen by the team), length of engagement, customer satisfaction, their response times and adequacy of response (Bengelsdorf *et al.*, 1984), their implementation of systematic procedures for risk assessment and management (NSW Health, 2001) and the proportion of their contacts with patients that take place in their homes and other normal life settings. Routine Australian data suggest that there are considerable variations among both specialist crisis teams and EHTs in the degree to which care is home based. Mobile 24-hour specialist crisis teams appear, however, to carry out more overnight home visits than either EHTs or those crisis teams that do not have full 24-hour availability.

Adding value as measured by the customer is crucial to a crisis service. Reviews of crisis intervention teams have found that this form of care and treatment is more satisfactory than a largely hospital-based service for both patients and families (Hoult *et al.*, 1984; Joy *et al.*, 2004). For some people, a relapse is inevitable. The team providing crisis care may build up a person's capacity to manage the next crisis, but the key to future interventions is confidence in seeking help early before the crisis is full-blown. Whether this is better provided by a specialist crisis team or an integrated team on the EHT model is a question requiring further research investigation (Chapter 5). Personal relationships are of great relevance to client satisfaction and retention in treatment; therefore, our impression is that EHTs in which patients' continuing therapeutic alliances with their case managers are the fulcrum of the crisis response have advantages over separate crisis teams in the domains of client satisfaction and engagement. The EHTs often assign as case manager the person who engaged and bonded with the patient in crisis at the time of their initial service contact, a relationship which then develops further during continuing case management. Therefore, it seems highly appropriate that this professional is also the main person to whom the patient is expected to turn for help in a crisis: such a system would be expected to facilitate prompt help seeking when a relapse occurs. It is also often hypothesized that there are fewer drop outs in the transition from crisis to case management phases with EHTs than with separate crisis and case management teams, though data are not available to confirm this. An advantage of integrated EHTs over case management teams is that they tend not to develop waiting lists. Where teams are separate, case management team waiting lists often result in the crisis response component of the service becoming blocked up with clients who cannot be referred for case management (see, for example, the section on Manchester, above).

Table 19.4 compares the advantages and disadvantages of specialist crisis teams (such as CRTs) and EHTs.

Table 19.4. Comparative advantages and limitations of extended hours combined crisis and case management teams versus discrete crisis teams

	Extended hours teams	Discrete crisis teams (e.g. crisis resolution teams)
Advantages of EHTs compared with discrete crisis teams	1. Greater ability to • engage in crisis phase and retain engagement rapport, trust and satisfaction with service into the follow-up case management phase with same service provider • provide seamless transition from crisis phase to continuity of care • utilise trust of case manager to ensure early presentation with early warning signs of subsequent episodes • retain client engagement in transition between crisis and following phases and in long term 2. Varied and satisfying range of work, with low burn-out reported, contributing to lower turnover 3. More interdisciplinary mix in teams, with cross-fertilisation of skills 4. A wide range of skills learned and employed in crisis and follow-up 5. Always busy; when crisis work is quiet, much continuity casework to do 6. Enhanced ability of team to regulate intensity of care and support according to assessed needs 7. Less likely to lead to waiting lists for case management	1. Lesser ability to • retain engagement and trust in transition between crisis and continuing care services • provide seamless continuity • utilise trust of case manager in early crisis response to ensure early access to care in subsequent episodes • retain client engagement in transition between crisis and following phases and in long term 2. Less varied work, but possibly equally satisfying, with low burn-out reported 3. More likely to be monodisciplinary/monocultural teams (especially nurses), but some interdisciplinary teams 4. Possibly narrower range of skills 5. 'Feast or famine' pattern: when it is quiet, two or three team members have nothing to do but when busy, demands may be very high 6. Lesser ability of team to regulate intensity of care and support 7. More likely to be associated with waiting lists for case management with consequent blocking of places for crisis response team

Table 19.4. (cont.)

	Extended hours teams	Discrete crisis teams (e.g. crisis resolution teams)
Limitations of EHTs compared with discrete crisis teams	1. Less able to drop everything and do daytime crisis home visits, though equally able to do evening and weekend home visits 2. Sometimes pulled in too many directions, between crisis phone intake, crisis home visits, emergency department and case management; when busy with crises, hard to maintain good quality service to service users 3. Depends on variable individual case manager strengths, as well as team culture 4. Harder to 'drop everything' and provide fast response, particularly in office hours 5. Disadvantaged by less-intense response than ideal in first few weeks, tempered by better follow through	1. More capacity and time to do crisis home visits, day and night, and more often organised to be able to do overnight home visits 2. More focused on crisis intake and intervention, though increasingly teams report feeling torn between being dragged more into hospitals to meet emergency department demands at expense of crisis home visits 3. Depends more on consistency and quality of team culture than on individual providers 4. More able to provide rapid response, though must still triage between phone intake, crisis community centre or home visits, and emergency department referrals 5. Advantage of more-intense crisis response in first few weeks, though possible loss of engagement in transition to follow-up

Key points

- The psychiatric EHT model combines two evidence-based components of a contemporary integrated community and hospital mental health service: crisis response, including home treatment, and case management.
- Such integration has advantages and disadvantages. On the one hand, continuity of care is improved by integration of crisis inpatient and continuing community care responses, with maximum use of strong therapeutic relationships with case managers. On the other hand, the intensity of the crisis response may be diluted.
- No rigorous studies have compared the EHT model with discrete CRTs.
- It cannot be assumed that one size fits all. Separate CRTs may be best in high-density urban catchment areas with high levels of social pathology and deprivation, where the isolation and complex needs of many service users mean that a very intensive crisis response is required to avoid hospital. The EHT may be more suitable for suburban and rural catchments, where clients are often more socially stable and a consistent relationship with a case manager may help them and their families to work towards minimising the impact of relapses, or even avoiding future crises altogether, through early recognition of and response to any early warning signs of relapses.

ACKNOWLEDGEMENTS

The authors would like to thank Sheila Nicholson, Vivienne Miller, Sonia Johnson, Graham Thornicroft, Fiona Nolan, Adrian Galloway and the staff of the integrated HTS, EHTs and CMHTs at Camperdown, Marrickville, Lower North Shore–Ryde and Hornsby in Sydney and Manchester, UK, for assistance with the content. Sylvia Hands and Anthony Tjia provided help with the manuscript.

REFERENCES

American Psychiatric Association Task Force on Psychiatric Emergency Services (2002). *Report and Recommendations Regarding Psychiatric Emergency and Crisis Services*. Washington, DC: American Psychiatric Press.

Bengelsdorf, H., Levy, L. E., Emerson, R. L. and Barile, F. A. (1984). A crisis triage rating scale. Brief dispositional assessment of patients at risk for hospitalization. *Journal of Nervous and Mental Disease*, **172**, 424–30.

Bentsen, H., Boye, B., Munkvold, O. G. *et al.* (1996). Inter-rater reliability of expressed emotion ratings based on the Camberwell Family Interview. *Psychological Medicine*, **26**, 821–8.

Glover, G., Arts, G. and Babu, K. S. (2006). Crisis resolution/home treatment teams and psychiatric admission rates in England. *British Journal of Psychiatry*, **189**, 441–5.

Hambridge, J. and Rosen, A. (1994). Impact of a mobile community intensive case management team in surburban Sydney. *Royal Australian and New Zealand Journal of Psychiatry*, **28**, 438–45.

Hoult, J., Rosen, A. and Reynolds, I. (1984). Community orientated treatment compared to psychiatric hospital orientated treatment. *Social Science and Medicine*, **18**, 1005–10.

Johnson, S., Nolan, F., Pilling, S. *et al.* (2005). Randomised controlled trial of acute mental health care by a crisis resolution team: the north Islington crisis study. *British Medical Journal*, **331**, 599–602.

Joy, C. B., Adams, C. E. and Rice, K. (2004). Crisis intervention for people with severe mental illnesses. *Cochrane Database of Systematic Reviews*, Issue 4, CD001087. Oxford: Update Software.

Meadows, G. (2003). Overcoming barriers to reintegration of patients with schizophrenia: developing a best practice model for discharge from specialist care. *Medical Journal of Australia*, **178**, S53–6.

NSW Health (2001). *Mental Health Clinical Care and Prevention Model: A Population Mental Health Model*, version 1.11. Sydney: NSW Health.

Rosen, A. (1997). Crisis management in the community. *Medical Journal of Australia*, **167**, 633–8.

Rosen, A. (2002). Integration is as important as balance. *World Psychiatry*, **1**, 91–3.

Rosen, A. and Teesson, M. (2001). Does case management work? The evidence and the abuse of evidence based medicine. *Australian and New Zealand Journal of Psychiatry*, **35**, 731–46.

Rosen, A., Parker, G., Hadzi-Pavlovic, D. and Hartley, R. (1989). The Life Skills Profile: a measure assessing function and disability in schizophrenia. *Schizophrenia Bulletin*, **15**, 325–37.

Slade, M. (1995). Mental health services on lower North Shore, Sydney. *Psychiatric Bulletin*, **19**, 108–10.

Thornicroft, G. and Tansella, M. (2002). Balancing community-based and hospital-based mental health care. *World Psychiatry*, **1**, 84–90.

Thornicroft, G. and Tansella, M. (2004). Components of a modern mental health service: a pragmatic balance of community and hospital care. *British Journal of Psychiatry*, **185**, 283–90.

Wing, J. K. (1989). *Health of the Nation Outcome Scales: HoNOS Field Trials*. London: Royal College of Psychiatrists' Research Unit.

20

Home treatment and 'hospitality' within a comprehensive community mental health centre

Roberto Mezzina and Sonia Johnson

In Trieste, Italy, intensive community management of crises is one element of the comprehensive service delivered by 24-hour community mental health centres (CMHCs). This chapter describes the local strategy for crisis intervention, which integrates crisis management into the work of these CMHCs, allowing maintenance of continuity of care and flexible access to a wide range of community interventions. Comparisons will be made between crisis care integrated in this way into a comprehensive community service and specialist teams, dedicated solely to the management of crises.

Trieste's mental health system: history and service structures

Trieste's service network was established in the 1970s (Bennett, 1985; Dell'Acqua and Cogliati Dezza, 1985) in order to replace the old psychiatric hospital with a radically different network of services. The hospital, which had 1200 beds in 1971, finally closed in 1980. Franco Basaglia, radical theorist and pioneer of deinstitutionalisation and community alternatives to institutions, worked in Trieste and initiated this system between 1971 and 1980 (Basaglia, 1987) and CMHCs are the central component. Today, the Trieste Mental Health Department serves a catchment area with 242 000 inhabitants. As well as four CMHCs, it has eight hospital beds, a rehabilitation and residential support service that provides 72 beds in small group homes, and a day centre where training programmes and workshops are available. It collaborates with 13 social firms run on a cooperative basis. Family and service user groups, clubs and recovery homes are also available. The workforce consists of 237 staff, of whom 180 are nurses and 28 psychiatrists. The Mental Health Department is organisationally part of the local Health Agency of Trieste, which also provides comprehensive community

Crisis Resolution and Home Treatment in Mental Health, ed. Sonia Johnson, Justin Needle, Jonathan P. Bindman and Graham Thornicroft. Published by Cambridge University Press. © Cambridge University Press 2008.

health services, sectorised and specialised, particularly for elderly people, adolescents and the disabled.

The community mental health centres in Trieste

The four CMHCs are the engine of the Trieste service system. They are designed to meet local needs in small catchment areas of about 60 000 people, with an average staff ratio of one professional per 1500 inhabitants. Each CMHC team consists of four or five psychiatrists, between 25 and 28 nurses, one or two psychologists, one or two social workers and one or two rehabilitation technicians. Originally, during deinstitutionalisation, CMHCs were developed to meet two needs: as a means of managing crises and reducing psychiatric hospital admissions, and as a system of rehabilitation and social reintegration, initially targeting the former inmates of the local asylum. As the latter have become a less-prominent target group, the CMHCs have evolved to meet the demands of new user groups, establishing wide community networks and partnerships. They provide the following functions and activities:

- overnight hospitality
- day care
- outpatient service
- home treatment
- individual and group therapy
- psychosocial support and work with social networks
- psychosocial rehabilitation
- support for group homes
- support in accessing education, vocational training and job placements
- social activities, self-help and leisure activities.

They also promote access for service users to programmes that are delivered centrally by the Trieste Mental Health Department, including training and vocational programmes, self-help activities and psycho-educational services for families.

The CMHCs are located in large houses and are open 24 hours a day. The atmosphere is friendly and home-like, and the service is open to everyone on a drop-in basis, usually aiming to respond immediately or within one to two hours. Staff take it in turns to provide a reception service, which includes service intake functions. Initial assessment is problem rather than diagnosis led and problems are classified as urgent if this is how they appear from the perspective of the service user or carer. The major principles underpinning the work of these CMHCs are outlined in Box 20.1.

At the beginning of the morning shift, the day's priorities are identified and urgent work fitted in with planned tasks. A couple of clinicians take care of tasks at the CMHC, including care of the 'guests' currently resident at the centre and those attending for outpatient appointments, more informal contacts or group

Box 20.1. Main principles underpinning the work of the Trieste community mental health centres

- The CMHCs aim to shoulder the whole burden of psychiatric morbidity within the catchment area they serve. The three core activities of prevention, acute care and rehabilitation are seamlessly integrated.
- The CMHCs work on the basis of a shared and collective team responsibility. The small catchment area makes it possible for most staff to have direct knowledge at least of the most complex cases.
- The CMHCs aim to be responsive and mobile. Intervention is as far as possible in the service user's normal environment: within their homes or in other places they frequent. Responses are quick and flexible, avoiding waiting lists and other bureaucratic obstacles to accessing services.
- The CMHCs are accessible and open to drop-in referrals.
- Fully multidisciplinary working is a central goal, including integration of social care and partnerships in care with other community services and non-professional and volunteer inputs. The aim is to formulate collective understandings of the situations of service users and shared therapeutic plans. Frequent on-site multidisciplinary training and other joint activities underpin this comprehensive team working.
- The services are value-driven, in that their focus is on:
  - helping the person, not treating an illness
  - respecting the service user as a citizen with rights
  - maintaining social roles and networks
  - fostering recovery and social inclusion
  - addressing practical needs that matter to service users.

meetings and day care. Other clinicians are engaged in community work. This involves carrying out urgent and pre-planned home visits, engaging with social networks, fetching service users and bringing them to the day service, or accompanying and supporting them in important tasks such as attending medical appointments or going to the bank or the workplace. This both ensures that service users are supported in important daily living activities and engages them in a collaborative therapeutic relationship. At the extensive meeting between morning and afternoon shifts, afternoon priorities are set.

Important aspects of meetings of the whole team are free sharing of information and open discussion of current problems and formulation of shared solutions. A balance is found between each worker having an autonomous clinical role and freedom to make decisions, and collective monitoring and decision making. The technical language of psychiatry, which reinforces hierarchies and traditional institutional practices, tends to be avoided in favour of language that is informal, practical and close to that used by service users and carers. Division of work tends to be horizontal, shared and interchangeable.

Crisis management within Trieste's community mental health centres

In many mental health service systems, crises are managed within a loosely interconnected network of services, in which psychiatric hospitalisation is the last resort. Home treatment teams, crisis houses and family sponsor homes are alternatives that, even when extremely effective, will be able to manage only a limited and selected range of individuals, often depending on treatability and on level of risk (Chapter 9).

Principles of crisis management

In Trieste, the aim is that crises should be managed within a comprehensive service in which service provision takes place as far as possible in a normal living environment and is centred on people and their experiences rather than on symptoms and risks. It was decided not to create separate crisis services but to integrate crisis intervention as part of CMHCs. The CMHCs were seen as tools against the asylum, and their mission was to deliver a flexible response, not only to specific illness presentations but also to the problems encountered across a whole lifespan (Mezzina, 2005). Integrating the crisis response within the CMHCs allowed them to draw upon their full range of resources, including social and welfare as well as mental health interventions. The working principles of crisis management in the CMHCs are described in Box 20.2.

Crisis management in practice: the service user's care pathway

The CMHCs are open for new referrals and self-referrals from 8 am until 8 pm. Crisis access outside these hours is via the casualty department. The CMHCs have a high profile in the local community. Thus their low threshold, access and responsiveness are intended to dismantle and deconstruct alarm mechanisms so that referrals involving emergency services such as the police and ambulance services are rare. Procedures for taking referrals are very informal and often involve long phone calls. Sources include family, neighbours, primary care or health districts, welfare services, community agencies and prisons. One principle is that referrers can become resources, taking an active part in the process of engaging and winning the trust of the service user.

Engaging the person in a direct relationship in which increasing trust gradually develops is a central priority for the service, and the flexible approach and wide range of resources available mean that usually engagement can be achieved and compulsory treatment avoided, even among those who initially resist contact (Dell'Acqua and Mezzina, 1988a,b; Mezzina and Vidoni, 1995). Our experience confirms that compulsory treatment tends to result more from the breakdown of

Box 20.2. Working principles of crisis management in the Trieste community mental health centres

Accessibility and mobility of services and the ability to respond to a wide variety of crises. Crisis management is not a special or separate programme but a basic function of the comprehensive service. Selection criteria based on type or severity of illness are not imposed to regulate access to the service, nor does illness of a particular type or severity automatically trigger hospital admission. Promptness of response to crises is very reassuring to referrers, such as family or neighbours, minimising the need to admit users to hospital or even to the CMHC.

Integrated and comprehensive response (social and medical). Therapeutic plans are based on individual history, needs and wishes rather than on a fixed therapeutic model. Establishing a relationship is the first priority, and basing plans on individual needs allows the service to obtain and maintain consent to and engagement in treatment by service users.

Continuity of care. This is a guiding principle and involves treating service users within the usual care system and maintaining them in their usual social context, thus avoiding de-socialisation and institutionalisation. Follow-up is provided wherever service users are, even in prison.

Avoiding hospitalisation. Most people remain at home, but when this is not possible the aim is to avoid hospitalisation in favour of more flexible interventions, such as 24-hour residence ('hospitality') at the CMHC.

professional and non-professional social support networks than from the clinical features of crises (Katschnig and Cooper, 1991), and that service mobility and flexibility are the keys to avoiding involuntary admissions.

With people who do not spontaneously come to the centre for their first contact, staff seek to approach them wherever they spend most of their time, mainly at home, or in other community settings such as in a bar or at work. Members of social networks can act as intermediaries in establishing contact. Staff presence 'on the spot' provides reassurance to family, neighbours and others in their environment, thus beginning the process of defusing the crisis and establishing the human relationships that are the key to providing integrated and non-institutional mental healthcare.

Other principles of engagement are to explore, as far as possible, the person's perceptions of the crisis and his/her needs, and to provide interventions that fit those perceptions; to follow service users' wishes regarding the time and place of meetings; and to avoid time pressures. The priority for team members is to listen not only to the person but also to others involved (separately if necessary). Even though their main role is to understand and advocate for the patient, team members often act as intermediaries in resolving current conflicts and difficulties in their social system. Informing and engaging relatives is often the key to reaching a consensus on a care plan.

Sometimes a crisis cannot be defused in this way, especially where people live alone and have very few resources and relationships with the outside world. A person in this situation can obstinately refuse contact and isolate him/herself still further. The variety and intensity of strategies for making contact are then increased to include telephone calls; messages under the door; involvement of others such as friends, colleagues, the priest, the local policeman or the plumber; and attempts to make contact in a variety of different places where the person is known to go or to negotiate a meeting in a public place of his/her choice where he/she feels safe and not entrapped. These repeated attempts clearly demonstrate the service's assertive attention and wish to help, with the aim of establishing a reciprocal relationship that, even if it is conflictual, may eventually engage the person in some kind of response to his/her difficulties and to the attempts to help that are being made. Even the dramatic and forceful act of 'opening the door' with the help of the police to reach the person may be the gesture that breaks the psychotic circle, with the entry of real faces ending the nightmare and finally initiating a discourse about the 'real' situation and an attempt to establish a trusting relationship, or at least some sort of partial agreement. The process of trying to reach a consensus on treatment is seen as an important therapeutic activity in itself. Compulsory treatment, which is seldom the outcome, is seen as a measure taken because strategies to establish a therapeutic relationship have failed, not because of the illness presentation itself.

The meaning of the crisis is understood through exploration of individual narratives. Using different places or types of contact and participants (especially the 'significant others') is helpful in reconstructing and understanding from different perspectives the person's life history and how the current crisis fits into this history and into his/her belief systems and explanatory models and those of his/her network. Relationships and conversations between staff and service users at the centre and elsewhere develop to a large extent on an informal basis, avoiding the use of formal psychiatric consultations mainly aimed at making a diagnosis. More formalised therapeutic contacts also take place, with meetings at a defined place and time at which individual and family therapies are conducted. The aims of these meetings include:

- facilitating the expression of the person's accounts of their experiences
- encouraging comparisons between perceived needs and the person's current life situation
- analysing how the onset of the crisis and of illness occurred in the context of the person's life history.

Rather than 'acting on patients', a central priority is to 'be with' them during the crisis and to ensure that their historical and existential continuities remain intact. This requires that important relationships are maintained and that links between the crisis and their life history and related meanings are identified (Dell'Acqua and Mezzina, 1988a,b). The crisis is seen in the context not only of the person's psychological development but also of their social relationships and material circumstances (Chapters 11 and 12).

The aim is that the crisis response should mobilise the full range of resources available to meet the identified needs. The interventions provided by the CMHCs, the mental health department, the health districts and the welfare services address:

- living situation (repairs to the home, maintenance and cleaning, looking for more appropriate accommodation)
- money (cash subsidies, use of the centre's safe, daily money management on a temporary basis, support in maintaining tenancies)
- personal hygiene (laundry, personal cleanliness, hairdresser)
- purposeful activities, education and vocational training, work opportunities (from simple tasks at the CMHC to job placements in a work cooperative or in an open market setting)
- leisure (workshops in drama, art, music and needlework, gym visits, day trips, holidays, parties, cinema and theatre trips).

Thus the CMHC aims at the time of the crisis, as at other times, to improve users' overall quality of life and to translate psychiatric technical terms into concrete problems in living and actions that address these problems. These actions contribute to the development of a trusting relationship with the service user and allowing him/her to progress towards re-empowerment and reacquiring a social identity.

Hospitality versus hospital: the environment for 'guests' at the community mental health centres

Crisis treatment at home and/or in other community settings is the first choice and is delivered with the support and involvement of the person's social network and involves mobilising a wide variety of CMHC resources. Consequently, the CMHC is generally a key component in the pathway to recovery. Sometimes staff will suggest that the person could or should stay at the CMHC as an overnight 'guest'. Criteria for deciding on a case-by-case basis whether people need to be invited to reside 24 hours a day at the CMHC include not only symptoms and risk but also the availability of social support, the nature of the therapeutic relationship, the service user's ability to take responsibility for themselves, and the need for a different approach in a case that has become 'stuck'. A relatively low threshold is adopted, with the aim of reducing the separation between care 'inside' and

Table 20.1. Hospitality versus hospitalisation

	Hospitalisation	Hospitality
Rules	Institutional rules	Consensual/flexible rules
Timetables	Institutionalised timetable and routines	Flexible timetable according to user's needs
Relationships	Institutionalised (ritualised) relationships	Relationships tend to break with rituals
Crisis care	Time of crisis disconnected from ordinary life and usual care	Continuity of care before/during/after the crisis
Stay	Inside to take on the patient role	Inside only for shelter/respite
Social contacts	Minimal inputs from social network	Presence and involvement of social network maximised
Freedom	Difficult to avoid locked doors, isolation rooms, restraint, violence	Open door system and no use of restraint
Approach to problems	Problems understood in terms of illness/symptoms/brain disorder	Problems understood in terms of crisis/life events and experience

'outside'. The principle is that the CMHC offers hospitality, which is distinct from hospitalisation in several ways (Table 20.1).

Reasons for proposing that someone stays at the CMHC are openly discussed. The services maintain open doors, indicating a strategy of positive risk taking and a welcoming approach, but sometimes safeguards are needed for service users who are experiencing severe or high-risk crises. For example, it may be agreed that they should have staff with them on a one-to-one basis, or that they will not leave the centre unaccompanied.

Just one night may be spent as a 'guest' at the centre or, where an impasse has been reached regarding other solutions, a stay may even last several months (the average is 10–12 days). A key principle is that people's links with their usual social environments should not be severed, so they are encouraged to continue their usual community activities and maintain frequent contact with friends and relatives, who are free to visit at any time. The overall aim in the CMHCs is to create an open atmosphere in which those currently receiving hospitality mix freely with staff and with service users visiting for other purposes. There is substantial living and social space, and only six to eight beds per centre. As far as possible, all staff and service users live together, eat together and share structured and informal activities. Service users participate in providing and managing the service in a variety of ways. Rigid distinctions are not made between space for staff and space for service users, and the development of interpersonal relationships, both with staff and other service users, is key to the way the centre works and to creating an environment in which the crisis can be resolved and re-socialisation take place. Relationships are based on negotiation, and service users are expected to take responsibility for their actions. Authoritarian or paternalistic attitudes are avoided, and reasons for the rare use of power, as when professionals make unilateral decisions in a situation where there are severe concerns about risk, are clearly explained.

Use of the hospital service

A central aim of the eight-bedded local general hospital unit is to operate as part of the community service and not as a separate hospital facility. People who present in the casualty department during the night may be observed and referred to the appropriate CMHC in the morning. They may stay at the general hospital unit for an extended assessment of up to 24 hours without being formally admitted. The CMHCs manage the unit and aim to activate a community response quickly, whenever possible within this 24-hour period. Thus hospitalisation always takes place within the continuity of the community interventions delivered by the responsible CMHC, and not as a separate intervention. The traditional rigid distinction between inpatient and outpatient status inherent in the medical model has thus been broken down in favour of a much more comprehensive and flexible variety of crisis responses. Hospitalisation is in any case quite rare, with nights spent at the hospital only being about a tenth of those spent at the four CMHCs.

Evidence on the management of crises within community mental health centres

Routinely collected data suggest that this comprehensive approach is effective in delivering crisis care that is largely community rather than institutionally based. All inpatient and community facilities have open doors and no use of restraint. Of a total expenditure on local mental health services of €15 million per year in 2005, 94% was spent in the community and 6% on hospital beds. When the system was first introduced, attendances at the casualty departments at the local general hospital declined markedly, indicated by a fall in contacts from 4250 in 1984 to 3397 in 1988 and then to 1960 in 2005.

The following changes have also been observed over 25 years:

- a reduction by 50% in people presenting to out-of-hours emergency services and the casualty department
- a reduction not only in nights in hospital but also in CMHC bed use, which has fallen to about a third of its original level
- fewer presentations of very disorganised and aggressive behaviours with acute symptoms.

Compulsory treatment also remains very rare, and by 2005 only 15 people were treated compulsorily, representing seven compulsory treatment episodes per 100 000 inhabitants, the lowest figure in Italy (the national figure is 25 per 100 000). The Barcola CMHC in particular, one of four in Trieste, has used no involuntary treatments for any of the population (65 000 people) over the three years between 2003 and 2006.

Even episodes of compulsory treatment take place in the CMHCs whenever possible: two thirds of the overall number of days of compulsory admission were at CMHCs in 2005. With a suicide prevention programme in place, the local suicide rate had fallen by 30% over an eight-year period (Dell'Acqua *et al.*, 2003). Likewise, none of the current inpatients of Italy's forensic hospitals originate in Trieste.

A longitudinal study by Mezzina and Vidoni (1995) investigated outcomes of crisis intervention with a mainly psychotic cohort of 39 people experiencing severe crises at the Barcola CMHC. Eighteen of them required 24-hour hospitality at a CMHC for an average of 7.9 days. After the initial crisis, 37 were followed for four years, of whom 16 relapsed, 9 requiring further 24-hour hospitality at the centre. There were no suicides, crimes or compulsory treatments, and at follow-up four years later, 20 had attained a good level of functioning.

In a subsequent multicentre study encompassing 13 different Italian services (Mezzina *et al.*, 2005a,b), there was evidence that crises resolved quickly in Trieste and in Settimo Torinese, Piedmont, which also operates a 24-hour comprehensive model. This seemed to be related to maintaining trusting relationships with service users, continuity of care and ready access to a wide range of community interventions.

Advantages and risks of integrating crisis management within a community mental health centre

Table 20.2 summarises some of the main features of the Trieste system for crisis management, its advantages and the risks that may arise from organising care in this way. A potential obstacle to implementation of this approach to care is the resistance that may be encountered among professionals moving from more traditional systems. Issues include fear of loss of the status associated with specialist professional knowledge, fear of closeness and reducing barriers between professionals and service users, fear of spending the night with people in crisis without the 'protection' of the hospital, and anxieties owing to a wider concept of responsibility in community settings.

In comparison with specialist models such as the crisis resolution teams, this comprehensive integrated service has a number of potential advantages and disadvantages (Chapter 19), which are described in Box 20.3. Overall, however, the Trieste model is of great interest in that it has been sustained and

Table 20.2. Advantages and disadvantages of the Trieste integrated crisis management system

Organisational features	Care processes	Benefits	Risks or disadvantages
24-hour availability	CMHC reception allows immediate intake to services Walk in access Low threshold	Round-the-clock response No waiting lists for crises High accessibility and user satisfaction (Vicente *et al*, 1993)	Currently no direct intake at CMHC for new cases at night
Single location for full range of services	Single point of contact for service users and referrers Service is a space for social relations as well as clinical care	Integrated response, with rapid access to rehabilitation and socialisation programmes even at the time of the crisis Maintenance and development of social skills at the time of the crisis	An active and flexible intake system must be organised Possibility of social over-stimulation for service users in crisis
Single multidisciplinary team provides full range of services	Integrated workforce Shared knowledge regarding service users with high levels of needs Maintenance of therapeutic relationships throughout different phases of care (prevention, crisis, rehabilitation)	Shared style of work, strategic vision Collective formulation and review of care plans Flexibility and therapeutic continuity Reduced use of involuntary treatment	The wide range of tasks and needs to be addressed may make it harder to maintain focus on particular types of work, such as home treatment for crises Complex group dynamics in the team, constant need to achieve balance between individual autonomy and interdependence
On-site availability of community beds	Alternatives to hospitalisation available Crises can be handled with an open door	Decreased hospital bed use More acceptable care Decreased involuntary treatments Timely admission, shorter crisis time Acute residential care integrated with other types	Risks of excessive bed use or persistence of a hospital mentality

Table 20.2. (cont.)

Organisational features	Care processes	Benefits	Risks or disadvantages
Staff combine internal (CMHC) and external duties	Rotation between reception, tasks within CMHC, and real-life settings Day care, crisis care and residential care provided alongside each other	Flexibility of programmes and ways of working Shared burden and reduction in burn-out Shared therapeutic culture	Complexity of work patterns may lessen focus on particular tasks Risk of confusion and loss of staff continuity Maintaining good balance between CMHC based and external activities is a challenge
Whole team approach to case management	Collective identification of high-priority cases Keyworkers are defined within the team Extensive sharing of information	Culture based on balance between collective and individual responsibility Team approach allows persistence with service users who are difficult to work with	Because of night shifts, less continuity in daytime staffing Individuals may avoid difficult decisions and delegate excessively to the whole team and to doctors as case managers

CMHC, community mental health centre.

Box 20.3. Potential advantages and disadvantages of the Trieste system compared with the crisis resolution team model

Advantages include:

Single point of contact.   Service users associate the CMHC with daily living and continuous support, not only with management of crises.

Immediate accessibility.   The service operates on a drop-in basis and referral to a distinct crisis team is not required.

Flexibility and continuity of care.   Staff who are already familiar to service users from the ongoing support they provide can also manage crises, maintaining continuity of care.

Lack of rigid boundaries between types of care.   The comprehensive system removes the rigid distinction between hospital and community care, providing intermediate types of care and enhancing continuity. Rather than specific clinical tasks, people and their narratives are placed at the centre of the intervention. This approach allows workers to develop a comprehensive vision of care and of the service user's needs throughout crisis and recovery.

Reduces delegation of responsibility.   The temptation to withdraw from responsibility for 'difficult cases' by delegating their care entirely to the hospital is reduced, especially as the team maintains responsibility for managing care throughout periods of intensive residential care.

Integration of crisis care with social and rehabilitative interventions.   Immediate access is available alongside crisis interventions to opportunities for recovery, such as job placement in social cooperatives.

Sustainability in terms of costs.   Fewer staff are required than when specific functional teams are set up.

Disadvantages include:

Lack of focus.   Crisis care may be more structured and focused when it is the sole activity of a team.

Demands on staff.   The wide variety of functions that team members need to fulfil create high demands, although this is mitigated by a cohesive team approach, high levels of support for staff and a sense of agency for each member of the team.

evaluated for about three decades, a substantially longer period than most specialist crisis services, and it appears throughout this time to have been associated with low levels of hospital bed use and compulsory treatment. Replication and evaluation in other settings have started in Italy (currently in the Friuli, Campania, Tuscany and Sardinia regions) and abroad (e.g. in Brazil), and there are plans to implement it in centres in England and Scotland. These applications have tended to show indications of comparable service improvements to those in Trieste, and their outcomes will be of considerable future interest.

Key points

- In Trieste, Italy, crisis care is integrated with the other functions of the integrated and comprehensive 24-hour CMHCs, which are the engine of the local mental health service.
- Service users in crisis have access to a full range of recovery-oriented interventions, and therapeutic relationships with a single staff team are maintained through all phases of care.
- This approach to crisis care is centred not on an illness model, but on service users' lives, their narratives and the meanings they attach to these.
- CMHCs have six to eight beds in which they can offer hospitality to service users in an open environment that avoids barriers, restraints and separation from usual living environments and social networks, but where even compulsory admissions can generally be safely managed.
- The Trieste model has now been sustained for about three decades, and evaluations suggest that it results in Italy's lowest rates of bed use and compulsory admission.

REFERENCES

Basaglia, F. (1987). Madness/delirium. In *Psychiatry Inside-out. Selected Writings of Franco Basaglia,* ed. N. Scheper-Hughes and A. Lowell. New York: Columbia University Press, pp. 233–63.

Bennett, D. H. (1985). The changing pattern of mental health care in Trieste. *International Journal of Mental Health,* **14,** 7–92.

Dell'Acqua, G. and Cogliati Dezza, M. G. (1985). The end of the mental hospital: a review of the psychiatric experience in Trieste. *Acta Psychiatrica Scandinavica Supplement,* **316,** 45–69.

Dell'Acqua, G. and Mezzina, R. (1988a). Approaching mental distress. In *Psychiatry in Transition. The British and Italian Experiences,* ed. S. Ramon and M. G. Giannichedda. London: Pluto Press, pp. 60–71.

Dell'Acqua, G. and Mezzina, R. (1988b). Responding to crisis: strategies and intentionality in community psychiatric intervention. *Per La Salute Mentale/For Mental Health,* **1,** 139–58.

Dell'Acqua, G., Belviso, D., Crusiz, C. and Oretti, A. (2003). Trieste e il suicidio: un progetto di prevenzione. *Quaderni Italiani di Psichiatria,* **XXII,** 11–23.

Katschnig, H. and Cooper, J. E. (1991). Psychiatric emergency and crisis intervention services. In *Community Psychiatry. The Principles,* ed. D. H. Bennett and H. L. Freeman. Edinburgh: Churchill Livingstone, pp. 517–42.

Mezzina, R. (2005). Paradigm shift in psychiatry: processes and outcomes. In *Mental Health at the Crossroads: The Promise of the Psychosocial Approach,* ed. S. Ramon and J. E. Williams. Aldershot, UK: Ashgate, pp. 81–93.

Mezzina, R. and Vidoni, D. (1995). Beyond the mental hospital: crisis intervention and continuity of care in Trieste. A four-year follow-up study in a community mental health centre. *International Journal of Social Psychiatry*, **41**, 1–20.

Mezzina, R., Vidoni, D., Miceli, M. *et al.* (2005a). *Crisi Psichiatrica e Sistemi Sanitari. Una Ricerca Italiana.* Trieste: Asterios.

Mezzina, R., Vidoni, D., Miceli, M. *et al.* (2005b). Are 24 hours community crisis interventions evidence based? Indications from a multicentric longitudinal study. *Psichiatria di Comunità*, **4**, 200–16.

Vicente, B., Vielma, M., Jenner, F. A., Mezzina, R. and Lliapas, I. (1993). Users' satisfaction with Mental Health Services. *International Journal of Social Psychiatry*, **39**, 121–30.

21

Crisis resolution teams and older people

Ciaran Regan and Claudia Cooper

Older people with mental disorders can potentially benefit from crisis and home treatment services in managing their frequently complex mental and physical health needs. If the principles of equity and the recent anti-age discrimination policies in the UK (Department of Health, 2004, 2005) are to be upheld, such services developed for people of working age should be made available to older adults with mental health disorders on the basis of need. This is not, however, currently the case in the UK. For older people with physical health problems, there has been considerable development in intermediate care services providing intensive multidisciplinary input to allow people who would otherwise be at risk of unnecessarily long stays to live more independently, typically in their own homes (British Geriatrics Society, 2004). However, those who also have comorbid mental health problems face barriers in accessing these services (Morris *et al.*, 2006). In this chapter, we first consider the challenges in developing crisis services for older people. We then examine the current extent and nature of crisis and home treatment services for older people, and review the three potential models of service provision: intermediate care, general adult crisis resolution teams (CRTs) and specialist teams.

Challenges in setting up mental health teams for older people

The configuration of specialist mental health services for older people in the UK varies substantially, with some based on the model usual in services for adults of working age (multidisciplinary community teams allied to inpatient units), while others are based on more traditional medical models of 'doctor led' assessment (Challis *et al.*, 2002). Some services are closely allied to primary care and social services; others have a distinct demarcation between services delivering

Crisis Resolution and Home Treatment in Mental Health, ed. Sonia Johnson, Justin Needle, Jonathan P. Bindman and Graham Thornicroft. Published by Cambridge University Press. © Cambridge University Press 2008.

specialist, primary and social care, or between care for people with dementia and for those with mental illnesses such as depression and psychosis. Add to this the traditional barriers between services for those of working age and those for older people, plus those between physical and mental healthcare, and the resulting map of required interfaces is both complex and daunting.

While it is generally agreed that holistic care by professionals skilled in physical and mental healthcare is required for old age crisis work, the reality is that most healthcare professionals receive the great majority of their training in one or the other, and feel de-skilled when faced with health problems outside their usual remit. With the advent of old age psychiatry specialisation, this is now also true for staff who train either in 'adult' mental health or in 'old age'. This can be compounded when working out of hours in the community, where staff need to feel confident in their own competence, since other advice is difficult to access. Staff in general adult CRTs that have a policy of accepting older people tend to be concerned that their lack of expertise in dealing with this group, especially those who have dementia, will be an impediment to working successfully with them. Our recent survey (Cooper *et al.*, 2007) found that one intermediate care team in England that managed mental health problems saw a majority of people with dementia-related problems rather than functional mental illnesses such as depression or psychosis. At the same time, CRTs for older people, with primarily mental health-trained staff, saw mostly older people with functional illnesses, indicating a gatekeeping policy in line with the teams' perception of their own skills. Training, review of staff mix, recruitment of team members with substantial experience with older people and liaison with other services are likely to provide some solutions to these problems.

There has been no UK National Service Framework specifically for the mental health of older people, which may explain why this service sector is comparatively poorly served by crisis services. Earmarked funding has not been made available, as it has for intermediate care for people with physical health problems. Despite this, dedicated crisis teams for older people have shown promising results and these are reviewed later in this chapter (Richman *et al.*, 2003; McNab *et al.*, 2006). In promoting equity between and within services, the question for healthcare providers is how to augment or extend current services to provide the best care for older people with mental disorders.

Providing a service for older people

There are some specific differences in providing care for older people with mental health crises. The presentation of mental health disorders, as well as their course, is distinctive. For example, self-harm is more likely to lead to suicide in older people. Studies of community-based samples of older people with long-term severe mental illness show that they frequently rely on family members, as opposed to mental health services, for the majority of their care and often do not seek help or support even when this is available (Meeks and Murrell, 1997). Supporting carers is, therefore, particularly important for crisis workers. Liaison with both primary and secondary care staff, educating them in recognising the salience of symptoms indicating mental illness, and promoting earlier referral should be important roles for the team, reducing carer burden and stress. At times, rapid simple interventions, such as liaison with primary care regarding treatment of urinary tract infections, can prevent an admission to hospital. Where the care recipient requires a care placement, supporting older people and their carers in the community while this is arranged may be an important way in which admission can be avoided.

Current provision of older people's crisis services

We recently reviewed the literature (up to April 2006) relating to older people's crisis provision and undertook a survey to find out about current provision of crisis resolution and home treatment services (Cooper *et al.*, 2007). We interviewed team informants knowledgeable about team policy and caseload over the last year in 79 (99%) of the 80 trusts providing acute mental health services in England with at least one CRT. We found that in 25 (32%) of the areas studied (which included one area from each trust), there was a policy of offering full CRT services to older people, either through a specialist team (seven areas), the adult CRT (17) or an intermediate care team that also managed mental health crises (one).

Crisis resolution teams specialising in older people

Two studies relating to dedicated older people's CRTs, both descriptive in nature, have been published. The first (McNab *et al.*, 2006) described a dedicated older people's CRT recently set up in the Central and North West London Mental Health Trust. This 'home treatment team' sets out to 'bring hospital to home', to provide support to carers in the acute phase of the illness and put patients in touch with local services such as primary care and social services. To date, the team reports high levels of patient and carer satisfaction with services, as well as a reduction in bed occupancy. The second study (Richman *et al.*, 2003) described a specialist mental health outreach support team that has been established as a crisis intervention team since 1999. Its remit was to provide additional support for the community teams when older adults were in crisis, reduce admissions to psychiatric beds and facilitate early discharge from inpatient units.

The patient group was selected from a waiting list for the inpatient unit. The team reported favourable outcomes in terms of preventing admission but did not give details on acceptability to patients or carers. Both of these teams saw people with both organic-related disorders, such as dementia, and functional mental illnesses.

In our survey, we spoke to the managers of both of these teams, as well as to five other dedicated older people's teams in England. These varied considerably in terms of staffing, hours and case mix. Two teams acted as gatekeepers to beds for older people and one planned to start doing so soon. They had a median current active caseload of seven (2–25) people without and nine (0–25) people with dementia. Staffing mix varied, with most teams including social workers, community psychiatric nurses, occupational therapists, physiotherapists and allied support workers.

Intermediate care teams

Current policy regarding the physical healthcare of older people in England prioritises provision of intermediate care, which is defined as services or activities concerned with patients' transitions between hospital and home: from medical and social dependence to functional independence. It is intended to prevent avoidable hospital admissions and promote early discharge (Steiner, 1997). Intermediate care was a central tenet of the *National Service Framework for Older People* (Department of Health, 2001) and attracted considerable investment. A report reviewing progress of this five years on (Morris *et al.*, 2006) found that a third of older people needing intensive daily help in England now receive this in their own homes rather than residential care, and delayed discharge from acute hospitals had been reduced by more than two-thirds. Less promisingly, the report concluded that care for older people with mental health problems was often hampered by the traditional separation of medical specialties from psychiatry, so they may benefit less from these service developments.

In our survey, one intermediate care team had been managing mental health crises for four years. It was seeing eight people for whom the main reason for involvement was mental health, six of whom had dementia. Their staff included a registered mental health nurse. They did not act as gatekeepers for older people's mental health beds or use intermediate care beds for mental health patients.

General adult crisis resolution teams working with older people

Prior to our survey, only one paper, to our knowledge, reported on the work of general adult CRTs with older people. This was a descriptive study, published by a team with no upper age limit for its service users, of its patients over the course of a year (Brimblecombe *et al.*, 2003). It reported that age was not related to outcome in terms of admission rates and concluded that the results 'tentatively suggest that older people may be as able to benefit from home treatment as an alternative to hospital as people aged under 65 years, at least in terms of their ability to successfully complete a period of home treatment'.

General adult CRTs had a policy of providing younger and older adults with the same service in 17 (21.5%) areas, but only five (29.4%) of these teams were currently treating any older people. None was seeing people with dementia, and all but two excluded people with dementia. Three of these teams had seen more than one older person in the previous week.

The limited numbers of older people seen by the adult teams was perplexing and we explored the attitudes of the staff towards managing older people with mental health crises. Generally, staff in general adult CRTs were positive about working with older people. Comments made by team members included, 'older people's teams are very good at managing crises and working jointly with us'. Some commented on the low rate of referrals from older people's service and some felt that this was an area of low need. Indeed, in one area, an older people's CRT had recently closed, a lack of referrals apparently contributing to this decision. There were concerns about working with older people because of a perception that crisis work could take longer and would, therefore, make heavy use of resources. Staff were particularly concerned that they lacked the necessary skills for managing people with dementia, and that appropriate training had not been provided. They also expressed a lack of confidence in managing physical health problems.

Therefore, despite explicit governmental policy, our survey found that fewer than a third of the areas studied in England had a policy of offering the same CRT service to both older and younger adults, and that, in practice, only one in six areas regularly provided crisis services to older people. Current practice is, therefore, contrary both to national policy and to the ethical principle of equity.

Recommendations for future practice

A more positive finding from the survey was that numerous services were considering or planning crisis service expansion for older people, which suggests that government guidance regarding age discrimination in services may be having an impact. Innovations being considered included introduction in various areas of all three main service delivery models already found in the UK, namely, dedicated older people's CRTs, extended general adult teams and intermediate care teams that include older people experiencing mental health crises.

Experience to date of mental health services in England suggests that a specialist team with a critical mass of workers trained in older people's mental and physical healthcare is the service model that can treat the broadest range of older people experiencing mental health crises. We suggest that these 'stand-alone' teams should consist of staff from disciplines including nursing, occupational therapy, psychology and social work. Mapping local needs through audit has informed decisions about staffing numbers and hours of operation of existing teams. Working a 24-hour day, the accepted model for CRTs, is successful in a London-based stand-alone team, but we also found examples of effective teams with an extended hours working pattern in areas where overnight demand for services was found to be low. Gatekeeping of psychogeriatric beds is in our view an important part of the standard CRT model that can and should be retained in specialist teams. Preliminary work indicates that older people's specialist CRTs may reduce admissions, so despite concerns regarding resource implications, expansion of services may well prove cost effective.

Expansion of adult CRTs to accept referrals from older people's services is the main alternative service model. Such a team is currently operating in Kent and sees over 20 referrals per month of people aged 65 or over. Effective leadership, an experienced team and adequate resources no doubt help in expanding generic teams for this role. We suggest, however, that there are potential problems with generic rather than specialist services undertaking older people's crisis work, including lack of specialist expertise (e.g. regarding older people's mental health, cognitive disorders and physical health problems), that can lead to generic crisis workers feeling that they lack skills required for managing older clients. A crisis team working with all ages would face challenges in managing interfaces with other services, an issue that is already daunting in its complexity for general adult teams in some areas. In many trusts, general adult and older people's services operate from different budgets, and we found that negotiations over team funding have been a critical obstacle to expanding existing CRTs in several areas.

Teams managing older people's mental health crises need to be able to assess promptly both older people experiencing mental health crises and people who present with acute confusional states (acute impairments of cognition, attention and orientation, thinking and perceptions that often result in severe agitation, incoherence and behavioural disturbance and frequently have physical causes). Treating common physical causes of confusion is a key role and requires effective, timely liaison with primary care, while access to psychiatric clinicians is important for managing mental health crises. Interfaces with social services and care agencies are also important in ensuring prompt access to extra services in order to prevent breakdown in care. Family carers often provide older people with most of their care, so supporting and working with them as partners in care is particularly vital in this age group.

Key points

- The development and expansion of crisis services for younger adults has not been matched by similar services for older adults. This is an issue of equity.
- There are currently few CRTs in operation that regularly see older people, and to date most successful teams have used a stand-alone model.
- No formal evaluations of this stand-alone model have so far been completed, but local audit results have been promising.
- Providing best and dignified care for older people should where possible include the option of being treated at home.

REFERENCES

Brimblecombe, N., O'Sullivan, G. and Parkinson, B. (2003). Home treatment as an alternative to inpatient admission: characteristics of those treated and factors predicting hospitalization. *Journal of Psychiatric and Mental Health Nursing*, **10**, 683–7.

British Geriatrics Society (2004). *Intermediate Care: Guidance for Commissioners and Providers of Health and Social Care*. London: British Geriatrics Society. http://www.bgs.org.uk/ Publications/Compendium/compend_4-2.htm. Accessed: 27 December 2006.

Challis, D., Reilly, S., Hughes, J. *et al.* (2002). Policy, organisation and practice of specialist old age psychiatry in England. *International Journal of Geriatric Psychiatry*, **17**, 1018–26.

Cooper, C., Regan, C., Tandy, A., Johnson, S. and Livingston, G. (2007). Acute mental health care for older people by crisis resolution teams in England. *International Journal of Geriatric Psychiatry*, **22**, 263–5.

Department of Health (2001). *National Service Framework for Older People. Standard Three: Intermediate Care*. London: The Stationery Office.

Department of Health (2004). *Securing Better Mental Health for Older Adults*. London: The Stationery Office.

Department of Health (2005). *Everybody's Business. Integrated Mental Health Services for Older Adults: A Service Development Guide*. London: The Stationery Office.

McNab, L., Smith, B. and Minardi, H. A. (2006). A new service in the intermediate care of older adults with mental health problems. *Nursing Older People*, **18**, 22–6.

Meeks, S. and Murrell, S. A. (1997). Mental illness in late life: socioeconomic conditions, psychiatric symptoms, and adjustment of long-term sufferers. *Psychology and Aging*, **12**, 296–308.

Morris, J., Beaumont, D. and Oliver, D. (2006). Decent health care for older people. *British Medical Journal*, **332**, 1166–8.

Richman, A., Wilson, K., Scally, L., Edwards, P. and Wood, J. (2003). Service innovations: an outreach support team for older people with mental illness – crisis intervention. *Psychiatric Bulletin*, **27**, 348–51.

Steiner, A. (1997). *Intermediate Care: A Conceptual Framework and Review of the Literature*. London: King's Fund.

22

Integrating day treatment and crisis resolution teams

Mary Jane Tacchi

For some patients, the provision of home-based treatment from a crisis resolution team (CRT) will not be an adequate or safe alternative to admission. Realistically, two or three hour-long home visits per day are the maximum that a busy CRT can provide on a regular basis. Hoult (1986) described an Australian service where, as a pragmatic measure, a patient could accompany a clinician travelling over long distances to the next home visit as a way of providing increased supervision and support. This, however, is not the norm in the UK. Home-based treatment must be flexible in order to meet the patient's needs, but resources are necessarily finite. Occasional longer visits from a support worker are useful but cannot be seen as a sustainable intervention. One could argue that if a patient cannot be contained or provided with sufficient support by home-based treatment then admission should be sought. This is often the case, but while admission should certainly not be avoided at all cost, there are circumstances in which alternatives are preferable. One potential way of bridging the gap between home-based treatment and admission is to use an acute day service or a partial hospitalisation programme as an element in CRT service provision.

Acute day hospitals to which patients can be admitted urgently as a substitute for inpatient care have a long history, dating back to the USSR in the 1930s. The 1970s were probably the time of their peak popularity in Western countries (Shepherd, 1991). Of all the alternatives to hospital that have been evaluated, day hospitals have probably the most robust evidence base, with several evaluations and two systematic reviews suggesting that they are an effective and cost-effective alternative to admission for some patients (Creed *et al.*, 1997; Horvitz-Lennon *et al.*, 2001; Marshall *et al.*, 2003). Despite this accumulated evidence for their effectiveness, day hospitals seem recently to have fallen from favour, receiving relatively little attention in policy making or in mental health services research

Crisis Resolution and Home Treatment in Mental Health, ed. Sonia Johnson, Justin Needle, Jonathan P. Bindman and Graham Thornicroft. Published by Cambridge University Press. © Cambridge University Press 2008.

(Marshall, 2003), although a recent national survey indicated that substantial numbers of day hospitals in the UK still aim to provide an alternative to acute admission and/or to shorten hospital stays (Briscoe *et al.*, 2004). As few of the published evaluations are very recent, uncertainties remain about how far day hospitals can contribute to avoidance of admission in a modern community mental health system, and diminished interest in them is likely to reflect an increasing focus since the 1980s on working with patients in home and community settings, targeting especially patients who are unlikely to attend institutional settings. As with crisis houses, an interesting possibility is that a combination of acute day care and outreach to patients at home by CRTs may be an effective way of providing comprehensive crisis care for patients whose needs in areas such as purposeful occupation and contact with others are not fully met by CRTs.

This chapter examines how acute day services can be integrated with CRTs, using as examples the development of two different services. These demonstrate how services evolve to respond to local needs and pressures, learn from mistakes and cope with the reality of working within limited budgets. Finally, the advantages and potential pitfalls of such service developments will be discussed.

The Home Options Service, Manchester

Harrison *et al.* (1999) described the extension of the existing acute day service in central Manchester. The day hospital was well established and focused on providing an alternative to inpatient care, operating between 9 am and 5 pm, Monday to Friday. Evaluation of the service showed it to be successful in its aims, namely: patients at the day hospital were as ill as those admitted (Creed *et al.*, 1989), 40% of those presenting for admission could be treated at the day hospital with few differences in clinical or social outcome (Creed *et al.*, 1990) and the day hospital cost less (Creed *et al.*, 1997). Limitations of the service were the restricted hours of opening and the need for patients to attend the unit for treatment.

In order to address these limitations, the Home Options Service was developed. Extra funding of £235 000 per year was identified and the day hospital began operating 24 hours a day, seven days a week, with full staffing provided from 9 am to 11 pm and two members of staff available on-call overnight. Staffing consisted of two charge nurses, eight staff nurses, three support workers, three occupational therapists, a technical instructor, an administrator, a manager, four consultant psychiatrist sessions, four specialist registrar sessions and five senior house officer sessions. The service provided 30 places for patients known to the service and suffering from an episode of acute mental illness that would otherwise have required hospital admission. Criteria were that the risk should be manageable and the patient willing to cooperate. Patients could attend the base for some aspects of treatment but could be seen exclusively in their own homes if they preferred. Most were seen in both locations. Patients and carers were given a 24-hour emergency contact number and additional support was available in the form of one-to-one monitoring at the base between 9 am and 10 pm, with the patient then being taken home, with night-time medication if required, to attend again the following day. The service also had exclusive use of a single respite bed in a self-contained flat, which could be used for up to two nights for patients requiring closer supervision for a limited period. Staffing for this intervention was provided from within existing resources. At the time of writing, the service continues to operate as described, with approximately 50% of contacts occurring at the day hospital base (J. Harrison, personal communication).

A partial hospitalisation programme, Newcastle

In Newcastle upon Tyne, high bed occupancy rates and increasing concerns over the quality of therapeutic work being undertaken in inpatient facilities led to the development of a partial hospitalisation programme. This was planned as an alternative to inpatient care with three main purposes: to divert patients from acute admission, to deliver transitional care for those about to be discharged from hospital, and to provide treatment and rehabilitation for those living in the community who had a history of repeated admissions for severe and enduring mental health problems. The premise on which the service was developed was that targeting these three patient groups would reduce acute admission rates and length of stay in hospital, and prevent repeated admissions. The partial hospitalisation programme provided 50 places to the population of west Newcastle (150 000). Staffing consisted of two occupational therapists (one senior and one basic grade) and two experienced nurses, with medical sessional time provided from within existing resources.

Evaluation of the first year's activities indicated that 60% of referrals were for people who would otherwise have been admitted; 90% had severe mental illness and 50% had previously been admitted. Over the course of the first year, requests for urgent referrals increased. It was demonstrated that the programme reduced the pressure on the inpatient unit, as evidenced by reduced occupied bed days, number of admissions and length of stay (Tacchi *et al.*, 2004). However, the programme seemed to delay rather than prevent admission for 15% of patients. The restricted staffing and medical input meant that it was not always possible to offer places to patients with the most acute problems, which led to a reduction in turnover and a rise in occupancy of the partial hospitalisation programme to 96%. This, in turn, led to reduced ability to offer a range of therapies and, ironically, problems started to arise that mirrored the difficulties on inpatient units which the programme was designed to address. It was felt that the programme had been devised to target three patient groups but increasingly was needed for people at immediate risk of acute admission and was unable to meet demand because of inadequate funding and personnel. As a result, it was decided that the service would develop in a different direction.

The next development was the establishment of a crisis assessment and home-based treatment service to provide an alternative to hospital admission and to support early discharge from hospital. The model adopted in Newcastle and North Tyneside was that of a separate crisis service serving a population of 450 000. The aim was to plan the local acute system as an integrated whole, ensuring continuity and effective communication between its components (Keown *et al.*, 2007). This crisis service led to a reduction in bed usage, which, in turn, resulted in a reduction in the number of beds available. To prevent the re-emergence of the original difficulties of the inpatient wards, the service planners developed the acute day service as a distinct function of the partial hospitalisation programme. The service was available seven days a week, from 9 am to 5 pm, and provided six to eight places for patients resident in Newcastle (approximately half the catchment area of the crisis service) who required extra support that could not be provided by home-based treatment. Funding was secured for additional staff, in the form of two trained nurses and two support workers, five sessions of staff-grade medical time and three sessions of consultant medical time, but the only staff recruited were one trained nurse, one and a half support workers and the medical staff. Referrals to the service came exclusively from the crisis service, which provided a gatekeeping function and ensured that all patients being treated in the acute day service were also receiving home-based treatment over a 24-hour period.

The acute day service was located in the partial hospitalisation programme, which was housed within the inpatient unit. This was physically separate from the CRT base, and liaison between the two services occurred via telephone twice daily and by regular meetings of the CRT members at the acute day service, at which they saw patients and liaised with staff. Initial evaluation of the service showed that all patients attending were judged by staff to be appropriate for the service and were suffering from severe mental illness: 71% of referrals were to prevent admission and 29% to promote early discharge from hospital. Of those who were assessed, 29% were offered places but refused to attend. In the first three months, 50% of patients were subsequently admitted under the Mental Health Act, and it was felt that the service had delayed rather than prevented admission of these individuals. The building was found to be inadequate as its use was not exclusively for the acute day service. There were competing demands for space and no facilities for patients to rest quietly or sleep, which was identified as an unmet need. It was noted that patients were reluctant to attend the base at weekends and seemed more comfortable doing so during the week.

It was concluded that the service was a worthwhile addition to home-based treatment and provided useful increased input for some patients, although for others admission seemed inevitable. It was felt that the liaison between the acute day service and the CRT worked well but that ideally these two services should be physically located together.

Integrated day treatment and crisis resolution teams

Advantages

The most obvious advantage of integrating the day treatment service and the CRT was the increase in flexibility of care provision, with a choice of venues for patients and the ability to provide extended hours of therapeutic input. This, in turn, increased safety, reduced risk and allowed alternatives to admission to be provided for increasing numbers of patients. Increased contact in a service setting made it easier to supervise medication and to carry out physical assessment and interventions, such as those required for prescription of clozapine. There is evidence that such services lead to a reduction in compulsory admissions under the Mental Health Act (Harrison *et al.*, 2001), since some patients who refuse admission are prepared to accept this type of service as an alternative.

Other advantages of the service are similar to those of home-based treatment in general, in that patients can continue to be involved with their social networks and maintain independence. The stigma of admission, either voluntarily or under the Mental Health Act, is avoided and a more accurate assessment of patient need can be made. Additionally, cultural traditions are not disrupted by hospitalisation and the involvement of carers is the norm rather than the exception.

Potential pitfalls

One of the pitfalls of integrating such services is the potential duplication of input. This is overcome by the service being managed as a whole, as in the Home Options Service, or if one part of the service acts as gatekeeper to the other, as in the Newcastle model. In separate services, the issues of integration, communication and responsibility must be resolved before such services become operational.

Other potential pitfalls are similar to those encountered by other alternatives to hospitalisation, in particular that carer stress may be increased (though the literature gives little evidence of this; e.g. Hoult, 1986), that some patients miss the asylum function of hospital, and that provision of such care can challenge some patients' and carers' expectations and beliefs. Staff burn-out is also a possibility, though again there is little evidence of this (Chapter 5), and in fact those services where staff have a clear aim and feel that they are succeeding in it show greater job satisfaction. Harrison *et al.* (2001) point out that staff may experience increased stress because, when serious incidents occur, innovative services are more closely scrutinised by the media. A practical issue in the provision of day treatment is the ability and willingness of the patient to travel to the service base. Providing taxis or staff to escort patients may be initial solutions to this and may increase the number of patients who can be engaged with this form of care, but patients being able to travel independently for treatment can also be used as a goal for treatment. Harrison *et al.* (2001) also noted that in some services a high proportion of patients are referred but not accepted, suggesting that referrers need further training in order to maximise efficiency. Finally, for some patients, providing an alternative to admission seems to delay rather than prevent admission. If such patients could be identified accurately it may be more appropriate for admission to be sought earlier (Chapter 8).

What can be seen is that the integration of day treatment and crisis services can bridge the gap between home-based treatment and hospital admission for some patients. The services described have been developed as a pragmatic response to local needs. They suggest that service delivery models can be adapted to suit circumstances and needs as long as a clear overview is maintained of the integrated functioning of the local service system. In Manchester, the day hospital extended its remit to provide home-based treatment for patients known to the service. In Newcastle, partial hospitalisation was the first development, but because of inadequate funding this was not robust enough to provide a sustainable alternative to admission. The crisis service was then established and acute day service care provided for a number of patients receiving home-based treatment, while the CRT went on to provide care for others and assess patients not known to the service. The outcomes for both services are similar, showing, perhaps, that a variety of approaches to delivering acute care may be effective in meeting local needs.

Key points

- The provision of acute day services can bridge the gap between home-based treatment and hospital admission.
- Successful services have integrated acute day service provision and home-based treatment.
- Advantages for patients are increased flexibility and more frequent contact with services, which increase safety, support and therapeutic input. Such services

provide a choice of venue for patients and maintain the advantages of remaining in the community.

- In order to maximise efficiency, further training needs to be provided for referrers to the service.

REFERENCES

Briscoe, J., McCabe, R., Priebe, S. and Kallert, T. (2004). A national survey of psychiatric day hospitals. *Psychiatric Bulletin*, **28**, 160–3.

Creed, F., Anthony, P., Godbert, K. *et al.* (1989). Treatment of severe psychiatric illness in a day hospital. *British Journal of Psychiatry*, **154**, 341–7.

Creed, F., Black, D., Anthony, P. *et al.* (1990). Randomised controlled trial of day patient versus in-patient psychiatric treatment. *British Medical Journal*, **300**, 1033–7.

Creed, F., Mbaya, P., Lancashire, S. *et al.* (1997). Cost effectiveness of day and in-patient psychiatric treatment. *British Medical Journal*, **314**, 1381–5.

Harrison, J., Poynton, P., Marshall, J. *et al.* (1999). Open all hours: extending the role of the psychiatric day hospital. *Psychiatric Bulletin*, **23**, 400–4.

Harrison, J., Alam, N. and Marshall, J. (2001). Home or away: which patients are suitable for a psychiatric home treatment service? *Psychiatric Bulletin*, **25**, 310–13.

Horvitz-Lennon, M., Normand, S. L., Gaccione, P. and Frank, R. G. (2001). Partial versus full hospitalization for adults in psychiatric distress: a systematic review of the published literature (1957–1997). *American Journal of Psychiatry*, **158**, 676–85.

Hoult, J. (1986). Community care of the acutely mentally ill. *British Journal of Psychiatry*, **149**, 137–44.

Keown, P., Tacchi, M. J., Niemiec, S. and Hughes, J. (2007). Changes to mental healthcare for working age adults: impact of a crisis team and an assertive outreach team. *Psychiatric Bulletin*, **31**, 288–92.

Marshall, M. (2003). Acute psychiatric day hospitals. *British Medical Journal*, **327**, 116–17.

Marshall, M., Crowther, R., Almaraz-Serrano, A. *et al.* (2003). Day hospital versus admission for acute psychiatric disorders. *Cochrane Database of Systematic Reviews 2003*, Issue 1, CD004026. Oxford: Update Software [DOI: 10.1002/14651858.CD004026].

Shepherd, G. (1991). Day treatment and care. In *Community Psychiatry: the Principles*, ed. D. H. Bennett and H. L. Freeman. Edinburgh: Churchill Livingstone, pp. 386–414.

Tacchi, M. J., Joseph, S. and Scott, J. (2004). Evaluation of a partial hospitalisation programme: good news and bad. *Psychiatric Bulletin*, **28**, 244–7.

23

Integrating crisis residential care and crisis resolution teams

Brynmor Lloyd-Evans, Sonia Johnson and Helen Gilburt

The advantages of treatment at home are described elsewhere in this book and there is substantial evidence that many service users prefer this. Recent English mental health policy reflects this in its central focus on diverting patients from admission by caring for them at home. However, home treatment is not always desirable. In this chapter, the circumstances in which residential acute care is appropriate are identified and the potential advantages of community residential services over hospital inpatient care are discussed. A summary of the development of residential alternatives to hospital is provided. Finally, three examples of how crisis residential care can be integrated with crisis resolution teams (CRTs) are presented and the benefits of such integration discussed.

The need for residential crisis care

Home treatment may be inappropriate in several crisis situations. Risk of harm to self or others may be too great for patients to be left for many hours without staff supervision. People who are severely neglecting themselves, for example by failing to eat and drink properly and care for themselves and their environment in basic ways, are difficult to manage with CRT visits alone. Some have no home or live in very poor circumstances, while others may live in a home environment that exacerbates their difficulties, for example because of an abusive relationship. Another impediment to home treatment is that carers may feel unable to sustain their role in supporting someone at home. When one or more of these obstacles to home treatment exists, it does not necessarily mean that acute hospital admission is required: community residential alternatives to hospital also have the potential to address the needs of some of the people for whom home treatment is unsuitable.

Crisis Resolution and Home Treatment in Mental Health, ed. Sonia Johnson, Justin Needle, Jonathan P. Bindman and Graham Thornicroft. Published by Cambridge University Press. © Cambridge University Press 2008.

Advantages of community residential settings

Potential advantages of admitting to community residential settings rather than hospital include acceptability to service users and maintaining social networks.

- Non-hospital residential care may be more acceptable to service users and be perceived as less stigmatising than hospital. This type of support may, therefore, be used more readily and at an earlier stage, allowing necessary treatment to be provided promptly and a more collaborative relationship to be maintained between professionals and service users. These benefits are especially great if the increased acceptability of community alternatives means that compulsory admission can be avoided.
- Community-based residential crisis services may be more able than hospitals to help service users to maintain contact with friends and family, and to remain engaged in their usual activities. Thus the risk of social networks and activities declining following an admission may be less in a community facility than in hospital, and strengths and coping skills may be better maintained.

The availability of different types of alternative to admission is also important for service user choice. In their absence, the introduction of CRTs and their gatekeeping role would mean that, unless the high threshold for hospital admission is reached, service users in crisis would have no option other than to cope with their problems at home, something they may feel especially reluctant to do if they live alone and have little support available other than the CRT's daily or twice daily visits.

Development of residential alternatives to hospital admission

Several forms of residential alternative to hospital have been described since the 1960s, though evidence regarding their outcomes remains limited. While many of the published descriptions and evaluations relate to stand-alone residential services, some residential services have operated in conjunction with home treatment teams. For example, the extensive network of community services established by Paul Polak in Denver, Colorado, in the 1970s included family sponsor homes, where acutely unwell patients could be placed for a few weeks. The families involved were carefully selected and were supported by members of the home treatment service, who could be paged at any time. They were paid a fee for receiving up to two patients in crisis as guests in their homes, and they were encouraged to involve them in the life of their households, for example through participating in household chores and joining family meals (Polak *et al.*, 1979). A similar network of family sponsor homes was established by Leonard Stein and his colleagues in Madison, Wisconsin, in the 1980s and is still operating (Stein, 1991; Bennett, 2002). The family sponsor home systems in Denver and Madison have involved placement of acutely unwell patients with selected families, who receive some specific training and have 24-hour support from the home treatment service. Stroul (1988) surveyed community-based residential crisis facilities in the USA and reported that such short-term housing and support at the homes of carefully selected families was the most widely available form of residential crisis care. Hoult *et al.* (1983) described agreements made with selected boarding houses in Sydney, Australia, that patients could be placed there urgently for respite, with support from the local home treatment team.

The only published description from the UK of a service of this type relates to the Accredited Accommodation Scheme in Powys, Wales, which aims to provide crisis care, although in practice it has often been used for planned periods of respite and rehabilitative social care (Readhead *et al.*, 2002).

Residential units in the community offering short-term emergency admission, sometimes known as crisis houses, are the residential alternative to admission that has received most attention in the UK (Davies *et al.*, 1994). A few descriptions and evaluations of such services have been published in the USA, though the model has not been widely adopted. These studies have usually been small and problems with study design have sometimes made the results hard to interpret, but overall their results have suggested clinical and social outcomes at least as good as for standard inpatient care (Bond *et al.*, 1989; Fenton *et al.*, 1998; Hawthorne *et al.*, 2005). Crisis residential services in the USA have varied considerably in the degree to which they adhered to conventional clinical practices and staffing patterns, or offered an alternative that was substantially different in philosophy and treatment approach from hospital services. Probably the best known of the more radical alternatives was Loren Mosher's Soteria service, which operated from 1971 to 1983 and aimed to manage first-onset schizophrenia in a community house, if possible, without recourse to antipsychotic medication (Mosher *et al.*, 1975; Mosher, 1999). A randomised controlled trial, finally published more than two decades after its completion, suggested better or similar outcomes for Soteria compared with hospitalisation, and lower subsequent use of antipsychotic medication, with 43% of Soteria residents identified as 'drug-free responders' who were well after two years without having received medication (Bola and Mosher 2002, 2003). The model had a few early replications in the USA, and more recently in continental Europe, especially the German-speaking countries, where the most renowned service based on the Soteria model is in Bern, Switzerland (Ciompi and Hoffmann, 2004). As yet there is insufficient research evidence for the effectiveness of this interesting model or to establish the groups for whom it is appropriate.

In the UK, investigations of the Drayton Park women's crisis house in Islington, North London, which is staffed 24 hours a day, have suggested that most women managed there have a previous history of hospital admission, and that it is highly valued by service users (Killaspy *et al.*, 2000; Johnson *et al.*, 2004). The women report that their recovery is promoted by a home-like environment, absence of disturbed male patients, ready availability of staff for talking through current and past difficulties, and good support from other residents. Admission to the house is often experienced as less stigmatising than hospital. Some crisis houses have adopted a user-led model of care, as in the residential crisis facilities supported and described in a report by the Mental Health Foundation (2002). In these services, crises have been understood in a social and interpersonal framework rather than in terms of illness. The enhanced ability to empathise with crises and the capacity to act as positive role models of workers who have themselves experienced and recovered from crises are mobilised. The emphasis in providing care is on the value of being with people during crises and helping them mobilise their own strengths and resources and engage in positive activities.

Another strategy for providing residential alternatives to inpatient care is to establish hybrid facilities that offer crisis admission alongside one or more other types of community care. Perhaps the most prominent examples are the community mental health centres (CMHCs) in Trieste, which combine crisis beds with a comprehensive range of other services (Mezzina and Vidoni, 1995; Chapter 20), and similar services that have been described elsewhere in Italy and in France (Katschnig *et al.*, 1993). In the UK, Boardman and colleagues (1999) have investigated beds integrated into CMHCs in North Staffordshire, with results suggesting greater client satisfaction and better outcomes on some measures for the group managed in the CMHCs than for hospital inpatients. Wesson and Walmsley (2001) have described a community-based unit in Southport that combines day care and crisis admission beds. These beds have a maximum stay of three days and are used for a variety of purposes, including as an alternative to hospital, for early discharge from hospital and for patients needing supervision when starting on new medications.

Thus a range of residential alternatives to acute hospital have been described, but relatively little is known so far about their clinical effectiveness and whether they manage crises of similar severity to those currently resulting in hospital admission. Most of the published literature relates to crisis residential services that operate independently of, rather than in conjunction with, a CRT or home treatment team. However, an ideal system for community management of crises should arguably include both a team providing intensive home treatment and residential alternatives to hospital. The extent to which synergy between these models might enhance the capacity of each to manage crises effectively in the community is worth investigating.

Integrating crisis residential care and crisis resolution teams: some examples

Current policy in England requires nationwide introduction of CRTs but not, as yet, of crisis residential alternatives. However, data from the Alternatives Study (Johnson *et al.*, 2007), which has involved surveying residential and inpatient alternatives throughout England, and in which the authors are currently involved, suggest that innovative ways of integrating CRT and crisis residential service provision are developing in some areas. Such service development seems to have been piecemeal and pragmatic rather than systematic, often depending on creative use of existing local resources. For example, voluntary sector hostels, temporary accommodation provided by local authorities and statutory sector respite care beds are all settings that may be used for crisis management, with additional support from CRTs. However, as CRTs become established nationally, many are creating more formal links and agreed working arrangements with residential services (Box 23.1). These links take various forms, including:

- the CRT managing and running its own residential crisis service as an integrated part of the team
- the CRT co-managing a residential service with another statutory sector agency
- the CRT having assured access to beds in an independently run and managed, often voluntary sector, service.

Some examples of how these arrangements can work in practice are provided as Case studies 23.1–23.3, below. Where residential crisis beds are incorporated as part of a CRT, continuity of care and the benefits of a coherent approach from management and staff are likely to be greatest. In a service such as Middlesbrough Crisis Beds (Case study 23.1), moreover, the physical proximity of the residential service to the CRT office helps to ensure that appropriate support can be provided very swiftly. A working agreement between a CRT and a completely independent service has different potential advantages; for example, the service can provide additional strengths to complement the input from the CRT, and may also be well placed to avoid a very medicalised or institutional environment and thus provide a genuine alternative to hospital for service users. In whatever form, a formal arrangement between a CRT and a residential service can provide a number of benefits to both (Box 23.1).

The development of community-based residential crisis services working closely with CRTs is a recent and largely uncoordinated innovation in England's acute mental healthcare system. Little is known about the effectiveness and acceptability of these residential alternatives; they do offer the possibility, however, of increased choice and a beneficial treatment option for people experiencing acute mental health crises.

Box 23.1. Benefits of formal arrangements between crisis resolution teams and residential services

Guaranteed or prioritised access to beds. Where a CRT has exclusive use of all or a number of beds at a residential service, crisis planning and prioritising need can be more efficiently managed.

Improved communication. Agreement can be reached in advance about what information the residential service requires when someone is admitted, so providing this becomes routine for the CRT. The CRT can also act as a clear, single point of contact through which the residential service communicates with other mental health and statutory services.

Guaranteed availability of support. Agreement can be reached in advance for the CRT to provide dedicated time at the residential service for specific care, such as a weekly visit from a psychiatrist or psychologist. By providing additional medical or nursing input and 24-hour access to additional support, a CRT may enable a residential service to offer a service to acutely ill people who could not otherwise be accepted. A close working link with the CRT may also make the process of hospital admission work more smoothly, if this is required; this again may give community residential services the confidence to accept severely unwell patients.

More coordinated management. The CRTs and residential services can agree policies or procedures together and cooperate over training and staff development. Clinical care can also be coordinated; for example, both services can use the same clinical assessment tools.

CASE STUDY 23.1. MIDDLESBROUGH CRISIS BEDS

The Middlesbrough crisis resolution and intensive home treatment team is based on the premises of a social services hostel in Middlesbrough and manages four crisis beds within it. The CRT acts as gatekeeper for all referrals to the crisis beds. Practical care is provided by hostel care staff, but CRT staff provide additional clinical care for users of the crisis beds, including dedicated weekly time from CRT psychiatrists and psychologists. The proximity of the CRT base to the crisis beds ensures that additional staffing needs can be met promptly. Many aspects of traditional acute inpatient care, such as nursing care, dispensing medication and taking blood tests, can be provided at the crisis beds. However, the service does not involve coercion: it is not locked and restraint and seclusion are not used. Nor can it admit detained patients. Organised social and recreational activities are not provided in-house, but service users can be helped to access what is locally available.

The service manager reports that most users of the crisis beds have a serious mental illness and are acutely unwell to an extent that would otherwise warrant hospital admission. A typical length of stay is seven days, and over 90% of people admitted are discharged home. The service has been running in its current form since 2003 and has contributed to a reduction in admissions to the local acute ward of about 30%.

CASE STUDY 23.2. THE CARE HOME AT 81 LOWTHER STREET, WHITEHAVEN, CUMBRIA

In Whitehaven, at 81 Lowther Street, there is a six-bedded residential care home that receives funding from the local primary care trust but is managed by Croftlands Trust, a voluntary organisation that also runs other supported housing services locally. The manager and deputy manager come from a nursing background, but most of the team are care staff without mental health professional qualifications. The local CRT, Copeland/West Cumbria Urban Crisis Resolution and Home Treatment Team, acts as gatekeeper for all referrals to 81 Lowther Street. Psychiatrists from the CRT have dedicated weekly time at the service and other CRT members can come into the service to provide additional support for service users when required. Information and a contingency care plan are provided by the CRT for all referrals. Despite close links with the local CRT, 81 Lowther Street operates independently. Staff will liaise directly with other mental health services and regularly refer service users for day care or a floating support scheme organised by Croftlands Trust. The service also offers out-of-hours telephone support for ex-service users at times of crisis.

Approximately three-quarters of people come from the community and are referred in order to avert hospital admission; the other quarter comes from acute psychiatric wards before returning home. The majority have a psychotic illness and all are people with severe mental illness who are acutely unwell. The nature of the building and the low night-time staffing levels do impose some limits on who can use the service, as constant observations or sustained one-to-one care cannot be guaranteed. Detained patients and people with a history of serious violence or arson are not accepted. Average length of stay is just over two weeks and nearly all service users return home. The success of the service in averting hospital admissions is one factor influencing current plans to halve the number of beds at the local acute psychiatric ward.

CASE STUDY 23.3. RIVERVIEW SOCIAL CRISIS HOUSE, NORTHEAST LONDON

The Riverview Social Crisis House is a three-bedded unit that serves residents of the northeast London boroughs of Havering and Barking and Dagenham. It is both a crisis and a respite unit for people with severe mental illness. The unit aims to keep people out of hospital who may have otherwise required admission, and it does not accept patients held under the Mental Health Act, except on Section 17 leave (a Section of the Act which allows patients temporarily to leave hospital).

The unit is funded by the North East London Mental Health NHS Trust and is run by the local social services department. It is staffed 24 hours a day by a team of 'support time recovery workers' (unqualified care workers employed to work collaboratively in direct contact with service users towards a goal of recovery) and managed by the manager of the home treatment team (HTT). It is independent of the HTT but a proactive link has been formed between the two services. People new to the service are assessed for admission to the unit by the HTT. Employing a psychosocial and medical model of care, the HTT assesses the nature of the mental health problem, current risk and any medication needs. Once individuals have been admitted to the crisis house, recovery workers utilise a social care model, working in partnership with the service users to identify their needs and the support required to meet these needs and help the individuals to return to the community. Where medical intervention is required, this is provided by the person's GP. Prior to discharge, the HTT works with the crisis house to put together a care plan within the community, putting the person in touch with a range of services, and on discharge, the HTT provides follow-up care. A clear understanding of the role of each service, a collaborative approach and joint management between the crisis house and HTTs allow people to benefit from a wide range of skilled staff and receive good continuity of care.

Key points

- Residential crisis services are developing and integrating with CRTs in England in a variety of ways.
- Service managers' reports suggest that these services are valued by service users and can reduce hospital admissions.
- Research evidence has yet to be provided for the effectiveness and acceptability of different residential crisis service models.
- Services of the crisis-house type are the most common in England. Other models, such as family sponsor homes or beds based in CMHCs, may also be worth exploring.
- The inability of most residential community crisis services to admit detained patients limits the extent to which they can provide an alternative to hospital admission. Exploring the feasibility of residential alternatives accepting compulsory as well as voluntary admissions is an important goal for future service development.

REFERENCES

Bennett, R. (2002). The crisis home program of Dane County. In *Alternatives to the Hospital for Acute Psychiatric Treatment*, ed. R. Warner. Washington DC: American Psychiatric Press, pp. 227–36.

Boardman, A. P., Hodgson, R. E., Lewis, M. and Allen, K. (1999). North Staffordshire Community Beds Study: longitudinal evaluation of psychiatric in-patient units attached to community mental health centres. I: Methods, outcome and patient satisfaction. *British Journal of Psychiatry*, **175**, 70–8.

Bola, J. R. and Mosher, L. R. (2002). At issue: predicting drug-free treatment response in acute psychosis from the Soteria project. *Schizophrenia Bulletin*, **28**, 559–75.

Bola, J. R. and Mosher, L. R. (2003). Treatment of acute psychosis without neuroleptics: two-year outcomes from the Soteria project. *Journal of Nervous and Mental Disease*, **191**, 219–29.

Bond, G. R., Witheridge, T. F., Wasmer, D. *et al.* (1989). A comparison of two crisis housing alternatives to psychiatric hospitalization. *Hospital and Community Psychiatry*, **40**, 177–83.

Ciompi, L. and Hoffmann, H. (2004). Soteria Berne. An innovative milieu-therapeutic approach to acute schizophrenia based on the concept of affect-logic. *World Psychiatry*, **3**, 140–6.

Davies, S., Presilla, B., Strathdee, G. and Thornicroft, G. (1994). Community beds: the future for mental health care. *Social Psychiatry and Psychiatric Epidemiology*, **29**, 241–3.

Fenton, W. S., Mosher, L. R., Herrell, J. M. and Blyler, C. R. (1998). Randomized trial of general hospital and residential alternative care for patients with severe and persistent mental illness. *American Journal of Psychiatry*, **155**, 516–22.

Hawthorne, W. B., Green, E. E., Gilmer, T. *et al.* (2005). A randomized trial of short-term acute residential treatment for veterans. *Psychiatric Services*, **56**, 1379–86.

Hoult, J., Reynolds, I., Charbonneau-Powis, M., Weekes, P. and Briggs, J. (1983). Psychiatric hospital versus community treatment: the results of a randomized trial. *Australia and New Zealand Journal of Psychiatry*, **17**, 160–7.

Johnson, S., Bingham, C., Billings, J. *et al.* (2004). Women's experiences of admission to a crisis house and to acute hospital wards: a qualitative study. *Journal of Mental Health*, **13**, 247–62.

Johnson, S., Gilburt, H., Lloyd-Evans, B. and Slade, M. (2007). Acute in-patient psychiatry: residential alternatives to hospital admission. *Psychiatric Bulletin*, **31**, 262–4.

Katschnig, H., Konieczna, T. and Cooper, J. (1993). *Emergency Psychiatric and Crisis Intervention Services in Europe: A Report Based on Visits to Services in Seventeen Countries*. Geneva: World Health Organization.

Killaspy, H., Dalton, J., McNicholas, S. and Johnson, S. (2000). Drayton Park, an alternative to hospital admission for women in acute mental health crisis. *Psychiatric Bulletin*, **24**, 101–14.

Mental Health Foundation (2002). *Being There in a Crisis*. London: Sainsbury Centre for Mental Health and Mental Health Foundation.

Mezzina, R. and Vidoni, D. (1995). Beyond the mental hospital: crisis intervention and continuity of care in Trieste. A four year follow-up study in a community mental health centre. *International Journal of Social Psychiatry*, **41**, 1–20.

Mosher, L. R. (1999). Soteria and other alternatives to acute psychiatric hospitalization: a personal and professional review. *Journal of Nervous and Mental Disease*, **187**, 142–9.

Mosher, L. R., Menn, A. and Matthew, S. M. (1975). Soteria: evaluation of a home-based treatment for schizophrenia. *American Journal of Orthopsychiatry*, **45**, 455–67.

Polak, P. R., Kirby, M. W. and Deitchman, W. S. (1979). Treating acutely psychotic patients in private homes. *New Directions for Mental Health Services*, **1**, 49–64.

Readhead, C., Henderson, R., Hughes, G. and Nickless, J. (2002). Accredited accommodation: an alternative to in-patient care in rural north Powys. *Psychiatric Bulletin*, **26**, 264–5.

Stein, L. (1991). A systems approach to the treatment of people with chronic mental illness. In *The Closure of Mental Hospitals*, ed. P. Hall and I. F. Brockington. London: Gaskell, pp. 91–106.

Stroul, B. A. (1988). Residential crisis services: a review. *Hospital and Community Psychiatry*, **39**, 1095–9.

Wesson, M. and Walmsley, P. (2001). Service innovations: Sherbrook partial hospitalisation unit. *Psychiatric Bulletin*, **25**, 56–8.

Section 5

Developing a local service

24

Planning and implementing a local service

Martin Flowers and John Hoult

This chapter is in two parts. The first provides guidance on how to plan and set up a local service, including the information requirements for effective planning; the preparatory steps that need to be taken, including consultation with a range of hospital and community agencies and service users; setting budgets; and the requirements for beginning to deliver a service. The second part explores the reasons why some teams fail to demonstrate their continuing effectiveness and identifies the factors that help a team to achieve success and sustainability in the long term.

Planning and setting up a team

The obvious needs to be stated: whoever sets up a crisis resolution team (CRT) needs to have a clear vision of the overall purpose of the team and what they want it to achieve. A team that will do predominantly crisis resolution/home treatment will have different staffing and organisational requirements from one focusing on carrying out all acute assessments in an area, and from one that has both expectations. This exact remit of the team needs to be decided and made clear from the start.

The most important steps in planning and setting up a CRT are summarised in Box 24.1 and described in more detail in the remainder of this section.

Visit other teams

It is important to ask around to find out what teams are operating in areas with similar characteristics to the planned area – especially teams considered to be operating successfully – and to visit them in order to learn about their methods and their problems. Networks of CRTs such as the regional groups operating

Crisis Resolution and Home Treatment in Mental Health, ed. Sonia Johnson, Justin Needle, Jonathan P. Bindman and Graham Thornicroft. Published by Cambridge University Press. © Cambridge University Press 2008.

> **Box 24.1. Key steps in planning and setting up a crisis resolution team**
>
> The following steps are expanded upon in the text:
> - visit other CRTs
> - determine the size of the team
> - get the support of the senior members of your organisation
> - get as much support as possible
> - consult service user and carer groups
> - secure funding
> - appoint a steering group
> - appoint the team leader
> - appoint the staff
> - set up the team's base
> - establish a medications policy
> - establish information and communication systems
> - liaise with local organisations
> - initiate training
> - establish the team culture.

under the auspices of the National Institute for Mental Health in England (http://www.nimhe.csip.org.uk) are often helpful sources of information and local contacts.

Determine the size of the team

It is vital that adequate numbers of staff are requested at the outset, since it will be much harder to request more staff later on and you will lose credibility if you do not do so because the team cannot be as effective. In determining the appropriate size of the team, you should take a number of factors into account.

The population size of the catchment area

The current guideline in England is for 14 clinical staff per 150 000 total population for an 'average' area. This seems about right for a CRT.

The characteristics of the area

The greater the social disruption of an area, the greater the need for staff. The bigger the city, the more social disruption there is likely to be in its centre. One inner-city London area that had a high level of homelessness, many immigrants from non-English-speaking backgrounds, many cheap hostels and boarding houses and one of the highest levels of deprivation in the country needed a team of 15 staff for a population of 70 000. At the other extreme, there are rural areas where the rate of severe mental illness and hospital admission is low. In such areas, the need for fewer staff is counterbalanced by the longer distances to be travelled on slow, narrow roads. One useful way of deciding on the size of the team is to look at the annual admission rate from the catchment area prior to the establishment of the team. As a rough guide, a team of 14 staff can usually deal with a rate of about 400 per year.

The task to be done

If a team is expected to do all accident and emergency department assessments and/or to be a common pathway for all referrals to the mental health system, then it must have additional staff to do these tasks so that the CRT function is not compromised.

The need for an adequately staffed rota

Team members have annual leave, study leave and sick leave. There should be enough staff to allow for these and to ensure that there are at least three people on each shift. Fewer than three rostered staff can incapacitate a shift in the event of sudden sickness.

Availability of senior staff

Senior members of staff should be available at all times throughout the rota to ensure that key decisions about treatment options can readily be made, and the team's finances need to reflect this. A CRT comprising relatively junior grades will not be able to act effectively or safely as gatekeepers to hospital beds.

Communication within the team

Too big a team can create communication problems, particularly at handover time. In some areas of England there are CRTs of over 30 staff but these only operate efficiently because the leader exerts iron discipline at handover time.

The amount of funding available

Sadly, money is too often the determining factor. It will be discussed below.

Get the support of the senior members of your organisation

The chief executive officer is going to have to fund and support this team, so securing their 'buy-in' is critical. The medical director and director of nursing also need to be convinced of the need for the proposed service. State clearly what the team will and will not do (avoid being the main provider of acute assessments in the accident and emergency department if you can) and make sure that the expectations of others are the same as yours: in particular, make sure that they are not expecting the CRT to do more than it can to solve their other problems. While you need to be enthusiastic about the proposal and emphasise the expected advantages, take care to be realistic and not to oversell the benefits. You should also ensure that the team's gatekeeping role is made clear.

Get as much support as possible

It is important to meet with organisations, both statutory and voluntary, whose work will be affected by the new service. Explain what you are planning to do and how it will affect them, and take note of any concerns. Talk to community mental health teams (CMHTs) and inpatient units and do all you can to get medical staff's support. It may help to bring in outside experts to meet with or address the various groups or to organise educational meetings about CRTs.

Consult service user and carer groups

Because treatment is being provided at home, carers will often express concern about the perceived burden that a CRT service may present to them. They will need a clear explanation of what the CRT can do and how it will deliver home treatment, including its role in working with the families and social systems of service users, how the team can be contacted, out-of-hours arrangements and referral pathways and systems. Service user groups are potentially valuable as a source of support for new CRTs, as they often very much welcome the availability of home treatment as an alternative to hospital admission.

Secure funding

You may have to lobby the organisation's management, who might well want to cut CRT staff numbers, or give it additional responsibilities. Resist this with all your might if you want to have an effective service. If you are forced to accept a reduced budget, endeavour to limit the population served so that your team will still be able to demonstrate an impact. An under-funded CRT with too big a task to do will face problems: it will probably change into a predominantly assessment-focused unit rather than a home treatment team, it will show little impact, and after a while people will start to question its value and staff on the team will lose morale.

There are instances in which management has linked the establishment of a CRT to ward closures in order to provide funding. Closing a ward before the team becomes operational has occasionally worked in localities with many beds and lax admission procedures, but it does have the potential to cause resentment towards the CRT. Unless there is a lot of slack, it should not be done.

Planning to close a ward within a very short time of the establishment of a CRT, on the assumption that the team will make a quick impact, is also a risky strategy. Some adequately staffed teams have made a rapid impact on admission rates, but it takes considerably longer for them to have an effect on bed occupancy. To be successful, this strategy requires good planning and a concerted effort by the ward and CMHT staff, as well as the CRT.

Life is not always easy, and the local health body may not have the resources to fund a CRT. There have been occasions, however, where outside bodies have provided funds to help to establish a team, for example if it is linked to a research programme. Do not, therefore, give up the quest for funds too readily.

Appoint a steering group

Once funding is secured, a steering group should be established to oversee the setting up and early development of the team. The group should certainly include representatives from the organisation that will run it (and someone from its finance department), together with the prime mover of the project and the proposed team leader. Service user and carer representatives should be invited. It is better to avoid too large a group, though local conditions may make it wise to include representatives from some services affected by the new team, such as inpatient wards and CMHTs.

Appoint the team leader

To be successful, a CRT leader needs, in addition to the usual desirable leadership qualities, to be flexible, adaptable, willing to tolerate risk and skilled at managing it. Usually, CRTs enjoy high levels of morale and most staff are willing workers who enjoy their jobs. However, the team leader still needs to be encouraging and to be able to balance trust in the staff with ensuring that they remain focused and clinically competent. A leader who is too anxious, rigid or controlling will damage a team's initiative and morale.

Appoint the staff

The team leader needs to be involved in appointing the staff both to secure a degree of loyalty and to ensure, as far as possible, that the recruits have the desired characteristics of flexibility and adaptability, as well as the necessary clinical skills. Further recommendations regarding staff recruitment are made in Chapter 25.

Set up the team's base

Once the team leader has commenced work, there are many tasks to be carried out during the recruitment process and initial operation of the team. A team base must be located and furnished. The obvious location is somewhere central in the area to be served, but in most cases location is dictated by what premises the organisation has available, and by costs. Some practitioners wish to avoid being located on a hospital campus, fearing that they will be too closely identified with the hospital or that the hospital culture will suck in its staff. In practice, however, there are quite successful teams based in the same building as the inpatient unit. Having adequate parking space is important. The team needs a meeting room large enough for all the team to gather for their daily handover, with a whiteboard displaying the names of their patients and details of tasks to be done for them. Only the team manager and secretary need to have their own offices; it is better for team members not to as this inhibits the important flow of information between them. Staff require desks, which can be in the meeting room, in order to use the telephone and write up case notes.

If a team is located in a hospital or CMHT base, then it does not need to see people at its own base since, on the few occasions where a patient comes to visit, the CRT can use the host's facilities. Free-standing CRTs may wish to have one or two interview rooms with lockable doors available. Security will need to be considered if office appointments are offered at times when few people are on the premises.

Having secured premises, the leader then needs to furnish them and obtain the necessary office supplies: a visit to one or more existing teams will reveal what is needed. The team's policies should be prepared at this time: usually, these can to a large extent be copied from those of other CRTs, but they should also give a clear description of the planned patient pathways through the local acute care system.

Establish a medications policy

All CRTs need quick access to medication. The team leader must meet with the chief pharmacist in the area to work out a policy for ordering, storing, dispensing and carrying medication. In England, there are national policies and guidelines about this, but they have not yet been adapted to include CRTs. Nevertheless, a practice has developed within CRTs themselves of storing medications in locked cupboards at the team base. Only nurses can dispense from original packets into containers for individual patients and label them, but any member of staff can deliver unopened, labelled containers to the patient. Only nurses and/or the patient can take the medication from the containers. Sometimes the local chief pharmacist expresses some concerns, but contact with pharmacists in areas with operating CRTs helps to allay these.

Establish communication and information systems

In order to become a well-integrated part of the local mental health system and to ensure continuity of care between different parts of this system, the CRT needs effective systems for communicating with other teams and obtaining and sharing important documentation, such as risk assessments. Early attention should be paid to establishing systems for record keeping, communicating with other services and transmitting information, with early discussions held with key departments such as information technology (IT) and medical records to ensure these systems work as effectively as possible. Use of email and electronic records is likely to be very helpful in ensuring that information is passed on as efficiently and comprehensively as possible, though the value of phone calls for establishing relationships with staff in other services and for informal discussions should be remembered. Systems need to be set up for record keeping within the CRT; again, use of electronic formats is likely to result in clear records that can readily be transmitted to other clinical services as needed. Plenty of computers need to be available for staff and IT training needs should be assessed and addressed if available electronic systems are to be used effectively. The potential advantages of using simple structured measures for recording patient characteristics and outcomes should be considered at this stage: this may be very helpful for the team in demonstrating what it is achieving.

Liaise with local organisations

During the waiting period, before the other team members begin their duties, the leader should liaise with all of the groups in the area that will be affected by the team's operations. It should be explained how the team will operate and how it is likely to affect them, and written protocols should be provided where necessary. Organisations to be visited must include the inpatient units, the relevant CMHTs, the accident and emergency department, the social services department and local service user and carer groups. The consultant psychiatrist attached to the team should meet with the other consultants working in the area and, if possible, with local general practitioners (GPs). The more likely it is that a group or organisation will be affected by the activities of the team, the more important it is to meet with its representatives.

Initiate training

Finally, the appointed team members present for duty. While they ideally should all arrive on the first day, usually only around three-quarters of them will be present. Nevertheless, the team needs to begin its work, so training should be initiated with those present. Staff training is dealt with in Chapter 25, but it is worth noting here that, during this time, new members of staff not only acquire knowledge but also begin the team bonding process. Staff come to realise that they need to rely on each other and learn new ways of coping with and managing patient crises.

Establish the team culture

A newly established CRT lacks its own culture but will develop one within a few months. The training period and the first few months are, therefore, critical; it is much harder to change the team culture later on. Principles and practices – such as the expectation of being able to treat each patient at home, positive risk management, frequent visiting, spending lengthy periods with patients rather than just monitoring medication, and intervening with social networks – have to be inculcated right from the start, during the training period, and then put into practice correctly. The team leader and the consultant psychiatrist must take the lead in modelling these practices for the team and in monitoring their implementation. Once the culture is established, new team members will fit into it.

Sustaining a crisis resolution team

Research evidence shows that CRTs can be effective and are generally preferred by patients and carers (Chapter 5). Given this, why have many CRTs in other countries not been sustained? Although there is little evidence about this in the literature, the likely answers are that they have not been seen as an integral part of the total service system and/or that they have failed to demonstrate their usefulness and effectiveness, thus becoming an easy target for cutting when times become difficult.

Teams that have continued to be successful over a period of years share some common features, which have helped them to remain focused on a model that enshrines the home treatment culture but allowed them to adapt to changes both in their community and in mental health services. In order to ensure long-term success and sustainability, CRTs should adopt a number of principles and patterns of working. These are summarised in Box 24.2 and described in more detail in the remainder of this section.

Be an integral part of the whole area mental health system

The CRT should have a clearly delineated role, backed by management and accepted by the rest of the service. Some services have evolved to include a home treatment function within a fully integrated acute service (Chapter 15).

Be helpful and useful to other parts of the service

New services are often seen as having been given the biggest slice of the cake and this can get relationships off to a difficult start. The team needs to be aware of this and should conduct its business in a sensitive manner. If a team is perceived as helpful by other components of the service, then they will not want to lose it. Exchanging staff for a time-limited period with other components can help them develop an understanding of the CRT's role and work (and vice versa).

> **Box 24.2. Principles for ensuring the sustainability of a crisis resolution team**
>
> A crisis resolution team should:
> - be an integral part of the whole area mental health system
> - be helpful and useful to other parts of the service
> - avoid unnecessary conflict with other parts of the service
> - work constructively with other components of the area service to improve service delivery
> - ensure continued support from within and outside the service
> - collect data about the team's activities and outcomes
> - make an impact
> - publish the data
> - undertake research
> - ensure effective management and leadership
> - provide continuing training for staff.

Avoid unnecessary conflict with other parts of the service

Conflict can frequently occur when CRTs reject referrals on insufficient grounds or with inadequate explanation to referrers, or when they fail to advise referrers on alternatives. Both GPs and CMHTs will not at first really understand how to use the CRT; such understanding only comes with experience developed over a number of cases, so tolerance is needed. It is better to accept an inappropriate referral, assess it and provide feedback and advice about what else would have been appropriate than to create conflict by rejecting the referral and then having an unhappy referrer complain to everyone about the uselessness of the team.

Not infrequently, CMHTs find that they have a patient (or carer) in crisis late on a Friday afternoon, usually one whom they have not seen for weeks. This is a frequent source of conflict and resentment between teams, and it is, therefore, helpful to have negotiated clear rules about such situations in advance.

The CRT set-up is particularly vulnerable to hubris and team members can be quite critical of the perceived failings of other components of the service. This naturally causes resentment and those in other areas will subsequently be more than willing to point out any defects in the CRT's work.

Work constructively with other components of the area service to improve service delivery

Given the nature of their work, CRTs can show up defects in the overall system. Examples include very soft admission criteria, unnecessary delays in discharging inpatients, long delays in having referred patients assessed and taken up by CMHTs, and patients not being seen for unjustifiably long periods. If they do encounter such practices, CRTs must resist the temptation to spread blame but should work constructively with the other teams and/or more senior management to improve things. Similarly, CRTs must be prepared to alter their own practices in the light of criticism from others.

Ensure continued support from within and outside the service

It is important to keep management informed about what is happening, especially if there are good outcomes to report. A good service should be delivered to patients and carers and data should be collected that reveal the views of service users and carers on the team. This information can be used to inform practice development. Efforts should be made to ensure good communications with other components of the service and links with the local community and voluntary sector partners. Effective CRTs depend on these links to plan creatively for home treatment and to identify relapse as quickly as possible, thereby lessening the effect of crises on service users and their social systems.

Collect data about the team's activities and outcomes

Data about activities are useful for auditing the practices of the team. Is it doing too little or too much work? Are some patient groups missing out? Are patients staying too short or too long a time with the team? Collecting such data can allow the team to make comparisons of their workload against other CRTs in the area.

Collecting outcome data is important for determining whether the team is making an impact. The only data that can be obtained easily and cheaply are those on admissions and bed use. An organisation's IT department will probably have this information, but experience shows that it can be exceedingly difficult to extract. If so, the team needs to collect its own data. Information on patient satisfaction can be collected with a little effort and this is certainly worth doing.

Make an impact

Data and good feedback will demonstrate the impact that the team is achieving. If a team has fidelity to the CRT model and provides a good gatekeeping function, it should follow that admissions will significantly decrease. Bed usage is affected by other factors, such as availability of supported accommodation for more disabled patients, but an impact should be apparent in this area as well. A combination of reduced admissions and bed use may then allow beds to close. The work of the CRT then becomes vital in preventing beds from having to re-open.

Ensuring a positive impact on service user satisfaction is also vital, and the team will need to adapt its practices to respond to any complaints or criticisms. The impact on carers is also crucial and the CRT needs to guard against the risk of increasing the burden on them. Using the existing Care Programme Approach and carers' care plans to gather information on their needs and views can form the basis for data collection.

Publish the data

Publishing the work you have done and the positive outcomes achieved helps to raise the profile of the CRT. This can help the team to make a case for investment to develop the service further and can attract money from other agencies to fund research. The morale and energy of the team can be sustained and improved by being a part of a service that feels proud of its work and is happy to share its outcomes. The publication of the team's work does not have to be in scientific psychiatric journals; a report in a publication such as the *Nursing Times* or the *Health Services Journal* is also useful.

Undertake research

A variety of important research questions about CRTs and their functioning within modern mental healthcare systems remain to be answered (Chapter 5). Benefits for teams of participating in research studies include raised team profile and opportunities to demonstrate benefits from the team's work. Carrying out large research projects, such as randomised controlled trials, requires considerable amounts of money, which, in the present climate, are often not very readily available, although establishing partnerships with local academics may be helpful in obtaining support for such projects. Lack of large-scale funding should not, however, deter CRTs from performing smaller-scale projects in order to inform practice. Satisfaction surveys, for example, are relatively straightforward to set up and can be based on information systems that are already in place, such as minimum datasets for local use. Local trainees placed in research posts or undertaking higher degrees may be valuable resources for such smaller projects.

Ensure effective management and leadership

The *Mental Health Policy Implementation Guide* (Department of Health, 2001) stated that leaders need to 'communicate a vision of the future system, engage key stakeholders across that system, and manage the organisational and structural changes required to reach the vision'. CRT managers should:

- provide leadership that clarifies the role and function of the team
- create an environment in which people can be creative and exercise judgement in their own practice
- encourage and support the team, since this is vital for maintaining morale
- be aware of current good practice applied by other services and attend CRT forums to discuss common difficulties and practice issues
- be able effectively to represent the service to higher management within the system, in order to safeguard its role and promote practice development.

Provide continuing training for staff

A very common sustainability issue for CRTs is the dilution of the model over time: teams often provide 'start up' training but the home treatment culture can become lost from view as people leave for new posts and their replacements do not receive the same level of training as was initially felt necessary. If such dilution takes place, then the impact of the team will inevitably diminish.

The community served by a CRT will have changing needs and these should be reflected in the practice of the team (common issues include working with interpreters and with drug and alcohol problems). Supervision and performance review systems need to be clear and effective to ensure that a team's practice evolves and that any deficits in knowledge can be quickly identified and relevant training needs met. Team members should be encouraged to enhance their clinical skills in areas where they have a special interest, though additional training should, of course, be in line with the needs of the service.

Key points

- Obtaining the support of senior managers, local service users and carers and other key stakeholders is crucial before the team is established. Enough funding needs to be secured for the team to carry out all its expected roles.
- Key tasks to be carried out during the set-up period include obtaining suitable premises, establishing medication policies, setting up communications and record-keeping systems and disseminating among other services an awareness of the team's role and operating principles.
- A team manager who is flexible, adaptable and skilled at tolerating and managing risk is required for team morale to be sustained and for good relationships maintained with other parts of the service.
- The team's culture tends to be established in its first few months and is subsequently rather hard to modify.
- Teams that survive and function effectively in the long term tend to be those that become an integrated and valued part of the local service system, and that maintain a clear vision of their aims and principles.

REFERENCE

Department of Health (2001). *The Mental Health Policy Implementation Guide.* London: The Stationery Office.

25

Recruiting, training and retaining an effective crisis team

Steve Ramsey and Warren Shaw

This chapter provides guidance on the recruitment, training and retention of a crisis resolution team (CRT) – on what does and does not work, and what clinicians need to know. These processes are of considerable importance, since the qualities and abilities of team members are the most significant components required to attain the results that CRTs have been shown capable of achieving. What follows is based on the authors' experience with more than 15 teams over 25 years, as well as on discussions with many people involved with these services.

Establishing a new crisis team

The first few months in the life of a new CRT are critical. This is the period during which clinicians are experimenting with new modes of working, trying new things and taking risks. With appropriate training and support, the new procedures required to ensure the success of CRTs can be firmly established, to the benefit of both staff and patients.

It is important to be clear about what CRTs are. They are sometimes described as a 'ward on wheels' or 'ward in the community' or, alternatively, as an extension of the work done by community mental health teams (CMHTs). While CRTs contain elements of both inpatient and traditional community services (Chapter 5), neither of these characterisations is accurate. Furthermore, assuming that they are can give rise to difficulties in the recruitment and training of staff and lead to expectations that are incompatible with effective service delivery. Successful services require that team members perform a broader and less traditional range of tasks than staff of either inpatient units or CMHTs.

While the normal staff mix of CRTs includes the disciplines found in other parts of the mental health service, such as consultant psychiatrists, nurses, allied

Crisis Resolution and Home Treatment in Mental Health, ed. Sonia Johnson, Justin Needle, Jonathan P. Bindman and Graham Thornicroft. Published by Cambridge University Press. © Cambridge University Press 2008.

health professionals and support workers, the roles of the various professions are different. These have broadened over time and are now much more team oriented, so people need to be prepared to work outside their traditional roles. These changes have important consequences for recruitment and training, as well as for continuing job satisfaction.

The key steps in establishing and maintaining a successful CRT are:
- recruit the appropriate people
- make sure that there are enough of them
- train them properly
- persist until the service is working effectively
- ensure that the team is working both with patients and with their social systems.

Recruiting the team

The staff selection process presents a number of challenges in achieving the desired team culture and dynamic. The authors have witnessed teams recruited by means of merit-based procedures and comprising senior clinicians that have nevertheless performed more conservatively and less effectively than teams largely made up of more junior staff. One possible reason is that more senior staff are generally less happy with shift work, are more rigid and comfortable in their approaches and have less need for the positive feedback that can be elicited within flexible, dynamic teams from both colleagues and the patient's social network. Experience has shown that a mix of senior, highly skilled clinicians and others with 'youthful enthusiasm', the right personal attributes and the ability to master specific skills, promotes the most dynamic and positive culture.

Desirable attributes, skills and experience

When recruiting staff to work in a CRT, one should consider candidates' relevant experience, skills and personal attributes. Experience in setting up, managing and reviewing many teams has shown that certain personal characteristics are important, both for the effectiveness of the service and for the satisfaction of the staff working within it. These personal attributes and skills are summarised in Box 25.1.

As for relevant experience, it is the range and diversity of this that is important, rather than its extent. It is neither necessary nor desirable that all team members have extensive experience, since flexibility in the team will be better achieved when staff do not continually rely on what has happened in the past. Job descriptions need to be written with care in order to avoid placing undue emphasis on length of health service experience.

Box 25.1. Desirable personal attributes and skills for members of a crisis resolution team

Personal attributes include:
- comfortable with high levels of personal responsibility and delegation from the team
- assertive
- decisive, but with the ability to review decisions in light of new information
- comfortable with scrutiny of their ideas and judgements
- sufficiently confident to avoid controlling behaviour (toward patients or colleagues)
- practical and solution focused, with an action-oriented attitude
- helpful and empathic
- honest and possess integrity
- persistent and optimistic
- motivated by positive reinforcement.

Desirable skills include:
- ability to represent the service effectively
- engagement skills:
  - the ability to operate in an informal style while respecting personal and professional boundaries
  - the ability to converse freely and be inquisitive without being inquisitorial
  - the ability to anticipate the approach that will elicit the optimal therapeutic alliance, and the ability to adjust to this approach quickly and subtly.
- ability to appear calm in anxiety-provoking circumstances
- ability to differentiate between types of risk, e.g. clinical, medicolegal and corporate
- ability to identify, manage and share risk (Chapter 9) by seeking (or imagining) an objective perspective on it
- ability to formulate cases using an approach that includes problem-oriented and solution-focused perspectives
- ability to construct and initiate a preliminary plan
- ability to 'sell' the plan to the social system (and to colleagues), using tools such as 'reframing' (achieving behaviour change by seeking to identify the positive intention that may underlie a problematic behaviour and then to generate other behaviours that could satisfy this intent)
- ability to adopt a clinical leadership and coordination role in relation to other agencies
- ability to elicit relevant information and construct a narrative for optimal information exchange and recording purposes.

The selection process

Although perhaps not the most effective method for choosing staff, the interview is the generally accepted method of selection in the public sector. Interviews should focus on attributes and skills rather than seniority or experience. There are a number of useful strategies that can be used to identify desirable characteristics of potential members of staff:

- create informal interview structures
- ask candidates to comment on multifaceted clinical scenarios that require them to address different components of crisis work, including decision-making processes
- ask for examples of formulations for cases they have been involved with
- present and ask them to discuss ethical and management dilemmas.

Applications are sometimes received from people who possess great skills and interest in areas not really required for CRT work, such as psychotherapy or dialectical behaviour therapy. While such skills can make a useful contribution, the team does not need specialists and consideration should be given to whether these people will be happy doing more diverse or generic work.

It is not always easy to identify staff who are ideally suited to working in CRTs. Furthermore, they appear to be a scarce resource. It is important to be flexible in terms of the final staff mix: one may have the ideal mix in mind but fail to achieve it. The ultimate goal, however, is a well-functioning team. The happiest of teams will still experience a degree of staff turnover, so there will be opportunity to adjust combinations of skills and attributes over time and recruitment should be practical.

Where possible, it is useful to talk directly to referees and to focus especially in these conversations on whether candidates possess the required personal attributes, as well as on validating the information presented in their curriculum vitae.

Training the team

Given appropriate organisational structures and human resources for the new CRT, the next priority is to ensure that staff members are adequately and appropriately trained to carry out the tasks required to achieve successful crisis resolution and community treatment. Training is expensive, so the first issue that needs to be dealt with is whether it needs to be provided. After all, when someone takes a job in an inpatient unit or a CMHT, they will (with luck) receive some orientation to that particular site or organisation, but not normally any training in how to do their job. There is an assumption that they will know this from their professional training or previous experience.

For most staff, crisis intervention work involves a major reorientation. As there is significant sharing of duties in such work, each team member must be prepared to undertake tasks in almost all areas of client management. There is ample evidence of services being ineffective when staff fail to relinquish their traditional roles.

Most existing CRTs have provided at least some training specific to their operation, and some have invested quite considerably in this. This is usually because they constitute a new service element for the area they will serve, and most new staff members will not have had any exposure to the CRT model in the course of their formal training. The fact that teams are commonly starting 'from scratch' makes training easier, since there is no existing service to be maintained.

What is the goal of training?

Staff training provides orientation to the CRT model and its specific roles, development of specific skills and a common knowledge base. When the members of a new team train together, it is also an excellent opportunity for team building: staff get to know each other and begin to form working relationships and to operate as a professionally and socially cohesive group.

Orientation to the crisis resolution team model

The model of care adopted by successful CRTs involves a paradigm shift for all staff away from their formal training and previous experience. In order to be motivated to follow the CRT model and to promote it to referrers, patients and their social systems, team members need to be familiar with the evidence for the effectiveness of CRTs (Chapters 4 and 5). This understanding needs to be shared by all team members in order to ensure that they present the team's work in a consistent way to referrers, patients and the general public. The model also provides the basis for the skills training that will need to take place. The investment in training can be justified on the basis that, if the CRT functions well, there will be a significant saving to the organisation.

Orientation to specific roles

The best teams manage to blend team working with individual responsibility, generally by allocating a team member (named worker/key worker/crisis coordinator) to each case. This role is a fundamental element in the success of CRTs, ensuring individual accountability for patient care and reassuring patient and family that one person within the team is overseeing their care. It also provides the opportunity for each coordinator to be acknowledged for innovative planning and comprehensive and effective crisis management by their team manager, team mates, clients and carers. Such acknowledgement contributes significantly to individual job satisfaction.

Development of specific skills and a common knowledge base

The development of specific skills and knowledge are essential for an effective crisis resolution and home treatment service. It is important that team members have a common understanding of and shared attitude towards the model and its operation, since they will be dependent on one another for its success. Inconsistency of response is a common source of complaints from patients and carers.

Team building

A further goal served by team training is team building: a cohesive and mutually supportive team with shared goals is vital to the success of the service.

What should be included in a training programme?

Because of the variety of staff disciplines and backgrounds, the training programme needs to include basic 'refresher' and 'bridging' material, as well as new knowledge and skills. The development of a common knowledge base and shared understanding of individual capacities helps to establish a culture that promotes quality and sustainability.

The orientation and background information which the training programme should cover is summarised in Box 25.2. The elements of the model that require the greatest shift in thinking are acute treatment in the community and social systems interventions (see Chapters 6 and 12).

Box 25.2. Crisis resolution team training programme: orientation and background information

- Overview of the classification of mental disorders.
- Theory and practice of crisis intervention.
- Social systems intervention model.
- Legal aspects of home treatment.
- Interviewing/comprehensive assessment/engagement skills.
- Physical illness that presents as psychiatric illness.
- Major psychiatric treatments, including:
  - medication
  - cognitive and behavioural treatments
  - counselling methods
  - evidence-based family interventions
  - early intervention
  - education for individuals and families concerning mental health problems.
- Problem identification and problem solving.
- Familiarisation with available community resources.

The implications of putting the theory into practice become clearer with further skills-oriented training. The clinical skills that should be covered by the training programme are:

- triage of referrals
- assessment
- care planning
- management of acute illness
- documentation
- communication
- interventions
- relapse prevention.

It is important to develop a common understanding and practice within the team, and to promote confidence in each other's abilities.

Experience indicates that, for staff new to CRTs, the most stressful aspect of crisis work is assessment and immediate action planning. If this is neglected then hospitalisation – as the 'safe' treatment option – will be used excessively. Carrying out exercises that address these topics is useful.

A training programme for a new crisis resolution team

The ideal minimum training period for a new team is four weeks prior to the commencement of the service and then, if possible, six weeks of 'on the job' training after the service has become operational. It is important that all team members are together for the initial training.

The new knowledge and orientation component of the training, which is largely theoretical, can be carried out by a combination of experts from outside the local system and people drawn from within local services. External providers, using techniques such as role-playing and small group discussions, are often best for the skills-based training and this will help to identify 'local champions' of the model for future individual training of new or replacement staff. To reinforce didactic training, all team members should be provided with key articles regarding the evidence on CRTs and on techniques such as social systems intervention and strategies for reduction of expressed emotion. If time permits, placement with operational CRTs is also recommended, since seeing at first hand the way in which a service works is very useful.

Once the team is operational, it is valuable to engage experts with extensive experience and clinical knowledge of such services to undertake further training of team members and work with them 'on the job'. The aims of this additional training are to reinforce the initial learning, provide further skills and support for staff, help to put theory into practice, solve problems that might derail the work of the team, build staff confidence and create a common understanding and approach within the team.

Training programmes can be structured in a number of ways. An example of a four-week programme is provided in Table 25.1.

Training for new staff in an existing team

The issue of how to provide training for new recruits to existing teams is also very important and a subject to which insufficient attention has been devoted. A few years into the operation of a service, staff turnover can easily lead to a situation in which the majority of the staff members have effectively received no CRT-specific training, a major issue for the durability of the model (Chapter 24).

There are a number of ways to induct new recruits. The team manager needs to assess the new team member's strengths, weaknesses and knowledge base, which will obviously vary from individual to individual. It is important that all new staff be provided with reading material, especially articles that give evidence about the model and that present key techniques such as social systems intervention. Also of value are the provision of a mentor to guide new staff, and a period of working as a supernumary member of the team in order to learn about the area, work with new colleagues and understand how the service operates. These elements all help to maintain the team culture. The team manager may also choose to provide specific training to address gaps in knowledge and/or to send individuals on specific training in areas such as social systems intervention or use of medications. Unfortunately, such training is rarely available when wanted, but making it available may be facilitated by establishing national or regional networks of CRTs, such as the regional crisis resolution networks supported by the National Institute for Mental Health, England.

Retaining an effective team

Once an effective team has been recruited and trained, the task is then to maintain that effectiveness (Chapter 24). The following factors required to achieve this all fall within the remit of management, but achieving the first five is a direct result of effective initial and ongoing training:

- active adherence to the CRT model
- clearly defined relationships with the wider network of care
- effective team working
- a shared definition of success and a mechanism for feeding back regarding team outcomes to the team
- a culture in which mistakes are to be learned from
- sufficient resources (staff, equipment, premises)
- support from management (both line and senior).

Table 25.1. Example of a four-week training programme

	Monday	Tuesday	Wednesday	Thursday	Friday
Week 1	Introduction: the rationale for community treatment	What comprises community treatment? Introduction to social systems intervention	Implications of CRT working for the role of the clinician (lecture and open forum discussion)	The issue of boundaries: 'alliance versus friendship'	Case scenario 1: setting the scene to illustrate the issues and processes, e.g. referral, triage
Morning tea	'Why community treatment?'	Uses of social systems intervention	'How is the role expanded? Is this my job?' (small group work)	'Becoming an actor': the importance of behavioural flexibility (open forum discussion)	Role-playing exercise on engagement and assessment
Lunch	'Why at home?'	Engagement; alliance forming; motivating clients	Engagement, rapport and the shift in power; making key relationships with patient and others	Exploring personal repertoires (small groups)	Managing the case – individual role and team responsibility – collective commitment; practical help and support
Afternoon tea	Research evidence and examples	Crisis intervention theory	Crisis intervention theory continued	Reframing: the art of using leverage without losing rapport (homework)	Reframing continued
Week 2	Differential diagnosis of psychotic illnesses: knowledge refresher	Triage; pre-assessment phase: what happens when it is not done well? How to refuse a referral	Acute management	Management techniques overview; perception of choice; using the crisis as an opportunity for change	The depressed person: management techniques

Table 25.1. (cont.)

	Monday	Tuesday	Wednesday	Thursday	Friday
Morning tea	Differential diagnosis continued	Assessment: initial clinical assessment of mental state and symptom severity	Home visiting: etiquette, risk, working in pairs, techniques, dangers of premature discharge	Schizophrenia: management issues	The unstable personality: management techniques; involving patients in development of written management plans
Lunch	Pharmacotherapy: knowledge refresher	Assessment: use of a problem-orientated focus to plan initial actions and interventions; what can happen if this is not done well	Plans (and what can happen if they are not made well); identifying issues and prioritising actions; selling the plan to the team; issues regarding particular types of patient; indications for reviewing/changing plans; written plans; working cooperatively with other providers	The paranoid person: management techniques and medication issues	*Titration of level of support:* tailoring level of involvement to the client's changing needs and social system; relapse profiles and prevention strategies
Afternoon tea	Legal aspects of crisis management: knowledge refresher	Risk management: managing risks, sharing them, being resilient	Examples of plans	The person with an elevated mood: management techniques	Feedback session: question and answer

	How do you organise the work of the team?	Talking treatments	Orientation to local services	Social systems interventions and family psychoeducation: further techniques and case examples	Visits to other crisis teams
Week 3	How do you organise the work of the team?	Talking treatments	Orientation to local services	Social systems interventions and family psychoeducation: further techniques and case examples	Visits to other crisis teams
Morning tea	White boards, files and other communication tools	Working with other providers (internal and external)	Continued	Continued	Continued
Lunch	Handover and the 2-minute story	Discharge planning and referral	Continued	Continued	Continued
Afternoon tea	Working as a team: collective commitment, mutual support, valuing quality in work, not tolerating substandard performance, rewarding initiative, importance of humour	Continued	Continued	Continued	
Week 4	Visits to other crisis teams	Visits to other crisis teams	Visits to other crisis teams	Team building	Feedback: question and answer

One of the characteristics of an effective team is a high level of morale. This is gained by knowing what you are setting out to do, being equipped to do it and knowing whether you are achieving it. There will inevitably be some staff turnover but, in our experience, this occurs within effective teams at quite a slow rate: most people leave for 'good' reasons, such as furthering their careers or starting new teams, rather than because they are dissatisfied with the work.

Key points

- Staff recruited to CRTs need to work in new ways, with roles that are broad and team oriented rather than narrowly defined by profession.
- A mixture of experienced senior clinicians and enthusiastic younger staff often works well.
- Staff should be positive, confident and assertive, but also empathic and flexible, with a willingness to review decisions and appearances when new evidence emerges.
- Desirable qualities include excellent engagement skills, ability to represent the service, to remain calm in anxiety-provoking situations and to identify and manage risk effectively.
- Initial whole-team training is important for establishing a team culture and developing a high-quality, sustainable service.

26

Operational management of crisis resolution teams

Stephen Niemiec

Clinical effectiveness is dependent upon effective operational management. Drawing on extensive experience in the organisation and day-to-day running of crisis resolution teams (CRTs), this chapter proposes practical solutions to the challenges of managing such multidisciplinary teams in a complex service system that increasingly involves other specialist teams, as well as established community, ward-based and emergency services. Good-quality management and leadership allows the strengths of individual team members to be used to best advantage and promotes the development of good-quality care and a positive team culture. The challenges for any team leader are to shape the efforts that each team member contributes into a clinically coherent service, to support the team effectively in its purpose, and to ensure that adequate infrastructure is in place for the team to fulfil its function. A modernised mental health service is a much more complex system with multiple channels of communication for teams and clinical pathways for patients and their families. The following issues will, therefore, be addressed: team composition and size in relation to its catchment area population, shift working and ensuring adequate clinical cover, communication and information sharing, balancing demand with capacity, and the team's interface with other services.[1]

Team size and composition

Within England, CRTs have developed at an unsteady pace and in a relatively ad hoc fashion despite attempts at prescribing team size and implementation principles in the *Policy Implementation Guide* (Department of Health, 2001).

---

[1] This chapter is based upon the assumption that CRTs follow fidelity principles as described in Niemiec and Tacchi (2003) and the *Policy Implementation Guide* (Department of Health, 2001). See also Chapters 6, 8, 10 and 24.

Crisis Resolution and Home Treatment in Mental Health, ed. Sonia Johnson, Justin Needle, Jonathan P. Bindman and Graham Thornicroft. Published by Cambridge University Press. © Cambridge University Press 2008.

There is considerable variation in team size and functioning and, therefore, in impacts on service users and the whole system of care (Chapter 3).

There are two main models of CRT implementation within the UK: the sector CRT and the non-sectorised or 'city-wide' CRT. The main difference between the two is the size of the population covered and the number of staff employed. Sector teams serve small populations of around 150 000 to 200 000, whereas city-wide teams have been shown to be effective in populations of up to 450 000 (Keown *et al.*, 2007). The *Policy Implementation Guide* formula of 14 clinicians per 150 000 people of working age is applicable to either type of team, except in areas of very high social deprivation. City-wide services may improve the cost–benefit ratio by utilising one base instead of many, and economies of scale allow for a single large team to operate with a slightly smaller staff-to-patient ratio, as has been demonstrated in Newcastle and North Tyneside since 2000 (Niemiec and Tacchi, 2003). However, issues of inter-service liaison and interconnectedness are more difficult to resolve in larger teams, and managing these can consume considerable time.

Multidisciplinary teams have been shown to be effective, but operationally managing such teams when they are operating 24 hours a day brings its own challenges. The team should include psychiatric nurses, psychiatrists, social workers, some psychology or psychotherapist time (usually sessions) and support workers, and it can include other health professionals such as occupational therapists (Chapter 25). To ensure effectiveness and coherence it is essential that all team members are more or less able to do the same job. Role boundaries within the medical, nursing, social work and occupational therapy professions have undergone a redefinition, giving rise to a generic role of CRT clinician that encompasses triage, assessment, taking histories, writing formulations and utilising interpersonal skills to communicate with patients and families. The development of such generic specialist skills overlays the professional skill base, and any therapeutic skills that are specifically applicable to crises sit on top. A hierarchy of skills built upon a professional knowledge base is developed, and it is important that any CRT training programme addresses the issues of interdisciplinary working, cooperation and effective working patterns (Chapter 25). Specific professional skills are utilised when individual team members are required to perform certain specialist tasks, such as functional assessment by an occupational therapist. A balance between generic and specialist skills is, therefore, desirable and, since role inflexibility will inevitably lead to conflict and loss of timeliness in interventions, a willingness on the part of all team members to work in new and different ways is crucial. A specific advantage of teams that work in this way is the sense of shared responsibility and accountability in areas traditionally the preserve of the medical profession, and this helps teams to develop a positive approach to risk taking.

Some services employ a single staff-grade psychiatrist as the senior medical practitioner within the team, and this appears to be more frequently the case for sector teams with close working relationships with other senior medical staff within the same sector. In this model, sector consultant psychiatrists will generally remain responsible for patients' medical care throughout their period of treatment with the CRT. This is not, however, recommended for city-wide services because of the higher volume of people seen, which creates the need for more regular reviews by senior medical staff and uncovers more risk. City-wide services will, therefore, normally require more than one psychiatrist, including a dedicated team consultant. After-hours medical input is usually provided by on-call registrars or consultants.

Informed service user advisors are in a good position to advise service designers and some teams have employed service user representatives. However, although this is not in itself a contentious issue, it is preferable to leave local implementation teams to decide whether this represents the best use of scarce resources.

Ensuring adequate clinical cover

Once the operational manager and/or senior clinicians have matched the team size to the population size and developed a picture of local demand, they can determine how many clinicians are required per shift, how many shifts the team is planning to cover, and how senior clinicians are to be distributed across the shifts.

Following the model specified in the *Policy Implementation Guide*, acting as gatekeepers to inpatient beds is a 24-hour a day function, so if the team is not operating 24 hours, consideration will need to be given to how access and gatekeeping will be provided out of hours. These issues are solved in city-wide models, since they work active night shifts. Sectorised CRTs will, however, need to provide an after-hours on-call service and, since it is often preferable for two clinicians to be in attendance, arrangements will need to include mechanisms for calling out more than one staff member. If 24-hour cover cannot be provided, the risk is that admissions out of hours will be arranged by other clinical staff for patients who might have been suitable for home treatment, negating the advantages that CRTs offer.

If the demand from accident and emergency departments for out-of-hours working is sufficient, then it is advisable to consider recruiting active on-duty clinicians to night shifts. These systems work well in large urban areas where multiple accident and emergency departments are covered and which are located in areas with high population densities. An active night shift may not be required for a smaller or rural CRT, but the team will still need to be contactable by means of an on-call system. One disadvantage of this is that if there are several call-outs during the night, then the staff will need to take time off the next day. This will reduce the availability of the team for that day and, unless planned for, could destabilise the home visit schedule and increase levels of stress among staff. It is, therefore, recommended that, as far as possible, active night shifts be worked.

As for carrying out assessments, two heads are, as a broad principle, better than one and single clinicians may be more likely to admit patients to hospital than those working in pairs. The safety of clinicians must also be considered, and two people are more able to deal with any difficult situations that might arise. Clinicians require safe and efficient means of transportation and communication, for example mobile phones or pagers. All the working tools of a CRT must be oriented towards the rapid transfer of information and effective risk management.

Information sharing and communication

Effective systems for communicating, recording and accessing information are crucial. The presence of whiteboards in a central meeting area is essential for communicating what is happening, and when. The team will probably need running sheets that organise the day's work so that each team member knows in advance what they will be doing. Patient notes should include a summary of what has happened with each patient and the purpose of the next home visit. This means that, even if the clinician does not know the patient, he or she will at least be clear about the purpose of the visit and the extent to which it will require in-depth knowledge about the patient. Continuity of information can compensate to a considerable degree for personal discontinuity.

The team's clinical meetings should be chaired by someone in authority, such as a nurse consultant, consultant psychiatrist or team leader. The team should meet at least twice a day so that team members on different shifts are kept informed about what is happening, and because the clinical situation can alter rapidly. Clinical team meetings should be limited to within an hour to an hour and a half; longer meetings may affect the overall responsiveness of the service and, in any case, people may well have stopped listening and contributing by that time. Special conferences sometimes need to be held to explore difficult situations, families or patients, and valuable team learning can occur at such times.

Any team leader responsible for a 24-hour service knows how difficult it is to communicate with all staff members. Notes from team meetings (as opposed to clinical handovers) should be written up and circulated, preferably via email.

When a large number of assessments are being undertaken (and even if not!), it is necessary to present the main facts about a case clearly and share relevant information as quickly as possible. All types of clinician should be trained in presenting formulations (Hopkins and Niemiec, 2006), in which 60 seconds are available to summarise the biological, psychological and social contributions to a person's mental health problems and the current precipitating, predisposing and maintaining factors of the episode. Such summaries tell the team a number of things, including the appropriateness of the referral, the state of health of the person or family involved, and any ongoing assessment or treatment requirements. Supervisors and experienced clinicians are able to recognise similar or atypical patterns and, provided that the histories and formulations are of high enough quality, are in a good position to help to decide what should happen next.

Balancing demand with capacity

All CRTs require a great deal of flexibility in order to manage the balance between capacity and demand while continuing to carry out their functions effectively. Patients receiving treatment from CRTs value their accessibility and responsiveness highly (Hopkins and Niemiec, 2006), and referrers also value accessibility. In general, a CRT will always assess more people than it treats at home, and the proportion of assessments that transition on to the home treatment board should be approximately 60% or more. Higher proportions are preferable since less time is then spent completing one-off assessments, which means that the numbers of patients treated at home can be increased. Referral systems and team criteria require review if only a minority of those assessed are accepted for home treatment. Not all adjoining health or social care providers will share this perspective, however. There will always be more demand, for several reasons:

- by virtue of the CRT's existence
- everyone has a different notion of what a crisis is
- clinicians (referrers) get anxious
- the current system of response is fragmented, and there may be patients who do not meet CRT criteria but would nonetheless benefit from some form of rapid response, for example if they need detoxification or help in a psychosocial crisis.

However, the opposite view also has a certain attractiveness, namely, that the more assessments the team completes and the more people avoid using secondary mental health services, the better the outcome. It is true that, during initial assessments, the crisis is sometimes resolved, just as it is true that the team will see people who are not in a psychiatric crisis. The issue of accessibility is fraught with difficulty, and each team will need to develop its own criteria for access and assessment acceptability that allow it to carry out its primary function, which is to treat individuals intensively at home who would normally have been admitted to a psychiatric bed. At times, it may become necessary to remind the whole system of care that undertaking a large number of inappropriate assessments will hinder delivery of home-based treatment. The CRT needs, however, to be flexible in how it manages its incoming referrals, and it is always a good idea to adopt the rule of thumb that it is better to go and assess the situation if there is uncertainty, the rationale being that seeing patients is more defensible than not seeing them. Relationships between community mental health teams (CMHTs) and CRTs, the reasons why disputes sometimes arise, and the path to resolving them are discussed further in Chapter 7.

Experience suggests the following formula for assessing how many people can be on the home treatment regimen at any one time: for every one clinician there should be approximately 1.2–1.4 patients. A team of 14, therefore, ought to be able to treat 16 to 20 people at home, though this will vary according to how much additional assessment work the team is required to complete. Approximately a third of the patients on the home treatment board will be acutely ill and require two visits or more per day. A further third will be recovering and be being seen between three and seven times a week, and the remainder will be being prepared for transition to other services over the following week or two, or for being discharged.

It is not necessary to have more than one clinician doing home visits unless there is a specific history or risk of violence from the patient or his/her social network, or unless the area in which the patient lives is especially hazardous. From time to time, special attention will need to be paid to the sex of home treatment clinicians, since some patients respond better to men or women.

Interface with other services

The CRT needs to be well integrated within the overall mental health service. Careful and well thought through patient pathways need to be developed and agreed to ensure that transitions between teams are as quick and seamless as possible, and that they respect the needs of the patient rather than those of the overall service (Hopkins and Niemiec, 2006).

Most CRTs work with people who are known to the mental health service as well as those who are not. If the patient is known to the mental health service, it is accepted best practice to undertake the assessment with the care coordinator present. If the assessment takes place after hours, then the outcome and plan of action should be faxed to the CMHT as soon as possible so that they are kept informed. Home-based treatment is most effective when those who know the patient best maintain contact with them, even if the CRT is seeing the person several times a day.

Afternoons are typically a busy time for CRT services, as other 9-to-5 services are closing. Requests for crisis assessments or continued after-hours care should always be accompanied by a plan prepared by the regular care coordinator. Transitions to the CMHT should be agreed within timescales that are acceptable to all parties, though it should be borne in mind that CRTs need to keep their point of entry to assessment and home-based treatment open at all times. This means that it is incumbent upon other community services to accept patients back from home-based treatment readily. A recent investigation by Hopkins and Niemiec (2006) indicated that for some patients the transition from CRT to CMHT is accompanied by significant anxiety. It is essential that transfer from one team to another during the post-crisis phase is communicated and managed by all parties involved.

Developing and maintaining working relationships with accident and emergency departments has proved invaluable. Regular debriefings and liaison meetings between senior clinicians and/or managers are helpful, as well as regular pre-organised orientations to the service at the change of junior medical staff, allowing a more managed referral rate from junior house officers.

Early discharge planning is an integral component of CRT care and regular attendances at ward rounds and patient reviews are very useful in identifying those patients suitable for home-based treatment (Chapter 15).

Key points

- Effective CRTs operate 24 hours a day, seven days a week and sustain adequate levels of staffing as described in the *Policy Implementation Guide* from the UK Department of Health (2001).
- Team responsiveness is increased and waiting times reduced when all workers possess a generic skill base.
- Sector- and city-wide teams offer alternative models for CRT delivery.
- It is important that portals of entry and exit for CRTs are kept clear. Throughput is important, but not at the expense of quality. Interlinking with other mental health services is, therefore, essential to ensure that a coherent clinical pathway exists for patients and carers.
- Transitions from CRTs to CMHTs need to be organised and managed.
- Providing or organising training, supervision and team support are essential components of leadership in CRTs.
- Communication with internal and external providers can be time consuming but it is essential for ensuring smooth operations.

REFERENCES

Department of Health (2001). *The Mental Health Policy Implementation Guide: Crisis Resolution/Home Treatment Teams.* London: The Stationery Office.

Hopkins, C. and Niemiec, S. (2006). The development of an evaluation questionnaire for the Newcastle Crisis Assessment and Home Treatment Service: finding a way to include the voices of service users. *Journal of Psychiatric and Mental Health Nursing,* **13,** 40–7.

Keown, P., Tacchi, M. J., Niemiec, S. and Hughes, J. (2007). Changes to mental healthcare for working age adults: impact of a crisis team and an assertive outreach team. *Psychiatric Bulletin,* **31,** 288–92.

Niemiec, S. and Tacchi, M. J. (2003). CRHT for inner city populations: the Newcastle and North Tyneside story. In *More than the Sum of All the Parts: Improving the Whole System with Crisis Resolution and Home Treatment,* ed. P. Kennedy. Durham: Northern Centre for Mental Health, pp. 12–20.

Index

accident and emergency department, *see* casualty
    department
acute care system 71, 188–9, 302
adherence, *see* treatment adherence
antipsychotic drugs 123, 131, 133
Asians, services for 24, 30, 206
assertive community treatment, *see* assertive
    outreach teams
assertive outreach teams (AOTs) 15–17, 92–3
assessment of crises *see* crisis assessment
Australia crisis resolution teams
    first implementations 17–18
    home treatment studies 38
    North Shore service, Sydney 236–50
Austria
    crisis intervention services 19

Barnet family psychiatric service 14–15
benefits 143–4
benzodiazepines 130, 133
Black British, Caribbean and African people 24,
    30, 206
    services for 24

capacity 25, 225, 296–7, 324
Care Programme Approach (CPA) 213–14
carers
    investigation of carer views 60
    involvement in assessment 103, 112
    risk assessment 112
    role in home-based treatment 171
    views about CRTs 57
    see also social networks
casualty department 107, 129, 187–9, 194
Charter of Needs and Demands 177
children of service users 148–9
CMHT *see* community mental health teams
coercion and compulsion 223, 231
    definitions 223
      compulsion 224
      inducement 224
      leverage 224
      persuasion 224
      threat 224

    ethical justifications 224–6
    practical application 226–7
      avoiding coercion 227
      force and legal compulsion 230–1
      inducements 228–9
      insight 227
      leverage 228
      persuasion 227–8
      threats 229–30
communications 92, 95, 190, 300–1, 322–3
community mental health centres (CMHCs) in
    Trieste, Italy
    advantages and risks 260–3, 261
    crisis management 254, 286
      hospital service use 259
      hospitality versus hospital 257–9, 258
      principles 253, 254–5
      service user's care pathway 254–7
    evidence for effectiveness 259–60
    history and service structures 252–3
community mental health teams
    (CMHTs) 23, 30
    integration with 235–7, 246–8, 260–3
    referral from 87–9, 303
    working with 77, 90–1, 324–5
compulsory admissions and assessments
    under the Mental Health Act 54, 56, 89,
    90, 101, 230
confidentiality 152–4, 75–6
continuity of care 94, 138, 172–3, 255
core model for CRTs 74, 82–3
    current status 80–2
    interventions 78–80, 79
      acute symptom management 79
      family education 80
      patient education 80
      practical support 79
      treatment plans 79
    organisational characteristics 76
    organisational features 75–7
    target group 74–5
crises
    definition 11
    distinction with emergencies 11–12, 238